# Bulimia

## A SYSTEMS APPROACH TO TREATMENT

# Bulimia

## *A SYSTEMS APPROACH TO TREATMENT*

Maria P. P. Root

Patricia Fallon

William N. Friedrich

W · W · NORTON & COMPANY · *NEW YORK* · *LONDON*

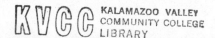

Copyright © 1986 by Maria P. P. Root, Patricia Fallon and William N. Friedrich

All rights reserved.

Published simultaneously in Canada by Penguin Books Canada Ltd, 2801 John Street, Markham, Ontario L3R 1B4
Printed in the United States of America.

First Edition

Library of Congress Cataloging-in-Publication Data

Root, Maria P. P.
  Bulimia: a systemic approach to treatment.

  "A Norton professional book"—P. facing t.p.
  Bibliography: p.
  Includes index.
  1. Bulimarexia.  2. Bulimarexia—Patients—Family relationships.  3. Family—Mental health.  4. Typology. (Psychology)  I. Fallon, Patricia.  II. Friedrich, William N.  III. Title.  [DNLM: 1. Appetite Disorders—therapy. WM 175 R783b]
  RC552.B84R66 1986      616.85'2      86–2354

ISBN  0-393-70024-0

W. W. Norton & Company, Inc., 500 Fifth Avenue, New York, N. Y. 10110
W. W. Norton & Company Ltd., 37 Great Russell Street, London WC1B 3NU

1 2 3 4 5 6 7 8 9 0

# Contents

Introduction                                                    vii
Acknowledgments                                                  ix

### I. BULIMIA: DEFINITION, ISSUES, AND EXPLANATIONS

1. Developing Bulimia                                            3
2. Sociocultural Contributions                                  20
3. Systemic Issues                                              32

### II. CONCEPTUAL EXPLANATIONS OF BULIMIA

4. The Bulimic Family System                                    39
5. Multigenerational Issues                                     52
6. The Family Life-Cycle of the Bulimic                         64

### III. THE FAMILY TYPOLOGIES

7. Eating-Disordered Families: Current Literature               79
8. The Perfect Family                                           83
9. The Overprotective Family                                    98
10. The Chaotic Family                                          112

### IV. THE TREATMENT OF BULIMIA

11. Assessment                                                  131
12. The Role of Consultation                                    150
13. Individual Systemic Therapy                                 161

14. Couples Therapy                                                     180
15. Group Therapy                                                       194
16. Psychopharmacological Issues                                        208

## V. TREATING BULIMIC FAMILIES

17. Principles in Working With Bulimic Families                         219
18. The Gems: Treating the Perfect Family                               226
19. The Longs: Treating the Overprotective Family                       249
20. The Weisfields: Treating the Chaotic Family                         267

## VI. PLANNING FOR THE INEVITABLE

21. Obstacles and Sabotage in Treatment                                 299

References                                                              311
Index                                                                   321

# Introduction

BULIMIA, COMMONLY REFERRED to as the binge-purge syndrome, is a major psychosocial health problem primarily affecting women.* Although it has existed for generations, bulimia has only recently been recognized as a significant clinical syndrome separate from anorexia nervosa.

It has taken a long time to define the syndrome of bulimia because it can be difficult to recognize. The professional needs to be able to distinguish between faddish, experimental binge-purge behavior, common binge-eating, and a clinically problematic binge-purge pattern. Unlike anorectics, whose emaciated appearance is a hallmark of the disorder, most bulimics are of approximately normal weight and appear, at least superficially, to be functioning well. The bulimic's secretiveness and denial of the problem contribute further to difficulty in professional detection of the disorder.

Bulimia is a complex, multidetermined disorder with social, cultural, familial, and individual contributing factors. As a result of this complex constellation of contributing factors, diagnosis, conceptualization, and treatment of bulimia are a challenge to the professional. Professional training in the treatment of bulimia has become more available following the recent inclusion of bulimia as a diagnosis in the Third Edition of the *Diagnostic and Statistical Manual of Mental Disorders* (American Psychiatric Association, 1980). Since 1980, inpatient and outpatient treatment programs have been developed throughout the United States, Canada, and Great Britain.

This book provides both an integrated conceptual basis for assessment and diagnosis of bulimia and an applied approach to treatment. The conceptualization of bulimia and subsequent treatment approaches offered reflect our blend of feminist and family systems theory. While some differences

*Subsequently, we will use the pronoun she throughout the book to refer to the bulimic individual.

vii

exist in the specific views of causality or locus of change between systems and feminist therapy (Libow, Raskin, & Caust, 1982), both views are strikingly similar in emphasizing a contextual framework for understanding symptoms. These two perspectives complement the deficiencies of each perspective alone. A family systems perspective complements a feminist perspective by conceptualizing symptoms as emerging from dysfunctional communication and relationship patterns, which are often multigenerational in nature. A feminist perspective widens our understanding bulimia by including a focus on the gender socialization process (Goldner, 1985; Hare-Mustin, 1978). Both perspectives are interpersonal and emphasize the need for restructuring relationships in order to eliminate the symptoms.

The information offered in this book is the result of our combined experiences in varied settings — inpatient, outpatient, community clinics, university counseling, and private practice. The book is divided into six sections which take the reader from a foundation for diagnosis and assessment of bulimia to treatment of the disorder. We start with a review of the literature and offer a psychosocial explanation for the prevalance of bulimia in women. The second section provides a synopsis of systems theory concepts relevant to the communication and interactional patterns observed in bulimic families, couples, and individuals. Multigenerational learning of dysfunctional patterns is also examined. In the third section we introduce a novel typology of the family contexts in which bulimia is developed — perfect, overprotective, and chaotic families. These family types point the way to better understanding of the age at which an individual becomes symptomatic, the function of the bulimia, and family coping styles around conflict, depression, and anger. Characteristics of each family type are highlighted through case illustrations.

The majority of the book is devoted to the treatment of bulimia. In the fourth section, the initial contact with the bulimic system is introduced through assessment and consultation (including consultation for medication). Individual, couple, and group therapies are discussed in separate chapters as viable modalities of treatment for bulimia. As illustrated here, "feminist family therapy" can be conducted in a variety of ways. In the fifth session three families, representing each of the family types, are followed through family therapy. The final section describes common obstacles in treatment posed by the client (individual, couple, or family), as well as by the therapist.

It is our hope that both new and experienced therapists working with eating disorders will find something of interest in this cohesive, feminist family systems conceptualization and treatment approach to bulimia, and that therapists will begin to utilize a variety of systemically appropriate interventions for a problem that is truly interpersonal.

# Acknowledgments

SEVERAL PERSONS MADE valuable contributions to this book on either a professional or personal level. In fact, the variety and sources of support have made this book what it is.

Without certain people this book would not have been possible. Susan Barrows, our editor, provided us with the opportunity to write this book. She was supportive, patient, insightful, and challenging. Special thanks goes to the individuals and families with whom we have worked, especially those persons who have allowed us to share their experiences of the recovery process in therapy. And last, but equally important, are the contributions our respective families have made to our understanding of human relationships and the complexity of family environments.

We thank three colleagues in particular: Dr. Donna Miller for her contributions to the pharmacology chapter and her willingness to allow us to quote her evaluation of a client referred for medication; Dr. Jean Rubel, whose articles in the ANRED ALERT provided many of the ideas for the guidelines for family members; and Dr. Alan Marlatt, whose work on relapse prevention provided a foundation for developing the section on "relapse, prolapse, and collapse."

Our research assistants, Cathy Reto and Jill Reule, offered extra hours to assist with literature searches, proofreading, and word-processing. We thank them for their support and enthusiasm.

Each of us grew professionally and personally during the process of working together to write this book. We appreciate each other's support, criticism, energy, and time, which made this book what it is.

# Bulimia

*A SYSTEMS APPROACH TO TREATMENT*

# PART I

# *BULIMIA: DEFINITION, ISSUES, AND EXPLANATIONS*

# CHAPTER 1

# *Developing Bulimia*

BULIMIA IS A SERIOUS psychologically-based disorder which usually starts in the late teens to early twenties (Abraham, Mira, & Llewellyn-Jones, 1983; Johnson & Berndt, 1983; Johnson, Stuckey, Lewis, & Schwartz, 1982; Pyle, Mitchell, & Eckert, 1981; Root, 1983; Rost, Neuhaus, & Florin, 1982) when the adolescent confronts the developmental task of leaving home. While bulimia often starts innocently, through the individual's own invention or through her reading or hearing about it (with a promise to use it "this one time only"), it can readily become a generalized coping response. Eating disorders usually begin subsequent to a period of dieting (Garfinkel, Moldofsky, & Garner, 1980; Root, 1983; Russell, 1979), moving away from home, the loss of an important romantic relationship (Johnson et al., 1982; Pyle et al., 1981; Root, 1983), ór an illness resulting in weight loss. Bulimia may start openly with friends or within sororities as a group activity. While some individuals are able to give up the behavior easily, others are not. We suggest that those who find the behavior difficult to stop come from families that, inexplicably, support the disorder. Over a period of time, the individual continuing to binge-purge becomes increasingly secretive, isolated, and desperate. Consequently, it often takes the bulimic and her family a year or more to recognize that the symptoms are out of control.

By the time she seeks help, she has usually tried to stop several times on her own. She has tried willpower, fasting (which actually increases the likelihood of a binge), reading books, and avoiding such binge situations (as studying at home or staying home alone); finally, she may have tried telling someone about her binge-eating in the hope that her disclosure would

3

shame her into stopping or provide the necessary external strength to overcome her bulimia.

When her secret has been discovered or disclosed, the bulimic feels disappointed and chagrined; even with other people knowing about her behavior, improvements in symptoms are often temporary. In fact, the symptoms often become worse as the individual feels watched and controlled by significant others. *Significant others usually interact with the bulimic in ways that exaggerate relationship characteristics that were present, but in more subtle form, before the bulimia was revealed.* The bulimia becomes a symptom around which the whole family revolves. The individual may increase her attempts to become more secretive (throwing up in pails, hiding vomit, sneaking binges, shoplifting food and laxatives) as she becomes more desperate. She makes and breaks promises to herself—"no more," "this is absolutely the last time," "if I do it one more time I have to seek help"—until she finally concludes that there must be something wrong with her mind, that she is going crazy.

*The family's involvement in the symptoms often mirrors what the symptomatic individual has been through.* Initially, the family members are not fazed by the problem and may optimistically rally to support their loved one. They read books, give advice, hide food, and attend support groups. These efforts are usually not enough to help their loved one overcome the eating disorder; then they feel scared and helpless. They may try with extra vigilance and determination to make available foods the individual likes and to set rules and limits; in frustration they may make threats. Increasingly, family life revolves around the symptomatic individual. Finally, the family is desperate. Depending on the type of family, they may reach out for help ("overprotective family"), disown the individual ("chaotic family"), or set up expectations so that the individual learns to hide her behavior even better and tells family members that she is cured when indeed she is not ("perfect family"). This response of initial support and encouragement followed by increased controlling efforts contributes to the interpersonal maintenance of the eating disorder.

*The bulimic may feel that there is no turning back; everyone in the family is overinvolved in her symptoms, even to the extent of feeling her pain.* She may seriously consider suicide as a way to end everyone's distress and pain. Discovery of a suicide plan or a suicide attempt may be the reason a family or individual enters therapy.

## STEREOTYPES

As a result of the sensationalizing of anorexia and bulimia by the media, stereotypes about bulimics have been accepted by laypersons, clinicians, and researchers. Four major stereotypes are associated with bulimia.

*The first stereotype is that bulimia is a female, heterosexual disorder.*

While females are most likely to develop bulimia, males, too, are capable of developing the syndrome. It is estimated that 5–10% of persons with bulimia are male (Pyle et al., 1981). Initially, there was clinical conjecture that bulimic males would be homosexual. This would be understandable, given the emphasis on body image in the gay male community. However, our experience is that heterosexual men are also capable of developing the full clinical picture of bulimia. At the same time, many of the bulimic men we have seen appear to be sorting out sexual identity issues. From our clinical experience, lesbian women are also vulnerable to developing bulimia, particularly if they have not resolved sexual identity issues.

*The second stereotype is that bulimia is a disorder affecting only teens and young women.* Bulimia is a new diagnosis which acknowledges the validity of a problem — a problem that can affect persons of all ages and has existed for years. While bulimia tends to develop at the age when an individual is leaving home, people do not tend to "grow out of it." It is not unusual for the bulimic to report a family history that confirms or strongly suggests that his or her mother and grandmother had bulimia. Most likely, these older relatives were bulimic all their life.

*The third stereotype is that bulimia is a white phenomenon.* For anyone who has worked extensively with people of color, this myth is soon dispelled. Bulimia affects all races. Neither color nor ethnicity provides a sure immunity to developing this disorder. While it is apparent that some ethnic groups, because of cultural norms, do not place as much emphasis on a thin body image, individuals who grow up in Western cultures are vulnerable to societal pressures outside the family; also, the family may adopt images and messages of the larger societal group.

*The last stereotype is that it is a psychological disorder which affects the upper and upper-middle class.* While research has indicated that anorexia nervosa is more often seen in the upper social classes (Crisp, Kalucey, Lacey, & Harding, 1977; Jones, Fox, Babigan, & Hutton, 1980; Morgan & Russell, 1975), recent research in this area supports the belief that eating disorders are increasingly occurring throughout all social classes. This may be due to increased public recognition of the disorder or to less stigma associated with seeking mental health services. Garfinkel and Garner (1982) offer an additional explanation — that attitudes towards weight and acceptable body image, which are a predisposing factor in the development of eating disorders, are becoming more evenly distributed among all social classes.

## DEFINING BULIMIA

Bulimia affects the individual behaviorally, psychologically, and physiologically. While it may appear to be the individual's problem, bulimia is a signal that the environment is not meeting her needs. A definition of bulimia requires an overview of the individual symptomatology and an

understanding of the general issues involved in the function of bulimia. We
also need to distinguish bulimia from other emotionally based eating disorders, particularly anorexia nervosa.

The definition for bulimia set forth by the American Psychiatric Association (1980) is met by compulsive eaters, yo-yo dieters, and bulimics without
distinguishing among them. The primary criteria are:

1) recurrent episodes of binge-eating;
2) recognition of bingeing as abnormal;
3) depression and self-criticism following the binges.

Using the *DSM-III* criteria, a wide range of clinical presentations fall
within the definition of bulimia. This in turn creates confusion about the
its prevalence. Many initial surveys used liberal criteria, e.g., "the individual
is distressed over binge-eating behavior which is cyclical." These yielded
estimates that 40–50% of men and 70–80% of women in college populations could qualify for the diagnosis of bulimia (Halmi, Falk, & Schwartz,
1981; Hawkins & Clement, 1980). The problem with using such criteria is
that distress over binge-eating is observed and reported in a wide variety
of clinical and nonclinical populations, including anorectics (Casper, Eckert,
Halmi, Goldberg, & Davis, 1980; Crisp, Hsu, & Harding, 1980; Garfinkel
et al., 1980; Garfinkel, 1981; Hsu, Crisp, & Harding, 1979; Russell, 1979;
Strober, Salkin, Burroughs, & Morrell, 1982), obese individuals (Edelman,
1981), and individuals with no history of obesity or anorexia nervosa (Boskind-Lodahl, 1976; Boskind-Lodahl & White, 1978; Crisp, 1981–2; Halmi
et al., 1981; Hawkins & Clement, 1980; Pyle et al., 1981; Russell, 1979;
Stangler & Printz, 1980).

Surveys using more stringent behavioral criteria yield much lower estimates of the incidence of bulimia. When both binge-eating and purging
behaviors are used as criteria, it is estimated that fewer than 5% of women
(Fairburn & Cooper, 1983; Pyle, Mitchell, Eckert, Halvorson, Neuman, &
Goff, 1983; Stangler & Printz, 1980) and .4% of men (Pyle et al., 1981) are
bulimic. Even with these conservative estimates, the actual numbers of persons who are likely to develop the symptomatic picture are large.

The American Psychiatric Association (1985) is considering a revision in
the criteria to address some of the aforementioned problems. The proposed
criteria listed below should yield a more conservative diagnosis of bulimia:

1) recurrent episodes of binge-eating occurring on an average of twice
   weekly for a duration of three months;
2) use of a method of purging to counteract the binges (self-induced
   vomiting, laxative abuse, or rigorous dieting).

## INDIVIDUAL SYMPTOMS

We define and diagnose bulimia according both to individual behavioral, psychological, and physiological symptoms and to family dynamics. In diagnosing bulimia, we use the more stringent behavioral criteria of both bingeing and purging behavior. In this section, we review the behavioral, psychological, and physiological criteria used to make the diagnosis at the individual level. Table 1 provides a summary of the symptoms. (Family dynamics are discussed extensively in Section II.)

### Behavioral Symptoms

Binge-eating and purging are the hallmark behavioral symptoms associated with bulimia. Several other behaviors develop or are concurrent with binge-purge patterns, such as substance abuse, excessive use of caffeine, shoplifting, suicidal gesturing, irritability, and mood swings. These latter, secondary symptoms are not essential to a diagnosis of bulimia.

BINGEING AND PURGING. The binge usually occurs over a period of less than two hours and may cycle repeatedly with purging behavior so that a whole day may be taken up with bulimic episodes (Abraham & Beumont, 1982). A binge does not necessarily involve a large quantity of food because the bulimic's definition of a binge is subjective. Binge-eating is precipitated by both physiological and psychological factors, such as restrictive dieting and stringent rules about eating (Wardle & Beinart, 1981), as well as by stressful events. Most often bulimics binge on food that they do not ordinarily allow themselves to eat, such as desserts and carbohydrates. Easily ingested, high calorie foods, e.g., ice cream, cookies, pudding (Johnson et al., 1982), are most commonly the target of binge-eating. A binge may also include nutritional foods in normal or vast quantities, e.g., vegetables, yogurt, cheese, meat (Root, 1983). The cost of a binge may be minimal to over $50.00 a day (Johnson et al., 1982; Root, 1983).

Purging behavior via abuse of laxatives, self-induced vomiting, or diuretics is often as important and as out-of-control as the binge-eating, though it may serve a different purpose. It often serves to undo the binge, reduce anxiety, and punish the binge-eater. Vomiting appears to be the most commonly reported method of purging, followed by laxative abuse (Johnson et al., 1982; Pyle et al., 1981; Root, 1983; Root & Fallon, 1985; Russell, 1979). In a study of 95 bulimic women reported by Johnson and Berndt (1983), 77% were self-inducing vomiting, 33% were using laxatives, and 25.7% were doing both.

SUBSTANCE ABUSE. This is a common concomitant of bulimia. Many individuals disclose a history of abusing alcohol, drugs, over-the-counter diet pills, amphetamines, and caffeine. Alcohol, drugs, and food can serve similar purposes in providing anesthetic relief from feeling.

Hatsukami, Owen, Pyle, and Mitchell (1982) compared the MMPI profiles of 52 bulimic women with 120 inpatient women being treated for substance abuse. Over one-third of their initial sample of bulimics had to be eliminated from participation because of alcohol and drug abuse problems. The MMPI profiles of the two groups were similar, although the substance abusers' profiles were more elevated. The two most commonly shared profiles between the groups were the 2-4-8 profile and a within-normal-limits profile. Over half of the MMPI code types observed in a bulimic sample analyzed by Root and Friedrich (1985) were profiles associated with alcohol and substance abuse.

As bulimia becomes more chronic and if the person has increasingly limited food intake when not bingeing, beverages containing caffeine may be consumed addictively. It is a familiar scene to see a client refilling a coffee mug several times a day or drinking one diet cola after another. These beverages provide a temporary relief from thirst, give an energy boost, suppress hunger, and provide a potentially unlimited quantity of sweetness (Sours, 1983).

SHOPLIFTING. Increasingly, bulimics are entering therapy through deferred prosecution and sentencing by the courts for shoplifting. Shoplifting may occur as the bulimia becomes more chronic (Crisp et al., 1980; Pyle et al., 1981; Weiss & Ebert, 1983), even in persons who have no history of shoplifting prior to the onset of bulimia. Shoplifting may become necessary to obtain food for binge-eating. However, shoplifting does not have to emerge in the chronic stage of the disorder. We have seen clients where it was the "cry for help" that precipitated treatment.

SUICIDE AND MOOD. It is surprising that suicidal behavior in the bulimic population has not been studied more extensively. Suicidal behavior (attempts and threats) is common with bulimia, with several researchers reporting that approximately one-third of their samples have attempted suicide (Hudson, Pope, Jonas, & Yurgelun-Todd, 1983; Russell, 1979). Root (1983) and Johnson et al. (1982) report lower rates, but still a significant incidence of 19.4% and 14.1% respectively, with their samples. In a recent study of 142 bulimic women, Reto, Root, and Fallon (1985) found that 49% of their sample had suicidal thoughts and 20% had attempted suicide. Suicide may be the most frequent cause of death with this population.

Irritability, depression, mood swings, and anxiety are commonly observed and reported in the bulimic. While these affective states do not necessarily predict suicidal behavior, they have been correlated with increased suicidal ideation and threats.

## Psychological Symptoms

The most common psychological features observed in individuals with bulimia include: a pervasive sense of powerlessness; numbness to feelings of anger, fear, and anxiety; depression and mood swings; low self-esteem, a poorly defined sense of self; hypersensitivity to approval and criticism; obsession and preoccupation with food, weight, and appearance; lack of close, emotionally intimate, and fulfilling relationships; and social withdrawal and isolation, particularly with chronicity. There are few psychological disorders in which the emotional and physiological symptoms are as intertwined as in bulimia. *All of the psychological symptoms are exacerbated by starvation.* This is supported by the University of Minnesota studies on human starvation, in which many of the men who volunteered to starve themselves, through gradual reduction in nutritional intake, experienced the vegetative signs of depression, e.g., irritability, difficulty sleeping, and social withdrawal, as their starvation continued (Keyes, Brozek, Henschel, Michelson, & Taylor, 1950). Moreover, these subjects became increasingly preoccupied with food.

We commonly observe many psychological and behavioral features in bulimics consistent with borderline personality disorder, such as impulsivity, anger, and lack of close intimate relationships. These features change markedly with recovery from bulimia for many women. Given the traumatic developmental histories revealed by many bulimics (Selvini Palazzoli, 1978), it is likely that there is a significant number of persons who warrant a dual diagnosis of personality disorder *and* eating disorder. Nevertheless, we strongly suggest that a diagnosis of a personality disorder be withheld unless the individual carries such a diagnosis prior to the onset of the eating disorder or until after the eating-disordered behavior is stabilized (Anderson & Mickalide, 1983). It is a good idea to wait until the eating behavior has stabilized in order to avoid making a diagnosis on the basis of behavior and psychological styles that are physiologically and psychologically transient. We will now discuss specifically the individual psychological symptoms mentioned above.

POWERLESSNESS. This is a pervasive feeling that the bulimic individual experiences within herself and her environment. Most often there are reasons why the bulimic feels so powerless. An exceedingly large number of bulimics have been victims of physical and sexual abuse, rape or battering. Root and Fallon (1985) report that 66% of 172 bulimic women reported having been victimized. As adults they may be in relationships in which they again sustain physical or sexual abuse. Others have been severely psychologically abused through parental manipulativeness, criticism, and unavailability. In other families, the rules have been so explicit and rigid that the individual has not had the power to choose. Indecisiveness and feelings of incompetency may accompany powerlessness. For other bulimics, the loss of loved ones through illness and death at critical times in their lives has contributed to a sense of powerlessness and inability to control one's life. Whatever the pathway, most bulimics have reached a point of personal resignation and hopelessness in relating to their environment.

Weiss and Ebert (1983) provide data that further support the observation that bulimics feel that they have little control over what happens to them. They noted that bulimic women exhibited lower internal locus of control scores than a nonclinical sample of women. In another study of bulimic women, Root and Friedrich (1985) noted low T-scores on scale 5 of the Minnesota Multiphasic Personality Inventory. Such a score is associated with behavioral characteristics of submissiveness, passivity, and lack of assertiveness. Traditional feminine sex-role behavior, such as dependency, unassertiveness, and an external locus of control, tends to decrease the individual's sense of self-efficacy and control within the environment.

Ironically, bulimia is often the individual's attempt to feel more powerful and in control. It becomes a costly way to structure predictability. Eating rituals and plans are established; when they are changed, the bulimic may be very upset, as she is once again reminded of her powerlessness. Repeated failure to control one's bulimia further contributes to a sense of personal failure, self-defeat, and ineffectiveness.

EXPRESSION OF FEELINGS. Depression is the most common feeling experienced and expressed by the bulimic. It is a major feature of bulimia, particularly with chronicity. This is certainly congruent with feelings of powerlessness. Also, there is no doubt that starvation increases an individual's vulnerability to depression.

Many bulimics have experienced losses of family members through illness, suicide, drugs, or accident. Often these families have not grieved openly. The bulimic may carry the family grief into a severe depression, with onset in childhood or in the teen years. This depression may not be observable to family members.

"Smiling depressions" are common in this population. This is not surprising when one realizes that bulimics often come from families where depression is not permitted. Tears can be streaming down the face of a young woman as she holds a smile on her face. Some families can talk of pain they feel or a loss they have experienced, while all the family members simultaneously smile.

Much of the bulimic's depression and irritability is the consequence of cognitive distortions resulting from a set of expectations and beliefs (Garner & Bemis, 1982). We contend that the cognitions that the bulimic individual holds, which contribute both to the bulimia and to the depression, are messages transmitted and reinforced by the family. Thus, the therapist can blend family therapy with cognitive therapy in order to address feelings, thoughts, and behavior.

Much recent research has focused on the possibility that bulimia is an alternative form of affective disorder (Herzog, 1982; Hudson, Laffer, & Pope, 1982; Pope, Hudson, Jonas, & Yurgelun-Todd, 1983; Walsh, Stewart, Wright, Harrison, Roose, & Glassman, 1982). Evidence for such a hypothesis is drawn from observation of the prevalence of affective disorders in first-degree relatives of individuals with eating disorders (Hudson et al., 1983); positive responses on the dexamethasone suppression test (Hudson et al., 1982); and the response of bulimics to antidepressants (Hudson et al., 1982; Pope et al., 1983). The results, while striking, are equivocal. A recent research study concluded that the prevalence of affective disorders among relatives is no higher than in the general population (Stern et al., 1984), and challenges the affective disorder/bulimia linkage. Responses to the dexamethasone suppression test may be correlated with low weight rather than depression (Gerner & Gwirtsman, 1981) or alcohol abuse (Swartz & Dunner, 1982). Lastly, there are well controlled studies which show that bulimics do *not* significantly respond to carbamazepine, a tricyclic medication (Kaplan, Garfinkel, Darby, & Garner, 1983), or that they relapse after a short period of time, despite initially promising results and continued medication (Brotman, Herzog, & Woods, 1984). We do not feel that an affective disorder-eating disorder connection exists in all of the bulimic clients we see. The affective disorder, as mentioned earlier, may be a transient physiological state. Yet chronic depression is very common in our clients. Medication as an adjunct to treatment is discussed in Chapter 16.

*Depression is linked with anger.* Depression may have been the only "safe" or "acceptable" feeling in the family of origin. Often, in initial interviews, the bulimic client will deny feeling anger. If the individual is not physically safe or permitted to express anger openly and directly, depression becomes a safer outlet; it is a way to direct anger towards oneself instead of others. In all three family types presented in Section III, anger is discouraged due to various family rules and injunctions. *Recognizing feelings of anger and learning to express them in a safe and appropriate manner are major issues in recovery from bulimia.*

SELF-IMAGE AND SELF-ESTEEM. A poorly defined self-image and low self-esteem are apparent in the bulimic's excessive need for approval and affirmation, as well as in her hypersensitivity to approval and criticism. Sometimes, more chronic clients are described as "hollow," reflecting this lack of a sense of self. Their relationships (or lack thereof) also reflect their low self-esteem. It is not only abusive families which foster low self-esteem; families expecting perfection can foster severe self-criticalness and a compulsion to do things "right" by others' perceptions, rather than one's own. Other families project an identification onto the developing girl of a hyperpassivity congruent with an ultrafeminine orientation, depriving her of opportunities to feel competent and establish selfhood.

Bulimics are often in search of an identity. They define themselves by their appearance, their achievements, and people's reactions to them. Therefore, criticism and approval are not merely feedback but signals of acceptance or rejection of their whole being. Definitions of self are largely external and easily shaken, even by a scale registering an extra pound. Much energy is spent trying to please and figure out what is the *right* answer, the *right* expression, or the *right* opinion. As a result, bulimics often confuse themselves further as to what they themselves believe or feel.

There is frequently a fear that if people really knew about them, these people would not be interested. Bulimics often excel at being tuned into others' needs while being unable to determine their own. This hypersensitivity is a frequent phenomenon and seems to reflect the extreme sensitivity some women have had to exhibit in reading subtle cues in their families (Friedrich & Pollock, 1982). They often end up knowing all about their "friends," but their "friends" know very little about them.

RELATIONSHIPS. Many bulimics are successful and well-liked and have friends; however, with increasing chronicity their social support system often becomes smaller and less accessible, especially as they become more secretive. While they want to have close intimate friends whom they can trust, many will have difficulty trusting people because of their developmental histories. In families where acceptance is dependent upon certain "appropriate" feelings and behaviors, intimacy may seem like dangerous self-exposure, since the "real self" may not be accepted. Where there has been abuse, molestation, and alcoholism, it is realistically hard to trust other people or rely on their availability. Bulimics learn to be social while keeping others at a distance. They try not to let people get too close, thus avoiding being hurt or violated.

Weiss and Ebert (1983) found that, while their bulimic sample was similar to nonbulimic controls, e.g., they held jobs, had friends, and were liked, on closer examination the bulimics had fewer close friends or relatives. Garfinkel and Garner (1982) observed that interpersonal relationships can fluctuate from superficial ones to intense, dependent ones leading to personal devaluation and/or anger.

Chronicity of bulimia is associated with increased withdrawal from interpersonal relationships and increased isolation (Root & Friedrich, 1985). Such isolation tends to be associated with idiosyncratic thinking, cognitive distortion, and hypersensitivity to criticism and feedback.

CONTROL. The bulimic's life alternates between extremes of being rigidly controlled and totally out of control. Out-of-control behavior can be manifested in binge-eating, excessive drinking or drug use, promiscuity, shoplifting, suicide attempts, and binge-spending. Excessive control is manifested in list-making, excessive covert rehearsal of interactions, restricted intake, restricted emotional expression, and rigid routines and rules. The excessive control the bulimic exerts can stem from learning to walk on eggshells while growing up in a physically abusive environment, being rewarded for manipulative behavior, or having to outmaneuver a parent who is particularly controlling. The bulimic tries to control whatever she can and concludes that the only sure thing she can control is herself or, rather, her physical appearance. Because the bulimic's self-image is so poorly defined, this obsessive self-control is superficial and unrealistic. Clients frequently report fearing vacations, regressing in coping skills during semester breaks, or living with a roommate because free time is more difficult to control.

Because relationships and circumstances (e.g., losses or victimization experiences) may be beyond control, bulimics soon focus on controlling their appearance. They become obsessed with what they eat or do not eat, their weight, and their physical appearance. They learn to do battle over the scale, feeling in control if they lose a pound or do not gain weight. Their preoccupation with food and weight becomes obsessional and consuming to the point that other things are secondary.

Binge-eating and purging become predictable and controllable. Even with the pain or exhaustion, the bulimic knows how bulimic episodes will go and so schedules them to experience control. The bulimic may panic when she cannot throw up one day.

While these symptoms have been organized under the heading of psychological symptoms, it should be remembered that all of the psychological symptoms are exacerbated by starvation and the physical experience of binge-purging. In many ways, the distinction between psychological and physiological symptomatology is an artificial one. Keeping this caution in mind, we now move to a discussion of the frequent physical effects of bulimia.

*Physiological Symptoms*

The physiological symptoms of bulimia are not well documented. The results of bingeing and purging can include such physical symptoms as cold intolerance (due to starvation and fat loss), painful digestion, parotid enlargement, dehydration, electrolyte imbalance, dental problems, and irregular menstrual cycles or amenorrhea (Root & Fallon, 1983). Death by physiological emergency is not the issue that it is within the anorectic population. At this time, the only documented irreversible consequences associated with bulimia are dental problems caused by increased vomiting and excessive carbohydrate intake. The other common physiological symptoms of bulimia appear to be reversible with recovery.

DENTAL SYMPTOMS AND CONSEQUENCES. The most common symptoms and consequences of bulimia are dental enamel erosion and increased cavities (Brady, 1980; House, Crisius, Bliziotes, & Licht, 1981; Hurst, Lacey, & Crisp, 1977). The effects of chronic vomiting (dental enamel erosion) are irreversible. Symptoms of enamel erosion are shortening of the teeth, increased space between teeth, and painful sensitivity to the temperature of foods when they touch the teeth. An increased number of cavities is attributed to increased carbohydrate intake during binges.

TABLE 1

Behavioral, Psychological, and Physiological Symptoms of Bulimia

| Behavioral | Psychological | Physiological |
|---|---|---|
| At least 90% of normal weight | Numbness and repression of feelings, especially anger | Menstrual functioning Irregular periods |
| Binge-eating | Depression, anxiety | Amenorrhea |
| Purging | Poor definition of self | Electrolyte imbalance |
| Vomiting | Low self-esteem | Muscle weakness |
| Laxative abuse | Hypersensitivity | Muscle cramping |
| Diuretic abuse | Hollowness | Dehydration |
| Regular cycling of bingeing and purging | Powerlessness | Dry skin |
| Secretive eating | Depression | Brittle hair/nails |
| Substance abuse | Victimization | Fainting |
| Amphetamines | Manipulativeness | Constant thirst |
| Street drugs | Impulsivity | Dizziness |
| Alcohol | Obsession with: | Dental problems |
| Caffeine abuse | Food | Enamel erosion |
| Shoplifting | Weight | Increased cavities |
| Suicidal behavior | Physical appearance | Parotid enlargement |
| | Control | Cold intolerance |
| | Superficial relationships | Fatigue |
| | Isolation | Cyanosis |
| | Secretiveness | Digestive problems |

MENSTRUATION. Irregular menstrual cycles and amenorrhea in bulimic women have been reported in the literature (Crisp, 1981; Johnson et al., 1982; Lacey, 1983; Pyle et al., 1981; Root, 1983; Russell, 1979; Weiss & Ebert, 1983). In three studies of bulimic women, 40–50% had irregular menstrual cycles (Fairburn & Cooper, 1982; Johnson et al., 1982; Root, 1983). When the percentage of body fat drops below a critical point, hormonal release is affected, which in turn results in amenorrhea. These investigators report only 7–20% of their samples having amenorrhea. It is our clinical experience that, while most women regain their menstrual cycle with some weight gain, other women may go years without menstruating. This observation is not well understood as yet. It is possible that poor nutrition, even at normal weight, and psychological development can affect hormonal functions.

ELECTROLYTE IMBALANCE AND DEHYDRATION. Purging behavior, particularly frequent vomiting, can result in electrolyte imbalances (the depletion of chloride and serum potassium) (House et al., 1981; Russell, 1979). Symptoms associated with electrolyte imbalance are muscle cramping and weakness. Extreme fluid loss as a result of vomiting, laxative abuse, or diuretic abuse also results in dehydration, as manifested by brittle nails, hair breakage or loss, constant thirst, and faintness when postural positions are suddenly changed, e.g., from lying to sitting or sitting to standing.

OTHER PHYSICAL SYMPTOMS. Cold intolerance, swollen parotid (salivary) glands, painful digestion, and poor circulation in hands and feet are reported in bulimia. Cold intolerance appears to be related to decreased body fat. Frequent vomiting is correlated with parotid gland enlargement (Levin, Falko, Dixon, Gallup, & Saunders, 1980; Walsh, Croft, & Katz, 1981–82). The explanations for parotid enlargement are equivocal. Walsh et al. (1981–82) suggest that a combination of severe and prolonged malnutrition with substantial binge-eating and vomiting increases the individual's risk for developing this condition. Painful digestion is related to abdominal bloating and gas. These symptoms usually subside as the individual resumes more consistent eating patterns, and the body relearns digestion on a regular basis. The reason for poor circulation in the extremities is not clear. While many women have poor circulation in their extremities, the bulimic's hands and feet appear redder or bluer at times when she is vomiting frequently.

Currently no research is available to document the pattern of physiological recovery. It appears that the chronicity of the bulimia is positively correlated with the time it takes to reverse the physiological sequelae. Informing bulimics of the potential physical sequelae of bulimia does not enable them to stop their bulimic behavior.

## A COMPARISON OF BULIMIA AND ANOREXIA NERVOSA

There is no question that a significant proportion of individuals with bulimia have a prior history of anorexia nervosa. Bruch (1978) estimated that 25% of anorectic patients evolved into a pattern of bulimia. Most studies providing this information yield estimates similar to Bruch's that 20–25%

TABLE 2

Comparison of Bulimia and Anorexia Nervosa

| *Anorexia nervosa* | *Bulimia* |
|---|---|
| 1. Refusal to maintain recommended minimal weight | 1. Normal or near-normal weight; may be above average weight |
| 2. Younger age of onset (early adolescence) | 2. Later age of onset (Late teens or early adulthood) |
| 3. Loss of menstrual period | 3. Menstrual irregularities are common. Menstrual period may be lost. |
| 4. Distorted body-image common | 4. More accurate perceptions of body-image |
| 5. Denial of food-related problems | 5. Acknowledgment of abnormal eating patterns |
| 6. Outwardly exhibits more self-control | 6. More impulsivity; alcohol and drug abuse common |
| 7. Anemia and vitamin deficiencies rare | 7. Anemia and vitamin deficiencies uncommon but not as rare |
| 8. Vomiting less pervasive | 8. Greater incidence of vomiting and laxative abuse |
| 9. Eating rituals | 9. May appear to eat normally when not bingeing and when eating in public |
| 10. Morality rate higher — death likely to be due to physical consequences | 10. Mortality rate undetermined — death likely to be due to suicide |
| 11. Treatment more commonly initiated by family and friends | 11. Individual more frequently initiates treatment |
| 12. Less commonly observed histories of substance abuse in family members | 12. Family histories commonly include substance abuse problems |
| 13. History of victimization less common | 13. Victimization experiences frequently observed (rape, molestation, physical abuse) |
| 14. Very low tolerance for intimacy | 14. More often in relationship or married though still has difficulty with intimacy |

Adapted from Neuman and Halvorson, 1983, p. 64.

of bulimics have a prior history of anorexia (Abraham et al., 1983; Mitchell, Hosfield, & Pyle, 1983; Pope et al., 1983; Root, 1983). Estimates vary greatly, from 5.2% of 316 respondents to a mail in survey (Johnson et al., 1982) to 60% of 30 patients observed by Russell (1979).

Several studies suggest that a previous history of anorexia nervosa may be correlated with the degree to which these individuals are currently functioning adaptively in their environments (Halmi et al., 1981; Pyle et al., 1981; Russell, 1979). Gwirtsman, Roy-Byrne, Yager, and Gerner (1983) suggest that " . . . the past incidence of primary anorexia nervosa in bulimic patients is lowest when the patients are relatively functional and not seeking treatment, higher when they are seeking outpatient treatment, and highest when they are dysfunctional enough to require inpatient treatment (p. 560)." Halmi, Goldberg, Casper, Eckert, and Davis (1979) offer two hypotheses for this relationship: 1) bulimia is a sign of the severity and chronicity of the same eating disorder as anorexia nervosa, or 2) bulimia represents a more advanced maturational state of psychological development than anorexia nervosa. This latter hypothesis is supported by the observation that, while bulimia develops in individuals who have previous histories of anorexia nervosa (Palmer, 1979; Russell, 1979), the reverse is clinically rare.

Levitan (1981) supports the hypothesis that the bulimia is a sign of the severity and chronicity of the same eating disorder as anorexia nervosa. He suggests that bulimic individuals with a previous history of anorexia nervosa represent a different subgroup of persons from those without such a history. The working criteria for bulimia being developed by the American Psychiatric Association for the next revision of the *Diagnostic and Statistical Manual of Mental Disorders* (*DSM-III-R*) result from an attempt to distinguish between bulimia with and without a prior history of anorexia nervosa. Those criteria may enable clinicians and researchers to further research these hypotheses.

*We find many "bulimics" who were previously at low weights and anorectic to still be "anorectic" in psychological presentation, even though they are of approximately normal weight and given the diagnosis of bulimia.* It is almost always the case that there was no time between a low weight and normal weight that the individual did not have an eating disorder. The diagnosis of bulimia is governed by the normal weight status and behavioral symptomatology, rather than psychological symptomatology, which may still be that of an anorectic.

Many differences have been cited between anorectics and bulimics. Demographic differences suggest that, compared to the anorectic, the bulimic is older and has been dysfunctional longer (Casper et al., 1980; Garfinkel & Garner, 1982), weighs more (Beumont, Abraham, & Simson, 1981; Garfinkel et al., 1980; Garfinkel & Garner, 1982; Herzog, 1982; Pyle et al., 1981; Russell, 1979), is more likely to have a mother who is obese (Garfinkel et al., 1980; Pyle et al., 1981), is more likely to be married (Herzog, 1982), and has a higher incidence of parental death or serious parental illness (Herzog, 1982).

Psychological differences noted between anorectic and bulimic samples suggest that, compared to anorexics, bulimics are more likely to enter treatment by their own initiative (Casper et al., 1980), are more extroverted (Beumont, George, & Smart, 1976; Casper et al., 1980; Garfinkel et al., 1980; Russell, 1979), more labile in mood (Garfinkel & Garner, 1982; Garfinkel et al., 1980), score higher on indices of depression and somatization (Casper et al., 1980; Crisp, 1981–82), and score lower on indices of obsessive-compulsiveness, somatization, anxiety, interpersonal sensitivity, and depression on the Hopkins Symptom Checklist (Johnson et al., 1982) (while Aono and Kumashiro (1983) conclude that bulimics display more manifest anxiety than anorectics on physiological measures).

It has been suggested that bulimics have a poorer prognosis in terms of recovery than anorectics (Beumont et al., 1976, Crisp et al., 1977; Garfinkel et al., 1980; Morgan & Russell, 1975). More recent research with group treatment suggests a more hopeful picture for bulimics (Boskind-Lodahl, & White, 1978; Root, 1983). In contrast to anorectics, bulimics report greater difficulty controlling their weight (Beumont et al., 1976), increased incidence of impulsive behaviors such as suicidal attempts and self-mutilation (Crisp, 1981–82; Garfinkel & Garner, 1982; Russell, 1979; Simpson, 1973), stealing, drug abuse, and alcohol abuse (Casper et al., 1980; Crisp, 1981–82; Garfinkel et al., 1980; Pyle et al., 1981). The differences between persons presenting with anorexia and those presenting with bulimia are summarized in Table 2.

There are many contrasts between anorectics and bulimics on demographic, familial, and behavioral levels that are qualitative rather than quantitative. While much of the early research suggested that bulimia has a poorer prognosis in terms of recovery, our clinical experience has been the reverse. This may be due to the fact that treatment programs have been in effect for a much shorter period of time for bulimia and, as the definition of the disorder and its causes have become clearer, treatment has become more effective.

Looking at symptoms and variables distinguishing bulimia from anorexia nervosa and from compulsive eating, we realize that bulimia is definitely more than a problem with food or self-esteem, and the problems in most cases are not simply individual problems. The symptoms of bulimia are reinforced by the culture in which we live and in which families are formed. The therapist working with individuals and families with bulimia must have an understanding of the way in which these three factors—the individual, the culture, and the family—interact to create a context for the individual's development of bulimia.

# CHAPTER 2

# *Sociocultural Contributions*

As FEMINIST FAMILY therapists, we feel that it is essential for the clinician working with bulimic individuals and their families to have an understanding of the cultural pressures that contribute to the development of bulimia. These cultural pressures are part of the larger system of the bulimic. While cultural contributions to the development of bulimia have been widely recognized by a number of researchers in the field of eating disorders, surprisingly little has been written about these influences by family therapists working with families with eating disorders. An understanding of the convergence of pressures exerted by society and by the family has a direct impact on the focus and course of therapy.

In this chapter we offer an overview of the research that illuminates the consequences of the socialization process for women, which increases their vulnerability to developing bulimia. Particular attention is directed to the sources and consequences of the cultural proscriptions of femininity and success, the processes that limit women's control and power in their lives, and the effects of socialization on women's body-image and self-image.

## LEARNING TO BE FEMALE

Equating femininity with adjectives such as "fragile," "thin," "small," "helpless," and "delicate" is in conflict with images of women as strong, powerful, and credible. The latter set of adjectives usually conjures up images for people raised in this culture of large women, not typically described as feminine. Bulimia symbolizes the particular pathology of the socialization process for females in Western cultures and certain family environments. Orbach (1978) emphasizes the importance of the nuclear family as the system

20

responsible for reproducing the societal expectations of women. The family is critical as a messenger of these societal expectations and determines how these social messages are incorporated into a woman's developing sense of identity, competency, power, and self-worth.

Women have long been reinforced for sacrificing their well-being in pursuit of approval for being feminine. For example, in the early 1900s women bound their waists with corsets so tightly that sometimes ribs were broken. Some women opted for surgical removal of lower ribs in order to achieve a more ideal "wasp-like" figure. Attainment of this ideal figure was so important that women would rather not eat than give up their corsets. Frailty was glamorized during a period when tuberculosis, a prevalent disease which resulted in the person's wasting away, was seen as a symbol of status and femininity (Sontag, 1978). As recently as 1975, *Playboy* magazine glamorized anorexia nervosa as the "Golden Girl's" disease. Such images of femininity were not restricted to Western cultures. The Chinese, for example, had an old custom of binding girls' feet to stunt growth and give the appearance of delicacy. Women compromised physical mobility and comfort for social approval.

Women are still raised on false hopes of power, led to believe that their power rests in their beauty and kindness. Romance novels perpetuate this notion with descriptions of heroines casting spells or rendering men powerless or speechless with their beauty. Fairytales promise women success, happiness, and love if they are beautiful, kind, and self-sacrificing (Kohlbenschlag, 1979). Limited, superficial means to achieve power (through beauty and kindness) are taught to young children. It is hard to challenge these messages when sex-role socialization starts as early as children are able to listen to fairytales like *Snow White*, *Cinderella*, and *The Little Mermaid*, which promote as positive characteristics of the female heroines passivity, beauty, and self-sacrifice.

This socialization process has a significant impact on how women subsequently learn to satisfy their needs. Women, reinforced to be passive in their developmental years, eventually wake to the harsh realization that passivity and self-sacrifice are not reinforced with an equal distribution of rights or power. However, at this point, many women do not feel they have the right to get their needs satisfied or to strive for power or control, much less to express anger directly — a way to feel more powerful.

## Women and Anger

There are few secondary rewards for angry women. In fact, women can be punished for directness by being negatively labeled — a "bitch." Consequently, women may learn to express anger passively and indirectly through

frowns, glares, and inflections of voice (Tavris, 1982). Then they are likely
to be seen as manipulative. An angry woman is negatively labeled whether
she is direct or indirect.

## Women and Depression

The social rules that discourage women from expressing their anger promote their vulnerability to further powerlessness in depression. As Chesler
(1972) observes:

> It is important to note that "depressed" women are (like women in general)
> only verbally hostile; unlike most men, they do not express their hostility
> physically — either directly, to the "significant others" in their lives, or indirect-
> ly, through physical and athletic prowess. It is safer for women to become
> "depressed" than physically violent. Physically violent women usually lose
> physical battles with male intimates; are abandoned by them as "crazy" as
> well as "unfeminine"; are frequently psychiatrically or (less frequently) crim-
> inally incarcerated. Further, physically strong and/or potentially assaultive
> women would gain fewer secondary rewards than "depressed" women; their
> families would fear, hate, and abandon them, rather than pity, sympathize,
> or "protect" them. (p. 45–46)

Far more women than men seek therapy for long-standing or recurrent
depression that seems to be linked to long-standing unhappiness (or powerlessness). Over several studies of women and men the observed ratio of
depressed women to depressed men is 1.6 : 1 (Weissman & Klerman, 1977).
Weissman (1980) cites three sources for the disparity between men and
women in rates of depression: genetic, endocrine, and psychosocial. While
she contends the rates are likely to be affected by both biological and psychological factors, she offers two explanatory pathways for increased rates of
depression in women. In the first pathway, the social-status hypothesis, it
is observed that real social discrimination against women which discourages
power and assertion " . . . lead to legal and economic helplessness, dependency on others, chronic low self-esteem, low aspirations, and, ultimately,
clinical depression" (p. 102). In the second pathway, the learned-helplessness
hypothesis (Seligman, 1974), it is proposed that the cognitive set taught to
women reinforces helplessness; "young girls learn to be helpless during their
socialization and thus develop a limited response repertoire when under
stress" (p. 102).

The most striking evidence in support of a psychosocial explanation for
women's increased vulnerability to depression rests in the finding that, while
marriage appears to provide a buffer for men against psychological dis-

turbance, the opposite is observed for married women (Radloff, 1975). Subtle forms of cultural bias, reflecting society's socialization process, are observed in the diagnostic system. If women are angry and do not know how to express it, except indirectly, they may receive a clinical diagnosis of passive-aggressive personality for this pattern of coping (American Psychiatric Association, 1980). Alternatively, they can end up feeling chronically depressed. The diagnosis given this reaction in *DSM-III* is dysthymic disorder (American Psychiatric Association, 1980). It is suggested that the sum of the differential socialization that men and women experience predisposes women to appear more depressed, neurotic, or unstable.

The emerging research on personality profiles of bulimics supports this conceptualization. It is no surprise, then, that the most frequently elevated MMPI scales for bulimic women, 2, 4, 6, and 8 (Norman & Herzog; 1983; Pyle et al., 1981; Root & Friedrich, 1985) in two-point code combinations, depict chronic depression, chronic anger, and passivity (Root & Friedrich, 1985).

Power or, rather, lack of power is a central issue for most bulimics. It is the lack of power in society and in the family that underlies the bulimics' intense anger, which is suppressed and emerges as depression. Because of developmental experiences in the family and in the culture, many give up trying to change their environments. Instead, their anger turns to depression and alternatively is directed inward through bingeing and purging, which function to establish some false, fleeting sense of control. Depression as a symptom in the bulimic syndrome is more significant when it is absent, since both symptoms—depression and bulimia—are a reaction to powerlessness. Bulimia is one more attempt to establish control over something—the body—in a way that is socially reinforced.

## Loyalty and Abandonment

The bulimic's relationship with his or her parents reflects another double-bind, whether the bulimic is female or male. The bulimic's family mirrors the inequity of power between men and women in society. The bulimic pursues joining with both parents, but at levels that are incompatible and raise a question of loyalty. The bulimic joins one parent (usually mother) in powerlessness, but attempts to join the other parent in powerfulness. Bulimia, at first seemingly an intrapsychic contradiction, becomes clearer in this light. The symptom provides a statement of powerlessness, as well as an attempt at personal mastery.

The relationship between mothers and daughters has received attention in a wide variety of literature (Chesler, 1972; Goldner, 1985; Orbach, 1978).

It is important for clinicians to observe the socialization process as it affects mother-daughter relationships and the development of bulimia. We observe two situations: 1) mothers overly involved with their daughters (Chesler, 1972; Goldner, 1985); and 2) daughters determined to create a life for themselves different than their mothers' lives.

The overinvolvement and enmeshment repeatedly observed between the powerless parent (usually mother) and the bulimic (e.g., daughter cries when mother is sad or is angry at mother for her father) are guided by the socialization process. "The overinvolved mother and peripheral father of the archetypal 'family case' emerge as products of a historical process two hundred years in the making (Goldner, 1985, p. 35)." Mother's role and identity have been invested in her children. As they attempt to leave home, the under-pinnings of her identity are threatened; she fears the emptiness (Chesler, 1972). A child's leaving home or increased independence poses little threat to father's identity, which is invested in his work. On the other hand, men may fear the emptiness of retirement and the loss of a work identity.

Further, daughters, particularly of the current generation, seem to be responding to their mothers' powerlessness. They search for success, often outside of the traditional home environment, but are often without the coping mechanisms, behavioral characteristics, and rights to effect a smooth transition and learn to operate as women in a man's world. Many bulimic clients who work in the business world by day recount their need to act assertively, boldly, and confidently. Their job may require managing people, solving problems, or making important financial decisions. Then they experience difficulty coming home and being accommodating and even seemingly subservient to their partner. Their bulimia serves to emphasize this paradox: "powerful" on the outside, "powerless" on the inside.

## WOMEN AND POWER

Society supports men in powerful places and discourages women from striving for positions of equality, although official statements from governmental agencies and politicians talk of equal rights and equal power. Traditionally, women have been seen as " . . . physically weak and politically powerless in a culture that values physical strength and its extended representation in the form of weaponry and money" (Chesler, 1972, p. 292). The family has mirrored this social inequity. Female children have been trained to have an external locus of control, which contributes to powerlessness, and to attribute success to luck or factors outside the individual. Such an orientation contributes to the perpetuation of an environment in which women are socialized to feel that they have little control.

*The Victimization of Women*

While women's attainment of positions of power in government suggests movement towards equality, underlying processes occurring in society suggest otherwise, as women are more frequently victims of physically violent crimes (rape, battery, assault, and molestation). It has been observed that violence against women benefits men *even if they do not engage in it themselves*, because women consequently are encouraged to seek men's protection (Walker, 1979). This vulnerability to personal assault (boundary violation), along with economic exploitation, and continued use of diminutive terms to refer to women (e.g., "honey," "dear," "doll," "sweetheart") powerfully communicate to women they they do not have equal power with men.

Women's realistic fear for personal safety requires a compromise on rights, such as walking at night, going places alone, or expressing feelings or opinions (Chesler, 1972; NiCarthy, Merriam, & Coffman, 1984). A social attitude still exists that victims of personal crimes "have asked for it" (Brownmiller, 1975). This attitude is striking, given that women are attributed blame (and assume fault) for an environment over which they are taught that they have little control. Such attributions reinforce women's pattern of socialization where they attribute success to luck (external locus of control) and failure to inadequate personal efforts or characteristics.

Being targets of personal violence more often than men has further perpetuated women's need for protection and reinforced a male-dominated society's control over women (Chesler, 1972; Walker, 1979). This mirrors the pattern some bulimics experience in their families, as they are overly protected or refused privileges for their own safety. Other women, victims of childhood abuse, carry a fear for personal safety into adulthood (Herman, 1981).

## THE SUPERWOMAN SYNDROME

The sociocultural system contributes greatly to definitions of masculinity and femininity, from appearance to expectations. Traditionally, women have been socialized to act more helpless, less competent, less intelligent, and less assertive than men. Women have been encouraged to be good listeners, kind, nurturant, considerate, giving, and understanding. The bulimic family's socialization process, like the larger culture, encourages women to be passive, helpless, and other-oriented (self-sacrificing) (Brodsky & Hare-Mustin, 1980). A double-bind is created for women because the behaviors and characteristics associated with desirable adult functioning are in conflict with the definitions of healthy adult female functioning (Broverman, Broverman, Clarkson, Rosenkrantz, & Vogel, 1970). Women can be

healthy and masculine or unhealthy and feminine; there is still not yet room
to be feminine and healthy. The findings by the Broverman team have been
referred to as the double standard of mental health.

A greater bind has been created in recent years, as additional expectations, diametrically opposed to the traditional model for women, have been
added to the definition of "successful female." The current expectations for
women include those traditional characteristics listed above *and* new expectations of women for success, intelligence, assertiveness, achievement, and
independence (Wells, 1977). In many bulimic families internal socialization
of female children supports these expectations. Women trying to fulfill both
sets of expectations become unhappy "superwomen" with impossible missions.

Given the increasing social recognition of superwomen, it is understandable that more women are striving for this recognition *despite the sacrifice
of their well-being and attention to personal needs.* The bulimic strives to
be a superwoman. She often has extra-sensitive antennae and is very other-
oriented. She has learned the cultural lesson well, often being socialized to
an extreme degree to demonstrate characteristics of the traditional female.
Personality studies using the Minnesota Multiphasic Personality Inventory
(Hathaway & McKinley, 1967) show a pattern consistent with this conceptualization, as Scale 5 is always the lowest T-score across studies of bulimies,
indicating high socialization to the feminine role (Herzog, Norman, Gordon, & Pepose, 1984; Pyle et al., 1981; Root & Friedrich, 1985).

## THE RELENTLESS PURSUIT OF THINNESS

Thinness is associated with favorable personality traits (Kurman, 1978);
it is also a ticket to social mobility (Schultz, 1979). In a review of several
studies on obesity and women (S. Wooley, O. W. Wooley, & Dyrenforth,
1979), it was shown that the preference for thinness begins at an early age.
Several authors have attributed women's increased vulnerability to developing eating disorders to "the relentless pursuit of thinness" in Western cultures
(Boskind-Lodahl & Sirlin, 1977; Bruch, 1978; Dally, 1969; Garfinkel &
Garner, 1982; Schwartz, Thompson, & Johnson, 1982; Selvini Palazzoli,
1978; White & Boskind-White, 1981).

Over the past several decades there has been a decided cultural shift to
a preference for the thinner woman. Garner, Garfinkel, Schwartz, and
Thompson (1980) identified changes in the ideal body image for women over
a 20-year period (1959–1978). Physical measurements and weights for two
symbolically ideal groups of women, Miss America contestants and Playboy
Bunnies, were compiled. Both groups of women demonstrated a statistically
significant shift towards a straighter silhouette, as evidenced by a decrease
in the average measurements for both bust and hips, while they gained in

height. For Miss America contestants, a significant trend in decreasing weight was confirmed. The highest average weights of contestants (89% of average weight for women according to actuarial charts) occurred in the years 1961, 1962, 1965, and 1966. Pageant winners weighed significantly less than the average contestant for all but four of these 20 years, and have weighed significantly less than the contestants since 1970 (82.5%). In 1978, the weight of the winner was 78% of the average weight for women according to the actuarial charts. This weight is perilously close to the weight at which a person is diagnosed as anorectic.

Another illustration of the cultural preference for increasingly thinner women was highlighted by a survey of visitors' preference for beautiful women at Madame Tussaud's Wax Museum in London (Wallechensky, Wallace, & Wallace, 1977). Elizabeth Taylor, an actress known for her buxom, well-rounded figure, was voted the most beautiful female figure on display in 1970; six years later, Twiggy, known for her stick-thin silhouette, was the most popular female figure. The preference for thin women is further reinforced by the thinness of the leading actresses of prime-time television (Kurman, 1978).

These findings are startling in light of the fact that the average woman has become heavier due to better nutrition. Thus, the American woman is faced with a dilemma. Because of better nutrition and increased height, she is physiologically predisposed to a higher weight (Society of Actuaries and Association of Life Insurance, 1979), which is in conflict with the idealized, thinner female figure. The gap between the culturally ideal woman and the average woman has increased dramatically.

## BODY-IMAGE, SELF-IMAGE, DIETING, AND BULIMIA

Messages about how to achieve approval, well-being, and acceptance are conflicting *except* for the message that everything will fall into place if you are thin (Orbach, 1978). It is no wonder that women, more so than men, become obsessed with their weight and appearance. The combination of cultural expectations regarding weight, cultural definitions of femininity, and family variables creates an atmosphere that promotes eating disorders in women much more so than in men.

The increasing obsession with weight control in our culture is reflected by the fact that the number of diet articles appearing annually in women's magazines doubled between 1959 and 1979 (Garner et al., 1980). It seems that each month the bestseller list includes a new diet book promising wonderfully quick, effortless weight loss. One of the most popular diets in recent years, *The Beverly Hills diet* (Mazel, 1981), advocates the mass marketing of bulimia (Wooley & Wooley, 1982). Mazel's diet is the result of her 20 years of fighting to control her body through the use of diet pills, diuretics, diets, and starvation. She advocates a life style requiring the individual to be obsessed with food and her body, as the bulimic is. Life is structured around food and the struggle against hunger and weight. She writes: "If you have loose bowel movements, hooray! Keep in mind that pounds leave your body in two main ways—bowel movements and urination. The more time you spend on the toilet, the better" (p. 79). Mazel, as well as proponents of other diets, contribute misinformation about physiological functioning and increase the individual's likelihood of developing bulimic habits.

As women have become increasingly preoccupied with their weight and controlling their appetites, a way of thinking has developed which is hazardous to women. The language of "dietese" equates being a good person to demonstration of restraint and an ability to deny hunger or physical cravings. Being bad is defined as showing a lack of control over one's appetite, giving into one's desires, and eating foods that are not allowed on the diet. With a very short leap in logic, a person comes to define herself as good or bad, okay or not okay, success or failure by what she has eaten, whether or not she has lost weight, and whether she has eaten forbidden foods. The definition of self and well-being becomes shallower and more tenuous as it becomes rigidly tied to external appearance. The dieter turns her power over to the diet industry and her scale.

### Body-image Dissatisfaction

Women are more critical of and more dissatisfied with their physical appearance than men (Klesges, 1983). Women tend to weigh themselves more often than men (Dwyer, Feldman, Seitzer, & Mayer, 1969) and are more likely to judge themselves as overweight when by objective standards they are not. In a study of sex differences in perceptions of desirable body shape, women perceived their current figure as heavier than both their ideal figure and their perception of the most attractive figure to men (Fallon, A. & Rozin, 1985) On the other hand, men perceived their current body shape as almost identical to their ideal figure and to their perception of the figure to which women would be attracted. A. Fallon and Rozin (1985) suggest that women's perceptions place pressure on them to lose weight and may be related to the greater incidence of dieting, anorexia nervosa, and bulimia among American women than among American men.

Consider the following statistics:

- The majority (63–70%) of high school females are dissatisfied with their bodies and want to lose weight (Huenemann, Shapiro, Hampton, & Mitchell, 1966).

- Sixty percent of women have been on a diet at some time by their senior year in high school (Dwyer et al., 1969).
- Of college women, as many as 77% diet (Jakobovits, Halstead, Kelley, Roe, & Young, 1977).
- In a study of college coeds, 58% of normal-weight women saw themselves as overweight; 32% of normal-weight men viewed themselves as underweight (Klesges, 1983).
- In another study of college women, 26% were significantly underweight, but only 5.3% perceived themselves as underweight (Halmi et al., 1981).
- In a recent survey by a popular magazine, it was determined that 95% of women used exercise for weight control (Gillies, 1984).
- In a study of female high school volleyball players, 81% were unhappy with their present weight and 73% wanted to lose weight (Perron & Endres, 1985).

The results of these studies dramatically emphasize that it has become the norm for women to be dissatisfied with their bodies. As a result of this dissatisfaction, increasing numbers of females have turned to dieting, so much so that dieting has become accepted as a normal, *expected* female behavior. Women diet more frequently than men (Gray, 1977), and 76% of women who diet do so for cosmetic reasons rather than for physical health. An incredible 90% of the victims of the diet industry are women (Wooley & Wooley, 1982).

*The Impact of Dieting*

Unfortunately, dieting and restrictive eating have been shown to contribute to the likelihood of binge-eating, regardless of weight classification (Polivy & Herman, 1985; Spencer & Fremouw, 1979), and to be precipitants of bulimia. For example, Pyle et al. (1981) reported that 30 of 34 bulimic females in their study reported a period of dieting just prior to the onset of their bulimia. This is consistent with other studies that have reported dieting to have preceded the binge-eating (Boskind-Lodahl, 1976; Boskind-Lodahl & Sirlin, 1977; Bruch, 1973). Normal-weight bingers also tend to report that they are dieters (Boskind-Lodahl, 1976; Boskind-Lodahl & Sirlin, 1977; Pyle et al., 1981).

Polivy and Herman (1985) convincingly argue that dieting precipitates bingeing by encouraging the development of a cognitively regulated eating style. Dieting as a solution to binge-eating simply continues the cycle and increases the likelihood of continued bingeing. A binge-maintenance cycle seems to involve, as a complement, regular periods of dieting. Polivy and

Herman conclude with a dramatic prediction:

> The pressures to diet that made anorexia nervosa the disorder of the 1970s may make bulimia the disorder of the 1980s. The continued perception of dieting as an appropriate reponse to bulimia — rather than as its principal cause — leads us to a pessimistic prognosis regarding the current epidemic of eating disorders. A dispassionate view suggests that perhaps dieting is the disorder that we should be attempting to cure. (1985, p. 200)

## THE MALE BULIMIC

It is estimated that only 5–10% of bulimics are men (Pyle et al., 1981). As a result, clinicians and researchers have far fewer insights and experiences to offer towards understanding the male's vulnerability to developing bulimia. It appears more difficult for the male bulimic to seek help, perhaps because the socialization of men discourages help-seeking and because bulimia has been described as a "woman's problem." A parsimonious conceptualization of bulimia, however, must be able to explain both the sex differences in the prevalence of this disorder and the occurrence of this disorder in males.

In general, our experience working with male bulimics shows that the disorder serves the same types of functions as bulimia in women, including:

1) avoidance of conflict;
2) expression of anger without risking physical violence;
3) repression of feelings;
4) barometer of family tension; and
5) detouring of dyadic conflict.

As will be discussed in Section II, bulimia in males, like bulimia in females, is symbolic of:

1) unresolved family-of-origin issues in a parent's family;
2) unresolved conflict in the family;
3) developmental stuckness in being launched; and
4) need for individuation and interpersonal boundaries.

### The Socialization of Men

While the social expectations of men are not without pressure, they are more consistent and have less to do with appearance than the expectations for women. Self-worth, identity, and masculinity are defined by job, intelligence, and power (Doyle, 1983). Power and control are demonstrated through a man's job status and material possessions. Men are expected to be aggressive, competitive, logical, decisive, and active; they are discouraged from being emotional, nurturing, and passive (expectations of women). While a feminist model of mental health would not propose these expectations for healthy adult functioning, they are more consistent with what people have viewed as healthy adult functioning (Broverman et al., 1970).

In contrast to women, men tend to be satisfied with their bodies. When men are dissatisfied with their bodies, they are more likely to perceive themselves as underweight with respect to objective standards (Gray, 1977). Men will attempt to alter their body size towards a larger figure congruent with the traditional definition of masculinity. Instead of advertising diets and weight loss programs, traditional men's magazines sport ads promising increased muscle mass. Men's "beauty" contests have focused almost exclusively on strength and power. Being large or "overweight" does not stigmatize as it does women, as evidenced by the presence of large — even obese — men in leading-men positions in both prime-time television and movies.

There are two aberrations in the socialization process which increase a man's vulnerability to developing bulimia. First, certain occupations or sports activities increase a man's preoccupation with weight; these include amateur wrestling (where it is advantageous to compete in the lowest weight category possible), jockeying, and distance running. In these sports, low weight is desirable and excessive dieting and binges after a wrestling meet or a horse race may be reported. Second, being gay adds the pressure of wanting to maintain a trim body-image and youthful appearance. While not all bulimic men are gay, it appears that most bulimic men are struggling with sexual identity issues.

Neither of the above factors in the socialization process of the male appears to be enough of a risk factor by itself to predict the development of bulimia. As with women, the family context is very important to understanding the need for a symptom which serves the purposes of bulimia.

# CHAPTER 3

# Systemic Issues

THE SYSTEMIC, DEVELOPMENTAL, family life-cycle issues associated with bulimia are not well documented, even though they appear as predictably as the symptoms of bingeing and purging. Since they are a salient factor in the development of the disorder, systemic issues must be understood if we are to formulate hypotheses about the purposes of bulimia.

Taking an inventory of "systemic symptoms" is not a part of conventional assessment and diagnosis. Minuchin, Rosman, and Baker (1978) suggest that the issues for eating-disordered families lie in enmeshment, inability to resolve conflict, rigidity, overprotectiveness, and the involvement of a child (the identified patient) in conflict-detouring. While we do not see these features in all of our families, many are present. We will present the variations we have identified in Section III on family typologies.

In this chapter we organize family symptoms by four general characteristics: 1) individuation and separation, 2) boundaries, 3) internal organization, and 4) expression and resolution of feelings. These characteristics enable us to discuss a multitude of issues in these families, such as leaving home, enmeshment, intrusion, victimization, control, lack of control, difficulty in expressing anger, multiple symptoms within families, family secrets, addiction, depression, grief, loss, lack of privacy, rigidity of rules, lack of rules, dissociation from feelings, and mistrust.

## INDIVIDUATION AND SEPARATION

Leaving home is generally considered the culmination of successful individuation and separation between parents and children. The experience and expression of anger between parents and children are markers of individuation. Without some capability to differ with and be assertive with one's parents, one cannot psychologically separate.

Years of preparation are necessary before parents and children are able to let go of each other. *Leaving home is more than the physical process of moving out; it is a psychological process enabling the individual to be emotionally separate.* Many bulimic families are characterized by the enmeshment that Minuchin describes; the individual is caught up in an invisible web that makes it difficult for her to determine who she is, what she feels, or what she wants when the persons with whom she is enmeshed are not around. Signs of this enmeshment are daily phone calls from an adult child who is away at school, intuition as to what is happening to another family member, or a mother's crying when her daughter tears up.

Some bulimic families have a very difficult time allowing the last child, particularly the youngest female, to leave home. These difficulties reflect the rigidity and overprotectiveness that characterize psychosomatic families. Separation by the last child launches the family into a new stage of development — one for which they may not be ready. It is a time for parents to become a couple again. This task may be avoided by the parents' adopting a baby or young child when the youngest is just moving into their teens; alternatively, when one child leaves home, another may return.

In other families children have not learned to trust themselves to take the step of leaving home. They feel either that they are personally incompetent or that they will be abandoning a parent. As the last child or the child with whom a parent is particularly enmeshed readies herself for launching, the parent may unintentionally become very ill; then the child feels she must stay. If she does not stay or return home from school or work, she feels incredibly guilty. Many children are kept younger than their chronological years by not being provided opportunities for age-appropriate responsibilities. Possibly their moves towards peers, dating, and experimenting with independence are obstructed through rules or guilt induction. As a result, many bulimic young adults or teens appear much younger than their age. They excuse themselves from certain responsibilities, seeing themselves as too emotionally frail or unsure of themselves.

## BOUNDARIES

The establishment of boundaries is also integral to the process of individual development and separation from parents. Boundaries are marked by physical space, implicit and explicit rules connoting personal respect, and tolerance of emotional distance. The quality of boundaries can be described by the terms "intrusive," "enmeshed," "permeable," or "impermeable." *All bulimics have personal boundary problems reflective of systemic problems. However, the types of problems vary.*

Some families do not provide for physical space and privacy, which are increasingly important as children grow up. These families may have an open door policy on the bathroom, parents' bedroom, or telephone conversations. People openly listen in on telephone conversations, borrow clothes without permission, walk into closed rooms without knocking, use the parents' bed as a lounging place for the whole family and even friends, or keep bathroom doors open beyond cultural norms. These situations signify absent boundaries or boundaries that are too permeable. These boundary problems are obvious to the outsider, though not to family members. Intrusive questions, violation of physical space by standing or sitting too close, or touching people one does not know well are all symptoms of these types of boundary problems.

Boundaries can also be too impermeable. This may happen through emotional cut-offs, lack of trust, parental unavailability, or intimidation. Powerlessness or resignation can be the feelings that follow. Impermeability is reflected in messages that each family member must take care of his or her own problems. It may occur when parents are alcoholic or otherwise compromised or when they are unpredictable, threatening, or intimidating. Signs of boundary problems of this type are varied; we have seen them not only in individuals who appear extremely needy and work hard for approval at the cost of self-respect, but also in those who do not reach out for social support under stress or during vulnerable periods.

Physical violation of boundaries is an extreme, though unfortunately common, example of intrusion. Preliminary data on a sample of 172 bulimics we have interviewed indicate that 66% have been victimized by rape, physical abuse, battering, or sexual molestation (Root & Fallon, 1985). Such intrusion violates both physical and psychological space and renders an individual powerless. All of these types of intrusion have lasting negative effects on the individual's sense of personal space, power, and self-esteem (Briere, 1984; Herman, 1981; Walker, 1979).

One indicator that relationship boundaries are lacking or violated is substance abuse in children, which enables them to create illusory boundaries. Other children have difficulty letting people get close and may create physical boundaries through weight gain, unattractive personal habits, or attempts to appear undesirable. Symptoms of powerlessness are compulsiveness in routines, addiction, and disorganization. The individual may attempt to establish a superficial control of the world through alcohol, drugs, or food.

## ORGANIZATION

All systems need organization or rules by which to regulate actions and expressions. Systems maintain organization through rituals, implicit and explicit rules, and the establishment of a hierarchy. The quality of family organization is important because it can either help the person establish her competence and self-efficacy or render her powerless. The extremes of organization obstruct personal development. Bulimic families often typify the extremes of organization: They are either rigidly organized or very disorganized; rules conflict with each other and are continually changing.

Rigid organization, with unchanging, explicit and implicit rules about family functioning, and enmeshment (as is always seen in these families) create intense family loyalty. Typical rules creating intense, potentially dysfunctional loyalty are: 1) Do not talk about problems outside of the family; 2) do not do things that will reflect badly on the family; and 3) think first of parental feelings. Unfortunately, these rules become dysfunctional when traumas occur for which the individual needs help. She feels she cannot go to her family for help, nor can she seek help outside the family, since that also would involve discussion of feelings. This type of family loyalty leads the bulimic to keep, for example, her eating disorder or an arrest for shoplifting a secret.

When the organization in the family fails or is unpredictable, an older child, usually the oldest daughter, precociously and implicitly assumes a parental role. Intense family loyalty can develop to create an illusion of family the child wants. This often happens when parents are ineffective as a result of severe depression, emotional abuse, substance abuse problems, or language barriers. Especially when alcohol is involved or a parent is emotionally unstable, unpredictability becomes the only rule. The individual becomes confused as to what to trust and may start to establish routines or rules for herself to exert some control in her life.

When an intense family loyalty exists, there are problems of emotional enmeshment, and a child may be taking care of parents, family secrets become more common. For example, we are amazed at the number of teenagers and women we have treated who have been raped but have not told their parents, primarily for fear of the pain the parents would feel. Without direction and support from the therapist, such incidents may never by discussed, even with the therapist, due to strict family loyalty.

## EXPRESSION AND RESOLUTION OF FEELINGS

All the bulimic families we have seen in treatment have had difficulty establishing a way to resolve and cope with intense feelings, particularly anger, resentment, jealousy, grief, depression, anxiety, and insecurity. This difficulty is reflected in the individual symptoms of bulimia. Without adaptive, constructive ways of coping with these feelings, stress either is discharged explosively or emerges in psychosomatic illness such as gastrointestinal problems, headaches, allergies, asthma, compulsive eating, and back pain.

*Families often determine which feelings are permissible and how and when one can express them*. Direct messages are, for example, "Of course, you can't possibly feel that, you're not that kind of person," "If you can't show a happy face, don't show your face at all," "People who are emotional are weak," or "Apologize for what you said (or did); you didn't really mean that." Indirect but equally powerful messages about expressing feelings are given through teasing, degrading a person for crying, or threats to physical safety. A child learns that expression of emotions correlates with a parent's becoming explosive or ill.

The atmosphere of the family may not appear obviously prohibitive of feeling, except in explosive families. Within families that initially look functional, it can be difficult to recognize the implicit rules of expressiveness. One signal of prohibition is incongruent smiling; for example, family members may continuously smile while tears are streaming down their faces, as they talk about the death of a son. Other symptoms are self-reports that people in the family never get angry or that people are strong because they can control their emotions.

Unfortunately, many bulimic families have sustained traumatic losses of family members through severe illnesses or deaths. These losses are naturally followed by grief, anger, sadness, and depression. The family can feel powerless to deal with these losses. If it is not okay for people to experience these feelings or if there is a rule about how long one can feel these feelings, the process of grieving is interrupted and may not be completed. As a result, many bulimics' symptoms seem to be related to an interruption of grieving necessary for themselves and other family members.

Understanding the salient systemic issues is necessary in order to formulate hypotheses about the psychological and ecological function of bulimic symptoms. Then the clinician can predict new symptoms in the family to replace the bulimia if the bulimic gives up her symptoms without resolution of the family issues. The number and complexity of the issues also explain why it takes time to recover from bulimia, why treatment can be difficult, why it is necessary for family issues to be addressed, and why the symptoms may be hard to give up. A more detailed discussion of systemic issues in bulimic families is found in Sections II and III.

# PART II

# CONCEPTUAL EXPLANATIONS OF BULIMIA

# CHAPTER 4

# The Bulimic Family System

IN THIS CHAPTER, WE introduce family systems concepts to illuminate certain relationship patterns observed in bulimic families. We are aware that the reader probably has some familiarity with family systems terminology, and our intent is not to provide an exhaustive primer of theoretical concepts pertinent to family systems. If that is your need, we refer you to several excellent sources, e.g., Benjamin (1983), Hoffman (1981), and Steinglass (1978). Our intent here is to discuss a number of family systems and family therapy terms and link them to actual case material from bulimic families. Our experience with bulimic individuals and their families solidifies our appreciation for a family systems approach to conceptualization and therapy.

The definition of a system that we use — "a set of people and the interrelationships between those people" — automatically forces us to think interpersonally, rather than individually. While we utilize techniques derived from individual therapy, we are convinced that successful treatment of bulimic individuals is done within an interpersonal context. Beginning with the first phone contact, we ask ourselves questions to illuminate the bulimic interpersonal system: Who are the people in the bulimic's family or peer system? What roles do they play? Who is part of the bulimia maintenance system? The set of people can be quite large if extra-familial relationships are considered and can include networks of loosely connected individuals (Speck & Attneave, 1973). We start by assuming a set to be the current members of a household, e.g., parents and children, and then add other family members, e.g., siblings, grandparents, and stepmembers, as needed or dictated by the circumstances of the case and by the degree of emotional involvement and the regular interaction that occurs among various family members.

Our including someone as a member of the system does not mean that he or she is automatically invited to therapy. Family therapy is not defined by the number of people in the room. The most typical family therapy situation involves treatment of a teenage bulimic, in that the members of her immediate household are certain to be considered as probable members of the therapy. It is exceedingly rare for us not to involve the immediate family from the beginning when an adolescent is living at home. However, the bulimic client who no longer lives with her parents presents a greater challenge to a systems theorist. It may be that, while not physically living at home, she still has her psychological residence there. The therapy system may be defined as the client and her mother and father, despite their physical separation. A sibling may also be involved, along with a partner or spouse.

For example, a recent consultation brought together a 16-year-old bulimic, her mother, stepfather, father, stepmother, one natural sibling, and two stepsiblings. In this case the bulimia seemed to reflect an ongoing post-divorce dynamic. The client, who was living with her mother and stepfather, had obvious emotional connections with her sibling, father, and stepmother. The two stepsiblings were included because they had conduct problems, and the therapist was looking for opportunities to "spread the symptom around" and treat the bulimia, as well as the conduct problems, truly systemically. The decision about who was invited to therapy was made according to what was operating in the system and how change could be maximized rapidly.

An advantage of a systemic conceptualization is the opportunity for a circular understanding of symptoms. In living systems, it is impossible "to assign one part of causal influence vis-à-vis another" (Hoffman, 1981, p. 8). This is an idea with extraordinary implications. Simple, linear explanations of etiology are not helpful clinically. The bulimic is not symptomatic because of a neurotransmitter imbalance or a bad mother. A circular conceptualization allows us to appreciate that a system is a large field in which family members, therapist, "and any member of other elements act and react upon each other in unpredictable ways, because each action and reaction continually changes the nature of the field" (Hoffman, 1981, p. 8). One event modifies another, which in turn modifies the first. In this process, there is no beginning and no end. This is especially clear when we look at multigenerational issues (see Chapter 5).

Yet our clinical conceptualizations also borrow heavily from Andolfi and his colleagues (Andolfi, Angelo, Menghi, & Nicolò-Corigliano, 1983), who, more than any systems therapists we know, put "at the center of the study of the family the individual and his/her process of differentiation" (p. 4). They use a relational theory (systems) to better understand human behavior and its development. We feel that the theoretical formulations we use allow us to still see the individual in the relational sphere in which we operate.

## TRIANGULATION

Family systems theorists have borrowed terms from cybernetics and physics, e.g., "feedback" and "entropy." Supposedly, "triangle" has been borrowed from engineering, where the triangle is considered the most stable geometric structure in building construction. The concept of triangulation is found in both psychodynamic family theory (Bowen, 1978) and structural family therapy (Minuchin, 1974). As early family therapists began to move away from considering only the dyad of mother and child, the two key players in double-bind theory, they began to look more closely at groups of three, or triads. Haley and Hoffman (1967) observed that in symptomatic families, a frequent triad was a coalition between two people at the expense of a third. This coalition usually cut across a generational boundary. The "perverse triangle," as they called it, has three characteristics: 1) Two people from one generation and a third from a second generation are involved; 2) a coalition is established between two people in different generations against the third person, who is excluded from the coalition; and 3) behavior that indicates the existence of the coalition is denied. This allows for covert violation of generational boundaries. They pointed out that in a family with two parents, two children, and four grandparents, any one person could be involved in 21 triangles simultaneously.

The importance of triangles in symptomatic families has also been emphasized by Bowen (1978), who believes that a dyad is possible only in a "conflict-free" environment. When the relationship between two people in a system becomes uncomfortable, one of them overtly, and the other more covertly, triangles in a third party. This can relieve tension between the two people (most frequently the spouses). In fact, triangling is a common method of system stabilization.

The emergence of perverse triangles in a system is a common phenomenon that allows for the detouring of conflict (Minuchin et al., 1978). Minuchin and his colleagues started with the premise that children could be used to obscure or deflect parental conflict. They developed a typology of "rigid triads" that systems could evolve for this purpose. Four different rigid triads were proposed: triangulation, parent-child coalition, detouring-attacking, and detouring-supportive.

When two parents are in conflict and each is actively pursuing the child's support against the other, the situation is called *triangulation*. A *parent-child coalition* consists of a parent's siding with the child against the other parent, with the other parent seen as quite peripheral. It differs from triangulation in that the parents are less overtly conflictual. The intense closeness of the child and the preferred parent can result in a lack of differentiation or an interruption of natural developmental evolution. As Andolfi et al. mention, "In a dyadic, exclusive relationship, it is not possible for differentiation to take place if neither of the two parties involved is able to establsih a relationship with a third party" (1983, p. 5).

The two types of "detouring triads" differ in their overt manifestation. In *detouring-attacking*, the child is viewed as bad or disruptive, and both parents are involved in a scapegoating process. The parents differ about how to handle the child and are frequently inconsistent, but both are highly controlling/rejecting of the child. The final triad, the *detouring-supportive*, allows for a sublimation of parental conflict via a combined focus on a child, who has been defined by the family as "sick." The parents show enormous concern and overt conflict is minimized. All four of these perverse triangles can be found in families with behavior problems or psychosomatic children. In addition, these triangles are seen to shift over time, and membership may vary from one time to another.

The parental conflict that is being detoured via a triadic process in the families of our bulimic clients varies depending on the type of the family. Most commonly, the parents in an overprotective family are continually grappling with fears of intimacy and closeness and seem to use triangulation, parent-child coalition, and detouring-supportive processes as a means of managing the conflict around these issues. Since there are restrictions on the expression of anger in the overprotective family, detouring-attacking is not very common.

The restrictions on the expression of "negative" affect in overprotective families inhibit affective expression and direct, honest communication, so the detouring of communication through the child, e.g., "tell your father that . . . ," provides an already established pathway for using the child as an exclusive confidant. The child is routinely more available than a spouse, and the risks are far fewer. Sometimes, from infancy on, the triangling process becomes more and more the pattern, and the "individual and family life cycle is arrested in a phase which corresponds to the overlearned solution" (Andolfi et al., 1983, p. 13).

Every change in the family seriously impinges on family functioning. These changes can be normal developmental transitions or crises of one sort or another. When the change challenges the family's flexibility, a possible reaction is to "select" a family member to "carry" the stress and tension that accompanies the change. This results in the child's demonstrating some symptom.

We use the term "select" in the previous paragraph somewhat loosely. It seems clear that with some families one child is more predictably symptomatic than another by virtue of gender, birth order, and circumstances in the family at the time the child was born. Our common observation that bulimics from overprotective families are typically youngest daughters is compatible with our understanding about the rigidity, overprotectiveness, and enmeshment seen in these families. The youngest child represents the last connection to a previous, very rewarding parenting experience, where the parent felt valued, appreciated, and connected to someone (a child) in a very special way. This is not easy to lose when there are no prospects for replacement.

Some of the most compelling evidence for the conflict-detouring role played by the child is derived from psychophysiological research reported by Minuchin and colleagues in *Psychosomatic Families* (1978). A group of diabetic children and their families were studied. Diabetics seemed ideal for study because emotional arousal is indicated by the presence of free fatty acids in the blood. A concentration of these substances has been linked to the onset of diabetic acidosis. Minuchin and colleagues reasoned that, if you were to measure the blood level of free fatty acids, you could learn what leads to those physiological changes linked to diabetic attacks. The free fatty acid levels in the child and parents were assessed during a structural family interview. Families with an asthmatic or anorectic or brittle diabetic were compared to control families with a child who had well-controlled diabetes. Half of the control families had a diabetic child with concurrent behavior problems. The addition of this behavior problem group was seen as important because the manifestation of behavior problems is thought to be a more "direct" expression of conflict, rather than an internalizing or "indirect" phenomenon like psychosomatic illness.

The children in the experimental group, i.e., asthmatic, anorectic, and brittle diabetic, all showed a greater rise in free fatty acids (FFA) than the control children during the family interview. Their FFA level had a greater amplitude and returned to baseline more slowly after the interview was over than that of either parent. Finally, when the symptomatic child entered the interview room where his or her parents were discussing family issues, his/her FFA level went up as the parents' FFA level went down. Somehow, in the symptomatic families, the child assumed the parents' emotional arousal. An additional finding was that in the experimental families the conversation routinely involved the child, whereas in the control families considerably more interaction took place between the parents. The structural family therapy approach espoused by Minuchin was directed at disengaging the child from his/her position between the parents or, in the term we are defining, from the triangle. Once the child is removed, the parents are forced to deal more directly with their conflict. Hoffman writes that these families are not characterized by "a simple triangle . . . but a complex force field" that is "strikingly conveyed by the lack of boundaries or appropriate status lines" (Hoffman, 1981, p. 154).

We agree that the word "triangle" does not capture the power and emotion present in the families we see. However, the essential points outlined earlier are clearly met, most commonly via the parent-child coalition version of triangling relationships. For example, a bulimic client from an overprotective family chronicled a three-generational history of unsuccessful emancipation by women in the family. Her grandmother for all of her married life lived next door to her own mother's (the client's greatgrandmother's) house. The client's mother moved away to get married but did so only while taking her older sister along with her. This older sister, to this day, maintains a room in the client's parents' home. The client twice dropped out from universities more than 500 miles from home but graduated with honors from the hometown college. When she moved 100 miles away to graduate school, she took almost six years to complete her master's degree and then promptly moved home for one year, during which time her bulimia went out of control and she began therapy.

This client described herself as "my mother's closest friend" and saw her mother and herself as "living inside each other's heads." During family-of-origin therapy, she initially attempted to sit between her parents and, during several early sessions, heard a variety of short lectures by each parent revolving around the theme of "considering your mother's feelings of loneliness now that you are out of the house and no longer in daily contact." Her father argued for the curative powers of daily telephone contact between mother and daughter and was absolutely sure that he could do nothing to alleviate his wife's loneliness. The depression in both mother and daughter stemming from the change in their relationship was very clearly evident.

What is clear in this family is a multigenerational history of parent-child coalitions and detouring-supportive triads. These cross the generation boundary, exclude the second parent, and capture a family in a frozen state of development, highly resistant to change. The primary affect was one of pleasantness; in fact, direct conflict emerged only with considerable prodding by the therapist. The conflict had deadly ramifications, including a mild heart attack in the father several days later. The client had developed several supportive relationships with older, maternal women as she inched out of her family in the early stages of therapy, but the disruption of the triangle activated a tremendous burst of growth, including a significant and positive heterosexual relationship.

What about chaotic families and their use of triadic relationships to stabilize the system or detour conflict? Clinical literature usually suggests that chaotic or centrifugal (Stierlin, 1973) families have rapidly shifting coalitions that reflect the general lack of consistency and sameness in the family. It is this lack of consistency that invites the triangulation of children in these families. The coalitions may be shifting but they do occur. This unpredictability fosters a precocious pseudomaturity; in addition, chaotic families seem to eschew attachment and cohesiveness, so that adolescents are expelled early from the family.

The triangling dynamics operative in a chaotic family are illuminated by the family of a client who was attempting to regain custody of her child and, during the evaluation, revealed that she was bulimic. This woman, the fourth of five children, had suffered a number of traumas: When she was 11, her mother committed suicide; when she was 15, her oldest brother committed suicide; her stepbrother was murdered when she was 16; and her boyfriend was murdered at 18. She had left home in her sophomore year of high school and lived with "friends." She denied any significant, close relationship with her mother, seeing her father as her anchor in the family. However, their relationship was volatile and physically abusive, and she never knew how he was going to greet her when she called. While intoxicated, he had attempted to rape her on one occasion. She seemed to shrug off this severe cross-generational violation. Her bulimic symptoms had recently increased when she began court-ordered therapy. The only enduring emotional triangle in her family was that including her mother, oldest brother, and father. The fusion between mother and son was reflected in their suicides four years apart. Currently, there seems to be a transient "conflict-detouring/scapegoating" triangle between the client, her father, and her older sister, who is in and out of alcoholism treatment. She and her father talk about the sister and ventilate with each other about how she has "ripped off" each of them; then a closeness develops as a result of the scapegoating process. However, she describes that as transitory and states "My turn to be on the outs will come again soon."

Triangulation is also seen in perfect families. It is not uncommon for these clients to have a history of anorexia, with the parent-child coalition that is associated with that history. As Hoffman (1981) describes the anorectic family in the initial lunch session used by Minuchin, "over and over . . . there is one authoritative parent who tries to force the child to eat and another who . . . attempts . . . to soften the other parent. The child is caught in the classic 'ballot box' situation: If he eats, he will be voting for one parent, and if he does not, he will be voting for the other" (p. 154). As outlined in Chapter 8, the perfect family focuses on appearance, family reputation, family identity, and achievement. Because of the few obvious signs of distress in these families, triangles may be hard to identify.

An example may be useful here to illustrate triangulation in the perfect family. One family included three daughters, each with an eating disorder, a controlling, highly successful father, and a mother who joined with her daughters primarily around issues relating to dress and appearance. The father's status was exaggerated and the mother's reduced, so that she was essentially pushed out of the parental hierarchy. She was more a sibling than a mother. She was not an equal partner in the parental or marital relationships; rather, she played the role of an older sister/fashion instructor. The mother-daughter relationships were not characterized by emotional intensity or desperateness, as is sometimes seen in overprotective families. Instead, the mother's emotional unavailability and difficulty with nurturing seemed instrumental in her daughters' development as precociously mature and successful young women who had considerable difficulty "feeling real" or getting close in relationships. In this family the triangles or, more accurately, parent-child coalitions seemed to primarily involve overly close father-daughter(s) relationships, with mother largely peripheral.

In summary, we routinely see triangular relationships in bulimic families. They seem to serve a primary function in the managing and detouring of conflict, but they also are expressions of the lack of differentiation and the "stuck" nature of these families. Lack of differentiation in a parent automatically invites his or her fusion with someone else with similarly poor personal boundaries. A child is a perfect option. When the parent has issues with food and appearance, equates food with nurturing, or is uncomfortable with intimacy, a coalition between that parent and a young child has a number of years to develop. A symptomatic child is certainly a possibility.

## ENMESHMENT

As mentioned in Chapter 3, all of the bulimic families we have seen have been enmeshed. A family is said to be enmeshed when the boundaries between subsystems and between individuals are diffuse. Family members are very reactive to each other and resonate emotionally; there is a definite lack of differentiation between individual family members. Enmeshed individuals lack the "I-position" that Bowen (1978) says is characteristic of mature individuals. Since enmeshment is a feature that allows for the development of triangling in families, many of the issues discussed in the preceding section apply here as well.

Another effect of enmeshment is:

> to weaken the boundaries that allow family subsystems to work . . . the boundary between the nuclear family and families-of-origin is not well maintained; the boundary separating the parents from their children is frequently invaded in improper ways; and the roles of spouse and parent are never clearly differentiated, so that neither the spouse subsystem nor the parent subsystem can operate with ease. Finally, the children are not differentiated on the basis of age or maturation level, so that the sibling subsystem cannot contribute properly to the socialization process. (Hoffman, 1981, p. 73)

We are most likely to use the term "enmeshed" to describe a simultaneous boundarylessness and overconnection. The chaotic family may not seem overly close but is characterized by routine boundary violations and reactivity among individuals to a degree similar to other bulimic families. Sometimes the enmeshment is reflected in incest. The differences are not in the underlying process, but, rather, in the style and content of presentation.

Since we discussed many of the principal features of enmeshment in our presentation on triangles, here we will discuss briefly only one special indicator of enmeshment, emotional resonance. We have been amazed at the degree of resonance described by our families. The following examples indicate the degree to which one family member's issues/feelings become the others'. One client said, "I would sit in the living room watching TV and feel the sad/bad/mad feelings my mother was having roll out the door onto me. She never had to say anything. I learned that the only way not to have those same feelings was to turn off my feelings." The act of purging for her was another way to turn off feelings. Another client described how she and her mother frequently would try to call each other at the same time and thus get busy signals. This would happen at all times during the day.

In terms of intervention, enmeshment is most routinely seen in sessions when one family member speaks for another and when children need to "check in" with a parent before answering a question. We try to point out and interrupt this pattern whenever it occurs and see reductions in enmeshing behaviors as signs of progress. For example, after some treatment the client described above no longer was able to predict when her mother's random telephone calls would come, and another client no longer reported that "when I'm with my father, I feel like I am two years old."

Enmeshment is a feature in rigid, change-resistant families and is difficult to interrupt. With a client who daily reported her bowel movements to her mother, weeks of simply discussing this activity, gaining insight into its origins, etc., did not seem to make a dent in the behavior. Finally the therapist escalated the intensity by prescribing and exaggerating the behavior, i.e., suggesting that the client weigh her bowel movements and report them in grams to her mother, along with urine volume and color. Thus, the therapist must be prepared to use a variety of means to interrupt such persistent, pervasive patterns.

## HOMEOSTASIS

The concept of homeostasis has had an interesting and very influential impact on family systems thinkers. Early theorists were impressed at the variety of "self-righting" mechanisms that systems utilized and likened this to a concept from physical chemistry, where a reaction achieves a balance or steady state. Family therapists commonly use the idea of homeostasis as a type of "governor" on the family machine. This belief gives rise to statements that "symptoms preserve the family homeostasis" and that the family vigorously opposes any evolutionary development.

Gregory Bateson (1972) was one of the first people to introduce the idea that a family might be very similar to a homeostatic system. Clinicians who worked with him emphasized the equilibrium-maintaining qualities of symptomatic behaviors in families. These symptoms were seen as analogous to homeostatic mechanisms, similar to psychodynamic defense mechanisms, and crucial in determining how a particular family deals with imbalance. Over a period of time families were seen to develop several repetitive, enduring interactions that maintained equilibrium in the face of stress.

Bateson's early research in this area illustrated that change in a family depended very much on a process families utilized to keep change or deviations from the norm within bounds. Family systems seem to possess limits within which the system operates. Limits are maintained through feedback that either preserves the status quo (negative) or promotes newness (positive). This has direct implications for therapy, which ostensibly should be positive feedback. How does one create an intervention that is truly positive? Hoffman (1981) states that an important factor in any family entering therapy is the "balance or imbalance of the system" at that time (p. 53). Apparently, the greater the imbalance, the more likely a system will change to a new style of interaction. This point illustrates the need, in many cases, to induce a crisis in the family so that positive feedback can activate the system to seek a new level of interaction. The behavioral change of one person in a family system will affect the equilibrium (homeostasis) of the system and cause an imabalnce to occur. When such an imbalance occurs, there is an extremely strong impulse on the part of the system to revert to its former homeostatic state, that which is known and customary. Whether or not the former homeostatic state is comfortable or painful is immaterial.

What keeps homeostatic patterns in balance? Why don't they break down when necessary and allow for evolutionary transformations? Some theorists "personalize" systemic properties and write "when . . . an imbalance occurs, there is an extremely strong impulse on the part of the system to revert to its former, homeostatic state, that which is known and customary. . . . A system would rather retain its familiar pain than subject itself to the vulnerability of change" (Okun & Rappaport, 1980, p. 81). This anthropomorphizing of systemic processes helps to make arcane systemic notions more understandable and thus serves a purpose. Another explanation is that the "balance" in the nuclear family serves to correct a complementary "imbalance" in the larger family-of-origin system, particularly along the dimension of closeness and distance.

When a child's behavior problems create a "diversion," this is essentially negative feedback that rebalances the family at its former level. It is customary for families to periodically become unbalanced. This is an automatic and natural byproduct of the shifts in status between generations or the various stresses that create problems interpersonally. Severely symptomatic families seem to repeat continually these vicious circles (homeostasis), without being forced into a change in structure or relational pattern; each time change threatens, the symptomatic pattern represented by an identified patient facilitates a return to a homeostatic balance.

The rigidity we see in bulimic families and the difficulties they have progressing successfully through each life-cycle phase underscores the usefulness of homeostatic principles. In bulimic families, there is a rich, unintentional tradition of utilizing a child to maintain homeostatic balance at the expense of her individual development. A marital system that is becoming increasingly distressed diminishes in intensity when the bulimic daughter becomes a focus of concern. The system initially became strained as the daughter moved into adolescence and was less emotionally present. A return to homeostasis afforded a truce. There are bidirectional relationships between marital discord, life-cycle pressures, and the emergence of bulimia. The multitude of interrelationships makes for a conservative system that readily returns to a former balance.

In later treatment chapters, we discuss the various systemic functions of bulimia. Each of these are homeostatic mechanisms, e.g., distraction, scapegoating, stabilizing a potentially runaway system. The concept of homeostasis has also given rise to one of the most important therapy principles ever: Systems have a strong resistance to change, despite spoken intentions to the contrary. *Being aware of this, the therapist of bulimic clients can appreciate their rigidity and slowness to change, as well as the sudden, discontinuous shifts that signal second-order change.*

## COMMUNICATION

Communication theorists, including Gregory Bateson, Jay Haley, and Paul Watzlawick, assume that you can learn about the family system by studying communication, both verbal and nonverbal. This assumption keeps the focus on here-and-now, observable behavior within the system and illuminates the process of family interaction. For communication theorists historical analysis of the individual family members is seen as unnecessary.

Communication theorists have developed a number of axioms that summarize their basic concepts. The first is that *all behavior is communicative.* Essentially, it is impossible not to communicate, since even silence indicates something about the relationship.

A second axiom is that *every communication has two components, a content/report aspect and a relationship/command aspect.* The latter aspect is usually a nonverbal message about the first aspect, that is, metacommunication. The nonverbal message may support the primary content that is being reported or contradict it, as in the case of the "double-bind." It is the degree to which these contradictions persist that contributes to "crazy-making" features in the system. For example, particularly in overprotective families, we see a lot of "smiling depression." This phrase is a contradiction in terms and is captured best in an exchange between a parent and bulimic daughter.

Parent: (Sobbing) I want you to grow up and be happy, even if it means
         leaving home. I'll be all right. Don't worry about me.
Daughter: But I worry about you.
Parent: (Sobbing) You have no need to worry.

A third axiom states that *relationships are defined by the command messages (metacommunications) identified in the previous axiom.* The concept of "punctuation" is useful here. The command messages are dependent on the "punctuation" of the communicational sequences. Each participant imposes her own "punctuation" on the ongoing system. Each defines his or her role and adapts to the other. The daughter may view her arguments with her mother as "I defy you because you nag." That is how she punctuates the relationship communications. The mother, on the other hand, views her arguments with her daughter as "I nag you because you defy me." Each punctuates the relationship in cause-effect or linear terms, ignoring the circularity of their connection. Misunderstanding and symptomatic behavior flow from punctuation difficulties and therapists find it useless to try to determine who is "right" in these circumstances, since that also fails to recognize the relationship's circularity.

A fourth axiom states that *communication is both verbal and nonverbal.* The verbal communication deals with the content of the message, whereas the nonverbal communication deals with the relationship dimension, which is often unclear and ambiguous (depending on punctuation). The meaning of the message *and* what it says about the communicator's relationship are of therapeutic concern.

The final axiom of communication theory presented here is that *all communicational interchanges are either symmetrical (equal and parallel where either can lead) or complementary (where one leads and the other follows).* This suggests that interactions are based on status differences and enables us to learn about the nature of the relationship between the communicators.

Let us now look at how these various communication processes are manifested in bulimic families. The first belief, regarding the impossibility of not communicating, brings to mind the subtle, almost imperceptible shaping the perfect family does regarding physical appearance and accomplishment. While it is true that the message may be clearly communicated in some cases, families in which overt communications are not evident still communicate expectations that can be destructive.

The way in which perfect families might communicate destructive messages, despite their overtly positive style, is best described in the second belief regarding the fact that communications have both content and relationship components. The father who speaks about everybody in the family being respected and appreciated belies that with a metacommunication which essentially states that this is not true for women. The metacommunication most frequently has a nonverbal component to it, underscoring the importance of the fourth axiom to bulimic families, i.e., communication is both verbal and nonverbal. For example, the nonverbal message attached to a family policy of "no knocking before entering" is a powerful commentary on the absence of personal boundaries. Or the sudden, painful look that slides across the father's face when his mother's name is mentioned gives lie to his statement that she "was a good woman." These discrepancies are routinely seen and train the child to selectively ignore reality, become confused, not know what she feels, etc. Punctuation differences also make for confusion in the family members. A parent may perceive her overly close relationship with her daughter as reflective of her abundant love for the daughter. The daughter perceives it as guilt-inducing and wants to flee from it. Both are left at odds, feeling totally misunderstood, because they are essentially punctuating the same behavior differently. As overt discussion of the discrepancy is not available to them, since the message "we love each other" carries with it the metamessage that "we show it in circumscribed ways that do not include assertiveness or forcefulness."

Regarding complementary or symmetrical relationships that characterize the interaction of the various family members, these are most evident in bulimic families in their difficulties with family hierarchy. Children who would benefit from a complementary relationship, where they follow their parents' leads, are either inappropriately elevated to peer status with a parent in an enmeshed relationship (symmetrical) or assume a superior role to the parent, a reverse type of complementarity. Even more confusing is a rigidly symmetrical parent-child communication pattern, with a metacommunication to take care of the parent because he or she is fragile.

The axioms from communication theory are very useful in understanding bulimic families. They force the therapist to listen to the communications and metacommunications operating in the family and to search for the relationship message that might be at odds with the actual content being expressed.

# CHAPTER 5

# *Multigenerational Issues*

WORKING WITH BULIMIC clients and their families continually reminds us that bulimia has multigenerational roots. By multigenerational, we mean that not only the preceding generation but also two, three, and four generations before that have had an impact on the identified patient. During the family history-taking, it is quite common for clients to report a "mother who had a very weak stomach," a grandmother "who would inform her husband how many times she had thrown up that day," or a preoccupation with food, dieting, and slenderness over several generations.

As we have seen in Chapter 4, strains in the marital partners are related to the emergence of symptoms in the child. We are also convinced multi-generational strains are related to the emergence of symptoms, including bulimia. As Hoffman (1981) points out about triangulation, " . . . there seems to be one common feature in all these cases: The symptom arises in a more expendable party when the relationship between at least two other parties—who . . . are . . . extremely important to the group—is threatened" (p. 178). This would also apply to a long-existing pattern of strain between parent and grandparent that involves the developing child.

This chapter extends our family systems approach into earlier generations. Discussing multigenerational processes enables the therapist to conceptualize family interaction and subsequent treatment recommendations.

Here we also help the therapist develop an understanding of how to use a multigenerational process in planning more effective treatment. For example, having multigenerational information on the family further spreads the symptom around the system, taking the focus off the identified patient as the "sick" one. It might provide the impetus for the parent to change a relationship with his or her own parent, with the subsequent effect rippling through the larger system. Also, a multigenerational perspective empowers

52

the therapist to look beyond the perfect family's presentation in the office. It is easier to intervene when it becomes apparent that there is a long history of unresolved losses or victimization. That may not be at all apparent in the family's presentation, despite the therapist's skillful questioning about what is going on in the here and now.

We begin by examining Murray Bowen's conceptualizations about families. Then we discuss bulimia in light of these formulations. Finally, a case that clearly outlines the importance of a multigenerational perspective is presented.

## MULTIGENERATIONAL TRANSMISSION PROCESS

A central figure in this area is Murray Bowen, who is categorized as a psychodynamic family theorist/therapist because of his strong roots in psychoanalytic theory. Bowen became interested in the degree to which individuals distinguish between the feeling and intellectual processes within themselves. He noticed that people differed in the degree to which intellect and feelings were fused or differentiated from each other. When the two processes were indiscriminable, the person functioned more poorly than when thinking and feeling could be distinguished. This balance between thinking and feeling parallels the developmental balance between differentiation and integration. Failure to achieve this balance or resolve this tension is carried to subsequent generations. In fact, Bowen (1978) has described a "multigenerational transmission process," which captures his belief in the transmission of irrationality across generations in general and his ideas about the development of schizophrenia in particular. (We see schizophrenia as only one outcome and include eating disorders as other possible outcomes, depending on a variety of systemic issues.)

For example, Bowen's early (1960) three-generation hypothesis was designed to account for the development of schizophrenia in a family. Apparently, he believes that it takes at least three generations of progressively less and less differentiation for schizophrenia to develop. The actual process, according to Bowen, depends on the least differentiated individual in each of several generations marrying a person of a similar degree of nondifferentiation. By the third generation, it is presumed that this results in a highly reactive, undifferentiated individual.

Bowen's writings, along with those of R. D. Laing (Laing & Esterson, 1964) and James Framo (1981), have provided the impetus for family-of-origin therapy addressing multigenerational issues. This basic concern with differentiation/individuation is found throughout this work. When we explore the bulimic client's family history, we also find evidence supporting a multigenerational transmission process, with the lack of differentiation culminating in the bulimic client.

*Undifferentiated Family Ego Mass*

Although the term undifferentiated family ego mass (Bowen, 1978) was
derived from psychoanalysis, it conveys an idea of a family emotionally stuck
together and operating according to a rule of maximizing emotional oneness.
Hoffman (1981) provides a perfect example of the undifferentiated ego mass:
the boys in Never-Never Land from the play *Peter Pan*, who had to all turn
over in bed whenever one turned over.

Bowen urges that each person can be placed along a continuum of individuation from this family ego mass. This continuum, which he has called
the Differentiation of Self Scale, is divided into quadrants and anchored on
one end by a theoretical position of an absolute lack of individuation or total
fusion. The person at this level is totally subject to the feelings of others, is
completely reflexive, and cannot maintain a sense of herself/himself as a
separate person, an "I." She is emotionally fused to the family and others.
In the second quadrant, there is more differentiation of self and less fusion
with others, but the quality of "stuck togetherness" still dominates. People
here function in a limited way because of their fusion and, while capable
of goal-directed behavior, undertake it only to gain approval of others. Those
in the third quadrant are more able to take an "I" position and rely less on
the judgments of others. Their thinking is sufficiently developed so as not
to be dominated by feelings when stress occurs, and they have a reasonably
developed sense of self. The final quadrant characterizes rare people who
easily separate their thinking from their feelings. These people base their
decisions on the former but are free to lose themselves in the intimacy of
a close relationship.

*Family Projection Process*

The importance of the theoretical concepts reflected in the Differentiation of Self Scale is manifest in a second tenet of Bowen's (1978) theory, the
family projection process. Considered a very common process, this tenet
refers to how the parental lack of differentiation is projected onto one or
more children. One child, the one most fused into the family system, emerges
with a lower level of differentiation than the parents and functions more
poorly than they do in their daily life. Siblings who are not fused, or who
are less involved with these parents, will do much better than the sibling
receiving the projection.

The family projection process results from parental immaturity and lack
of differentiation. However, why a particular child is projected onto in a
given family may not be readily evident. Although Bowen (1978) stresses
the parents' sibling position in their own families of origin as clues to which
child is chosen, a variety of potentiating factors exist. Sometimes it may be

that the child activates a projection process because of her appearance, birth position, or sex. For example, the mother of a bulimic patient was the oldest female sibling, as was the client. The mother had a history of overinvolvement with her own mother, the client's maternal grandmother, that was continuing even at the time the client came into treatment. The developmental stage of the marriage may also be a key determinant. Parental fusion with the youngest child may be a way to delay the transition out of the child-rearing life-cycle stage and to keep from mourning the loss of the grandparent.

Bowen writes that the child chosen will be the " . . . one most emotionally attached to the parents, and the one who ends up with a lower level of differentiation of self" (1978, p. 122). This child finds it more difficult to "escape" from the family because she is more involved in it. The qualities of adhesiveness and overcloseness will be more evident in her than in her siblings.

## MULTIGENERATIONAL FOCUS ON BULIMIA

We are interested in the multigenerational roots of bulimia for at least three specific reasons. First, the existence of multigenerational patterns in the family of a bulimic client allows us to understand more about the etiology of bulimia. In addition, when the behavior clearly has multigenerational roots, this information can be used to reduce the self-blame of the client and "spread the symptom around." This can make the case for family treatment more compelling to the immediate family present in the therapist's office.

Second, a multigenerational focus allows for secrets and emotional issues that have dictated the behavior of the bulimic client, her siblings, and her parents to be exposed and worked through. We are stuck by how nodal events will alter a family's organization or process and gradually cripple the family's functioning. Although a strict systems theorist may object to our describing a family secret as an "emotional block," we find it useful to frame it that way to family members and enlist their support in its resolution.

Third, a multigenerational focus allows for a variety of options for therapy. These include everything from involvement of parents and grandparents in the therapy to borrowing metaphors from the family of origin to reframe the family's interaction. For example, in a session with a bulimic client and her father, it became clear that he was responding to his daughter as if she were his mother. His awareness of this led him to spend some time getting clearer about his anger towards his mother, and this interrupted the projection process. While he was working on this, his daughter occasionally felt compelled to remind him that she was "not Grandma Mabel," which was enough to effectively circumvent the old way of interacting.

*Identifying Multigenerational Patterns*

The most immediately identifiable patterns in families with bulimic clients revolve around food, dieting, and weight. For example, Carol's mother reported in a family session that in times of stress, particularly when thinking of visiting her mother, she would "throw up." She also stated that women in her family had weak stomachs and disclosed that her sister had severely restrictive dietary patterns, e.g., she ate only certain vegetables, consumed no dairy products, and had only one meal per day. Carol was bulimic, her mother was very slender, and her two sisters were considerably overweight.

Elaborate food rituals across generations are common. The cumulative tension that these create in relation to food consumption can be enormous. The bulimic learns that food is approached ambivalently and thus it is an arena in which the messages may be conflicting. The family may use food as an expression of love, but yet also view eating too much as reprehensible and grounds for exclusion, at least temporarily, from any expressions of love or concern. Or, the consumption of food may be an arena where the battle for control is fought, with the child initially learning that fighting mom about food does not work. However, at a later date, the battle may be refought, with the daughter coming out "the winner."

Dieting also results in a pattern of food restriction that is frequently multigenerational. In many situations dieting creates a dilemma when it is obvious that a svelte look is genetically not possible due to bone structure, etc. It is more than dieting per se, however, that creates the issue. (Recall the discussion in Chapter 3 about personal boundaries in these families.)

A family-of-origin session with a perfect family allowed a firsthand look at how these issues operate. Present at the interview were the bulimic daughter, her father, mother, and one sister. The father, with whom the bulimic daughter identified, was gaunt, apparently as a result of a daily, rigorous running program and a decades-old dietary plan. His personal presence in the room was extremely compelling and hard to resist. He intruded on everyone in the room via touching, interrupting, speaking for someone, and several other mechanisms. The experience of a young child, growing up in that environment, would not be conducive to the establishment of a personal identity or boundaries.

The daughter had described in earlier sessions how she emulated her father and would wince whenever he decided that she was a pound or two overweight. Not surprisingly, she had become anorexic at 13 and bulimic at 22 (a change in symptomatology reflecting pseudo-resolution of the family issues). Thus, in this family, the daughter identified with the central figure in the family, the father, and yet was more severely restrictive than he was, thus "besting" him. The "control" she exhibited, first with anorexia, then bulimia, also created personal boundaries that were not presented in this family.

Therapy for her and her family initially focused on the example she was setting, by personal sacrifice, in order to teach personal boundary establishment to the rest of the family. The positive connotation of her behavior had a powerful effect, early on, of pulling her out of the sick role and creating a context for family therapy.

In chaotic families, the patterns of interaction seem to be more shifting and projections across generations are also more likely to shift. However, multigenerational family tolerances of alcohol abuse, physical violence, and spousal battering are common. These are patterns that are well learned in our clients from these families. Sometimes they express amazement that they are currently drinking too much and in a battering relationship. The client says something like, "This happened to my mother (or father) when I was growing up. I made a vow not to ever let this happen to me, but here I am. What do I do?" When we see this replication from one generation to the next, despite a person's conscious effort to reverse the pattern, we are reminded of Ritterman's (1983) belief in the hypnotically inductive capacities of all families. A violent, boundary-violating family induces a family hypnotic trance for many years. The inductions utilized in one family seem to be similar to those learned in another, providing an explanation for the recurrence of patterns and relationships from one generation to the next.

The power and persistence of these inductions are well documented by our clients' relapses when they visit their families. One client, who had been free of bingeing and purging for several months, went to her sister's wedding and purged immediately upon arriving at the airport in her family's home town. Another client binges and purges only when she visits her mother's house for their once-a-week get-together.

Carter and McGoldrick (1980) discuss the life-cycle of the family as progressing along a "horizontal" path through a series of essential transitions. There are "vertical" stressors at each stage that affect the resolution of each transition. Reflecting their influence by Bowen, they state that among the most powerful and insidious of these vertical stressors are multigenerational projections. These projections will reflect an area or several areas lacking resolution in the family-of-origin. The child may be viewed as if she were a junior representation of a sibling of the parent, or even the parent himself/herself. In another situation, the bulimic woman, named after her father, was viewed by him as a facsimile of his own mother, a chronically depressed mental patient. Despite the client's impressive strengths, her father admitted his fear that his daughter would also "go crazy." Other clients are more clearly identifed as "just like your mother (grandmother)." The type of self-fulfilling prophecy this sets up is quite compelling.

Walsh's (1978) study of the relationship of the birthdate of schizophrenics to the death date of a grandparent seems particularly relevant to this understanding of how patterns operate in a wide variety of families. Essentially, she found that schizophrenics were much more likely than nonschizophrenics to have been born close ( ± 2 years) to the death of a grandparent. This was not just any grandparent, but a grandparent about whom the parent had considerable unresolved feelings and conflicts. Walsh's contention is that a recently born child was the most convenient recipient of family projections that stemmed from the unresolved feelings. For example, if the parent-grandparent relationship was characterized by fusion, the parent would move to fuse with the young child as a way of dealing with the loss and also as a continuation of behavior that was perfectly acceptable in the family of origin. Or the parent may have been particularly estranged from the grandparent, whose death makes resolution of the estrangement quite difficult. This may activate depression in the parent, making her less available to care for the child. The depression may alternate with angry rejection so that the child becomes a scapegoat. We are convinced that many of these various mechanisms are operative in the families of bulimic clients and contribute to patterns and structures that are involved in the maintenance of the symptoms.

*Secrets*

The concept of family secrets is akin to a phenomenon Ferreira (1963) discusses, that of family myths. Secrets are a function of an ever increasing discrepancy between the inner self and outer public behavior. This creates confusion both in the person and in people exposed to the duplicitous behavior. The unresolved molestation many of the mothers in overprotective families experienced in their own family is ignored publicly. Yet, on nonverbal levels it is communicated as unexplained fear to the child. What the child experiences is someone else's (the mother's) attempts to regulate or control the inner life of her child in order to preserve her own inner life (Laing, 1969). The female child grows up publicly appropriate but privately fearful about relationships in general and intimacy in particular. This phenomenon explains what seems to be a "repetition compulsion" across generations, e.g., mother molested = child molested; mother miscarries = child who bears burdens of unborn children in addition to her own.

The majority of bulimic clients in our practices have reported being molested, battered, or raped. Most have not confided this to family members. When you add to that experience the fact that bulimics usually hide their symptoms, it is clear that a pattern of secretiveness is operative. This suggests multigenerational secretiveness, again a phenomenon that is evident. We have found that mothers of bulimic clients have been molested at a much higher rate than expected, often by the client's grandfather or uncle.

We offer several examples as illustrations. Becky's mother miscarried four times prior to giving birth to Becky. This fact was never mentioned, nor did Becky's mother ever resolve this series of losses. Becky's upbringing was characterized by extreme overprotectiveness, and she regularly experienced school phobia and subsequent periods of school absence through the sixth grade. As expected, Becky's "leaving home" was protracted and required two hospitalizations of her mother. To what degree this secret contributed to systemic interactions that evolved into Becky's becoming bulimic is uncertain. However, when Becky and her mother were in therapy together, the fact of the miscarriages came out, and Becky's mother sobbed for several minutes. The next several conjoint sessions involved grief work with both Becky and her mother — Becky for a lost childhood and her mother for the miscarriages and her own unhappy marriage, which had ended with Becky's father's death in an industrial accident when Becky was 12.

Despite lack of any precise understanding of their impact, these secrets serve to organize how family members perceive each other and their relationship to the outside world. The fact that most are related to a loss adds difficulty to any developmental task that exacerbates a sense of loss, change, or movement. This makes understandable the overprotectiveness and rigidity that we often see, or even the lack of protectiveness in the chaotic families, where the individuals might be incapacitated in their protective functions.

Secrets can continue to have an impact even when they have been disclosed. The reason for this is that *disclosure does not equal resolution.* The therapist of these families may hear much disclosure, because perfect and overprotective families are very willing to be "the best clients you ever had." Yet frequently there are rules pertaining to talking about the secret or the feelings associated with it.

For example, a family with an 18-year-old bulimic began therapy and was quite impressive in its seeming candidness in the first several sessions, with the mother disclosing several major traumatic issues in her life that she felt had had a direct impact on the development of an eating disorder in her daughter. The therapist was initially puzzled by the family, since family members appeared to be open and to have resolved the issues. Yet the openness was actually indicative of boundary permeability in the family, and there were a number of unspoken indicators that the resolution was not as complete as it seemed. First, the client's mother was unable to talk about the issues with her mother and was quite estranged from her. Second, the frequency with which she discussed her traumas with her children communicated analogically to the children the fact that these traumas were not resolved. One would expect a gradual decrease in discussion over time, and this was not true in her case. Finally, the manner in which the mother reported her losses fit her demonstrative, effusive style and was not convincing. Thus, there were still secrets on one level in the family between her mother and herself. Their continued presence was dictating her behavior more than she was aware.

*Therapy Issues*

We are convinced that interrupting the "inherited-by-learning systems" (Headley, 1977) that clients present benefits both the individual and her parents. The most efficient way to describe this is with a case that eventually involved four generations. The genogram in Figure 1 outlines the major players in the Manahan family. The reader may become as confused as the therapist with the similar sounding names of the family members.

Jo was 24 years old when she first contacted one of the authors for help with her five-year-old daughter, Jen. She and her husband, Bob, differed

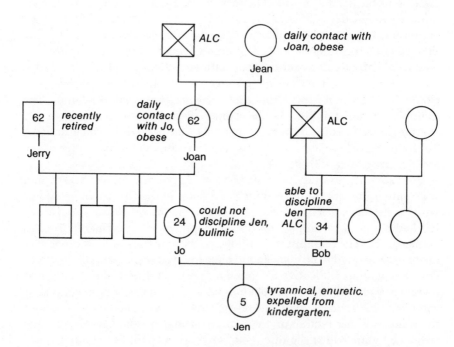

*Figure 1.* The Manahan Family

intensely on how to parent Jen, who was reported to be very tyrannical, going to bed when she felt like it, eating only sweets, and yelling at her mother frequently. In addition, Jen was enuretic and had been asked to leave a prestigious kindergarten because of her behavior problems.

At the first interview, it became apparent that Bob was the only parent who could consistently get Jen to behave. Part of Jo's problems seemed to be related to moderately severe depression of several years' duration. Jo had given up trying to discipline Jen and used her mother, Joan, for this whenever Bob was not around. The day after the first appointment, Joan called the therapist, offering to help "in any way I can." Joan and Jo had daily contact, and Joan was also successful disciplining Jen. The therapist declined Joan's offer, but told her she might be invited later, if Jo and Bob and the therapist saw fit.

By this time, the therapist had enough information to realize that Jo, as the youngest, least differentiated, and only daughter of four children in an overprotective family, was continuing to be inadequate raising her daughter, requiring the help of her mother and husband. This position between two people was familiar, with Jo and the maternal grandmother Jean being in a coalition against Jerry, her father. Jerry had always worked long hours and was only a minor figure in the family while Jo was growing up. His recent retirement had activated the long dormant marital discord between Jerry and Joan, pulling Jo back into her family of origin.

Her three brothers were quite a bit older and not as available emotionally or geographically. Bob, an oldest and only son, had acted as a surrogate father in his family of origin, replacing his own alcoholic father in the family hierarchy. So "taking care" of Jo was a natural extension of his role in his family. He and Jo had married when she became pregnant with Jen. Jo did not tell her parents about the pregnancy; rather, she married Bob, who was ten years older than she and whom she had never really loved.

The initial sessions focused on parenting Jen. Jo began to use some techniques and was somewhat effective. It was at this time that Bob informed the therapist that Jo was bulimic, that her behavior disgusted him, and that he thought she needed hospitalization. Jo was bingeing/purging at a rate of three to four times per day and had been for the past five years. It had begun when she was trying to lose weight after her pregnancy with Jen. The therapist suggested a change in treatment focus, from family to marital, and Bob and Jo agreed.

Several events occurred in quick succession. Jo began to work as a clerk and this added immensely to her self-confidence but intensified the marital conflict. Jo was more successful with Jen during this period, also. Bob began an affair, when Jo discovered it, she kicked him out of the house. Jo lost her job almost simultaneously with this and moved in with her parents.

When the therapist discovered this at the next session, Jo appeared very depressed, was bingeing and purging at her previously highest level, and Jen was again extremely aggressive with her. After a few sessions of this, with Jo becoming increasingly depressed, the therapist invited Jerry and Joan in for several sessions with Jo. The goals for these sessions were to remove Jo from between Jerry and Joan and to get them to support her parenting of Jen. Jo became suicidal at this time, however, and the plan changed to involving Jerry and Joan in keeping Jo from harming herself and meeting more frequently until the crisis passed.

The crisis persisted, as Jo began to lose weight and Jerry and Joan's marital conflict emerged fully. The sessions for over two months had a combined focus of Jerry and Joan's marital conflict and Jo's severe depression. Jerry was quite eager to make some changes, but Joan was angry and tired after 41 years of marriage. At this point Joan moved in with her own mother, Jean, and refused to move back home until she could "do some thinking." With her mother out of the house, Jo rebounded dramatically, but Joan, who was still coming to sessions, became extremely depressed and was now suicidal. Joan and Jean were quite conflicted but still enmeshed and, like Joan and Jo, overly close.

Using the metaphor of "going home to get sick," the therapist got Jean, Joan, and Jo to come in for a series of sessions, where they talked about their disappointments in life, particularly with men, their own loneliness, and their regrets at seeing their children grow up. The similarities across the generations were striking, including problems with eating for each woman, and moved the women towards making some real changes. Over the next four months, Joan moved back with Jerry and went on a long vacation with him. Jo got another job, moved into her own apartment with Jen, and filed for divorce from Bob. Jean even reported an increase in involvement with her same-age peers. Jen's behavior was markedly better at the time of termination, and Jo had not been symptomatic for four months.

The entire treatment course extended over 14 months from the first to last contact. During the therapy, the problems Jo was having as a parent were traced to the perpetuation with Bob of the relationship she had had with her mother, Joan, and the relationship Joan had had with her own mother, Jean. The mother-daughter overinvolvement had extended across all three generations, as had eating problems (e.g., compulsive dieting, obesity), suicidal gestures, and a history of depression. In each generation the husband had had at least one affair that had seriously affected the marriage.

By remaining focused on the systemic issues and not fearing to involve the appropriate systems members, the therapist was able to catalyze this family into making what appeared to be second-order changes or true structural changes in the entire system. Even though bulimia was not the presenting complaint, it was certainly a symbol for Jo's efforts at establishing some control in a system where she felt out of control. During the session in which Bob had informed the therapist that she was bulimic, Jo had stated, "It's the only thing that is my own. . . . It's like it stops all the pressures on me, at least for a bit."

What the therapist can derive from this example is support for expanding the focus in treating bulimia. Personally, for the therapist, the task of therapy became exceedingly more difficult. However, the continuing chaos in the system, when not amenable to a narrower focus, required an expanded focus. The addition of a variety of other individuals presented some unique opportunities for intervention and resolution.

# CHAPTER 6

# The Family Life-Cycle of the Bulimic

TOO OFTEN THERAPISTS, particularly those who work primarily with adults, ignore developmental issues. Consequently, therapists tend to approach the change process with a static conceptualization of individuals and systems. Treating bulimic families and individuals necessitates a movement away from this traditional framework. In fact, Benjamin (1983) writes that one of the seven characteristics of general systems theory is the concept of time. He states, " . . . all family processes exist in real time" (p. 56). In support of this, Dell (1982) argues that pathology is nothing more than a state of stuckness along a developmental course.

An awareness of the developmental issues operative in family systems is a necessity for the therapist working with bulimic individuals. In fact, as we discuss later in this chapter, it seems that part of what discriminates bulimia from anorexia is the developmental stage at which families get stuck.

While it is true that stage theories can be too simplistic, the concept of a family life-cycle or a patterning of predictable processes for families and individuals (Carter & McGoldrick, 1980) is very useful. All families face predictable stages of family life, though not all families successfully negotiate these stages.

Growth is an undeniable component of any system and its individual members. Developmental theorists (Kegan, 1982) discuss development as the continual interplay of two complementary processes, *differentiation* and *integration*, present at each life-cycle transition. To us, differentiation connotes the establishment of interpersonal boundaries and the maintenance of interpersonal distance and autonomy. Integration complements the separation and definition established through differentiation. Integration connotes movement towards closeness and intimacy, with the subsequent establishment of richer and more complex relationships between members of the system. For example, newly married spouses need to establish a series of patterns that allow them to function as a couple (integration). In addition, they need to foster a boundary between them that provides a sense of themselves as separate persons (differentiation).

Each stage of the life-cycle presents a new series of tasks that require mastering. Table 3 summarizes the family life-cycle, with special note of the tasks required of the family and the difficulties at each stage that bulimic families may have. Families will differ in how and when they traverse these predictable stages, but they cannot skip stages. Family development theorists suggest that there are consequences to how well or how poorly the family manages each transition. Essentially, a poor resolution at one stage will make the resolution of subsequent stages more difficult. Subsequent transitions become "pseudo-transitions." Typical problematic patterns indicate that the new stage is not being handled well by the family. For example, if, soon after the birth of the first child, the husband leaves the family, this signifies an unsuccessful transition from being a couple to being parents. We cannot emphasize enough'that *the majority of marital, family, and individual problems is related to derailments at specific stages of family development.* Successful life-cycle transitions require "second order change," a change in the system itself.

The two most frequent ages of onset for bulimia are during adolescence and young adulthood. Family life-cycle theorists discuss two very important transitions that occur at these stages of development. The processes that are operative and are in a dynamic tension are those of autonomy and intimacy. These complementary processes need resolution at a new level for each of these stages.

However, the stages of adolescence and young adulthood are preceded by several other life-cycle transitions that require negotiation. Our experience strongly suggests that bulimic families also have difficulties with these earlier stages. Consequently, we will examine each of these life-cycle transition points in order to understand those developmental processes that seem to be related to the onset of bulimic symptomatology. These stages include marriage, birth of a child, family with young children, adolescence, and launching.

## MARRIAGE

From a life-cycle perspective, the family begins as soon as the two future spouses leave their own families of origin and form their marital relationship. That this is indeed a struggle has been underscored by Stanton and Landau-Stanton (1984), who stated that families will fail unless the young

TABLE 3
Family Life Cycle of Bulimic Families

| Stages | Necessary tasks | Points of breakdown |
|--------|-----------------|---------------------|
| Marriage | Detach from family of origin | Failure to detach |
| | Move towards each other | Failure to integrate as a couple |
| Birth | Maintain marriage | Marital strain |
| | Expand into parental role | Parenting not accepted by both partners |
| Young children | Child develops autonomy | Precocious or delayed autonomy |
| | Appropriate parental expectations | Inappropriate expectations |
| | | Deepening enmeshment |
| Adolescence | Strengthen parent-adolescent boundaries | Marital relationship dissolves |
| | | Deepening enmeshment |
| | | Precocious "launching" (Chaotic) |
| Young adulthood | Family releases young adult | Marital relationship dissolves |
| | | Delayed launching |

couple receives permission to marry. This permission is either overtly or covertly received from the young people's parents. The marriage ceremony, hopefully, allows the potential spouses to receive this "permission" and consolidate their relationship.

Carter and McGoldrick (1980) identify several major tasks of this stage. The two most important tasks highlight the simultaneous resolution of differentiation and integration. Both partners need to detach from their families of origin (differentiation) and move towards each other (integration).

With this first task of differentiation, the spouses need to restructure their relationship to allow for greater independence from their parents, but still maintain ongoing loyalty and availability. Boundaries must be established between families of origin and the marital relationship. The parents of many bulimic clients appear to have had difficulty with this initial step in the life-cycle. For example, Terri's mother had a conflicted, ambivalent relationship with her parents that preceded her marriage and persisted long after. She still cannot speak to her mother without getting ill and asks Terri to visit her instead. The mother of another client, Lisa, refuses to visit her father, currently in a nursing home, and feels she has always let him down. He provided large sums of money to his daughter, Lisa's mother, to help his grandchildren attend private school. This "gift" further estranged father and daughter because of the strings that were attached.

This transition in the family life-cycle at this stage can evolve into problematic patterns (Karpel & Strauss, 1982), including: 1) rigid alliance of one spouse with his or her family of origin against the other spouse; 2) the assumption by the parents of major responsibilities, e.g., financial, of the couple's daily life; and 3) severing all ties with a family of origin.

In chaotic families emotional cut-offs are common and alliances can shift rapidly. In overprotective and perfect families there is more likely to be overinvolvement between the parents and new spouse. Sherri's father, for example, was still quietly angry at his mother 40 years later for her mental illness and was guilt-ridden about his relationship with his father, whom he placed in a nursing home. Meanwhile, his wife was overinvolved with her own mother but sent her husband to visit her father in a nursing home because she was still fearful of him.

The other task is integration. How do the two newlyweds move towards each other? McGoldrick (1980) writes that a basic dilemma in the coupling process is the "confusion of closeness with fusion" (p. 96). In this case, fusion would mean the loss of a sense of a separate autonomous self due to a merger with another person. In perfect families the spouses appear to have a satisfactory relationship, but close examination frequently reveals that it is non-egalitarian and the husband is both dominating and very narcissistic. Overprotective families commonly have spouses who are fused with each other. In chaotic families the spouses' relational style is more centrifugal or distant, although the outbursts of violence that commonly occur may be due to intense, sudden oscillation between distance and fusion.

In summary, the parents of many bulimic clients have difficulty in this first life-cycle stage. Oftentimes, they cannot leave their own family of origin, and when they do, the new relationship seems to be either overinvolved or overly distant. This does not create the type of marital union that will facilitate the successful negotiation of the transition into parenthood, the task of the next phase.

## BIRTH OF THE CHILD

The addition of a child to the marital dyad demands changes in the system. The parents must attempt to integrate their developing relationship with the infant with their ongoing marital relationship. Consequently, the system is being challenged to create new roles for all members. Along with these new roles, new boundaries and subsystems are also established. For example, the marital dyad must also become in part a parental dyad. The test of the new parents is whether they can have not only a marital relationship but also a parental relationship.

When individuals who are emotionally needy or depleted get married, there is a potential for distress in the relationship. The addition of a third member exacerbates this potential and threatens the ability of the system to successfully move into this new phase.

The picture we have of the parents of a bulimic client at this stage varies from one type to the next. If we imagine that this infant will become bulimic, our understanding of the family system when she presents in therapy at adolescence or young adulthood helps us extrapolate what was happening or failing to happen at her birth.

The marked tendency towards enmeshment, personal boundary violation, and triangulation in bulimic families would clearly suggest that marital, parental, and individual needs/wishes were not being balanced or met. Sometimes, particularly in chaotic families, the parents provide insufficient attention to the child. This could reflect depletion in the parents or an enmeshed, stormy marital relationship that cannot tolerate a consistent parental function. Conversely, a common pattern is for one spouse to become overinvolved with the infant (a natural phenomenon at first) and the other to become more peripheral. The longer this style persists, the more rigid the system becomes and the harder it is to make later, necessary transitions. It is much more common for the mother to become overly involved as the father becomes peripheral. The infant can be used early on by both parties as an obstacle to closeness and intimacy.

It is not uncommon for the mother to become depressed at this point. Her own lack of differentiation within the system and the helplessness that ensues render her more vulnerable. Her depression is accompanied by isolation from both spouse and infant. When she does get over her depressive episode and begins to attach to the infant, her early unavailability will often make for the development of an ambivalent mother-infant relationship. This can fluctuate widely in intensity and frequently will persist on the fused end of the spectrum.

The addition of the child to the marriage may temporarily stabilize it, with the mother-child dyad becoming overinvolved and thus lessening, for a time, pressures on the marital relationship. Yet this temporary stabilization lays the framework for continued rigidity, enmeshment, and lack of successful conflict resolution, and maintains the marital relationship as less than adequate. The balance needed between differentiation and integration (Kegan, 1982) is not reached, with overinvolvement between parent and child and a cut-off between spouses. At this early stage, however, there may be few visible signs of distress.

## THE FAMILY WITH YOUNG CHILDREN

Karpel and Strauss (1982) identify two major tasks for the family system moving through this stage. The first task requires yet another balancing act—balancing the child's developing autonomy with a sense of connection and belonging to the family. This is a tightrope; without an appropriate balance, the family could sacrifice autonomy for belongingness, or vice versa. Each has its consequences.

The second major task also requires balancing, this time involving expectations placed on the child. The family can either expect too much of the child, asking her to perform perfectly or be in subliminal tune to a parent's needs, or expect too little and not allow for the development of a sense of purpose or competence. These expectations can take many forms. Externally directed expectations would be such things as academic accomplishment or career choice, whereas more internal, family-directed expectations involve the expression of feelings, weight maintenance, etc. When expectations do not co-evolve, with both the parents' and child's developmental needs being respected, this is an indication of the absence of the firm and clear boundaries that should be emerging during this phase.

This is an important stage to examine when discussing the evolution of bulimia in the family. The balancing acts outlined above sound a great deal like the balancing acts the bulimic client is attempting to manage. The perfect family, for example, could simplistically be characterized as emphasizing pseudo-autonomy and rigid expectations. The chaotic family could be characterized as emphasizing precocious autonomy and as having few expectations. The overprotective family seems to emphasize belonging and no expectations. Problems arise when expectations are rigid and extreme; the child does not learn the balance between expectations and tolerance. Similarly, problems arise when belonging *and* autonomy are mutually exclusive. In these cases, the developing child is not able to have the advantages that belonging *and* autonomy bring, nor the benefits of expectations *and* acceptance.

Self-reports from clients about this time in their life clearly identify these precursors. One client reports, for example, how her mother told her how to gracefully decline any proffered emotional support. She credited this for the overcompetence she demonstrated, but the consequence was an underlying fragility and inability to receive support in relationships. A second client reiterated how "my mother's feelings of mad and sad would roll like a wave out of her bedroom door. I can remember being five years old, and I'd be sitting in the living room watching TV and start to sense them. I wanted to leave the house but then she'd be hurt. I don't think I learned how to have my own feelings, although I did learn to have hers. And I learned how not to have feelings."

Another woman, the youngest in her family, developed a persistent school phobia. Her parents kept her out of school, and she was tutored by her schoolteacher-mother until the fourth grade, when financial circumstances forced her mother to return to work. Imagine also how another young child learns the priority of obeying family expectations rather than allowing for one's own needs when the child is an intermediary between one parent and the grandparent. Rather than visit her mother-in-law, one woman sent her very young daughter to visit every summer. At the end of the summer, when she returned home, the child was placed on a diet, regardless of her weight, because "your grandmother uses so much grease in everything." This is a compelling message about body-image!

It is not surprising, then, when the bulimia emerges in the next stage. The affective intensity of adolescence activates patterns that have been in place for a long time. The family's efforts towards homeostasis do not allow for the second-order change needed to allow for a reversal of the bulimigenic patterns. The child in her family has not learned to balance autonomy with belonging and expectations with acceptance.


## ADOLESCENCE

Although bulimic families have difficulties with earlier transitions, it is in adolescence that stuckness is seen most clearly. For anorectic families, the stuckness is actually earlier, with more pronounced difficulties during family formation and school age. Bulimic families seem to have more familiarity with both closeness and distance and the balancing of the two, while anorectic families seem more one-dimensional.

Life-span developmental psychologists describe the typical parents of an adolescent as negotiating their own "mid-life crisis" (Kegan, 1982). Change appears to be the necessary order of the day in this phase. The adolescent's personal growth and increasing autonomy need to be responded to by the family's increasing boundary flexibility. A possible and positive means is for the parent-child relationship to shift in the direction of allowing greater autonomy and responsibility with less control. As Kegan (1982) has stated, the job of the adolescent's parents is to be left by the adolescent.

It is this loss of the child that Karpel and Strauss (1982) speak of as the most common and significant issue presented to the parents. The shared participation and enjoyment derived during earlier years are not as frequent, and parents come face to face with their own aging and mortality. Unresolved loss is a common theme in bulimic families. Loss at a later date reactivates earlier unresolved losses and activates loss prevention mechanisms. "You can't leave me" becomes a common, overt/covert refrain. Other issues specific to the parents are also operative. For many years, the marital relationship has had a secondary focus; now it comes back into the foreground. This can be due to the parents' responding to the adolescent's sexual development, which highlights their own problematic functioning. The increased conflict generated when parenting an adolescent also highlights tension in the parenting dyad, as does the fact that allowing an adolescent to leave home forces the parents to rely on each other again for purpose, focus, and meaning in the relationship. This is particularly true with the last child, and we see many youngest children as bulimics in our practices.

Unfortunately, many parents find that the marital relationship does not stand up to this close scrutiny and major marital problems emerge. This invites triangulation and, particularly when the family has a long history of boundary violation, it becomes easy to do more of the same. The emergence of bulimic symptoms effectively distracts the needed focus on the marital relationship. The end result is an unsuccessful negotiation of this life-cycle transition.

*The strengthening of adolescent-parent boundaries is the fundamental family system change needed during this stage.* The strengthening of the hierarchical boundary between the parent generation and the adolescent allows the adolescent to horizontally expand her participation in the peer system. Yet as the shift for separateness begins in the system, a countershift towards more inclusion and control of the adolescent is frequently activated in the bulimic family.

Negotiating adolescence is very difficult for bulimic families. In the words of Laurie, a 19-year-old bulimic, "Everything went to pieces. My parents divorced suddenly when I was 14, and my father remarried eight months later. My mother needed us kids desperately for the two years after the divorce because she was always having problems with her boyfriends and needed advice. And then, just when I finally made some real friends in high school, my dad moves to the east coast and insists that I go along—that it would be good for me and give me a break. But then I was in the middle of his problems with my stepmom — I didn't need them to be doing all those crazy things at that time in my life."

Laurie became bulimic at age 16. Ostensibly, she used purging as a way to remain slender. She felt that being slender would be the best way to keep the friends she had just started to make again after her return from the east. However, her behavior also resulted in her parents' communicating more. When her mother discovered her purging in the bathroom, Laurie responded, "If you want to know what's happening to me, ask dad." In addition, her stepmother resolved to remain in the troubled marriage so she could help Laurie with her "problem." In this young woman's family the systemic implications far exceeded the individual implications of maintaining thinness. The original family was temporarily restored, and her father's troubled second marriage was stabilized.

When Laurie presented as a client at the age of 19, one of her most pressing concerns was to resolve her conflicted relationship with her parents. Both still used her as a confidant and, by each implying the other should give her money for college, confirmed the triangulation and maintained her in a dependent child role.

For Laurie, the parents' marital breakup occurred while she was at a critical developmental stage. Just as she was beginning to strengthen her own boundaries by developing a set of outside social relations, her parents' divorce forced a turning toward the family again. More limits and more expectations were being made of her at a time when the opposite was necessary.

We are not implying that the family's breakdown during the adolescent phase in its life-cycle causes Laurie's bulimia. Her vulnerability to developing bulimia had been evolving over a number of years, as she played the role of mother's closest confidant and was subject to her father's self-centered, controlling style, which did not validate her own emerging opinions and needs. Laurie's developmental needs were subsumed by the emotional needs of her parents. Having learned no direct way to assert herself or deal with the frustration of having to continually stifle the expression of her own feelings, she found that bingeing/purging provided some relief and hurt no one but herself. This reinforcement, coupled with the social/familial approval of slenderness, made for rapid learning of a habit. Her bulimia provided some autonomy to balance her parents' incredible need for her to stay young.

In summary, while adolescence appears to be the time period when bulimic symptoms emerge for a large percentage of our clients, the issues that operate in adolescence are not that different from those in other phases the family has tried to negotiate. They are related to balancing autonomy with belonging. The additional stressors of adolescence, in addition to threatened alteration of the family, are too much for many families. This seems particularly true for overprotective families. Of the three types, they seem to be the most distressed by adolescence, as the child needs less protection. When the parents' developmental needs are considered (mid-life crisis), we see that two life-cycle transitions are occurring simultaneously and the entire family system is influx. The cumulative effects of previous difficulties in family evolution finally catch up with the family and one or more members become overtly symptomatic.

## LAUNCHING

Failure to leave home effectively inhibits individual development. Successful launching (or leaving home) is more psychological and emotional than geographical. Tasks that must be accomplished in this life-cycle phase include the parents' releasing the young adult children into work, college, or marriage. Basically, this requires the family to allow separation without cutting off the relationship. This goal again requires achieving a balance between autonomy and closeness. The recapitulation of this theme characterizes the entire family life-cycle. The family's resolution of the launching stage becomes problematic when either end of the balance is ignored. For example, a precipitous and angry departure emotionally "cuts off" the person from the family, effectively inhibiting future emotional development (Bowen, 1978).

The parents need to prepare themselves for the emotional issues revolving around the increasingly longer exits and increasingly shorter reentries into the family. As the young adult prepares herself to invest in an independent life and work of her own, she maintains an emotional investment despite distance. It is important for the family to maintain a supportive home base. Or, as Kegan (1982) would put it, the "holding" environment of the family must remain in place. This allows the young adult to leave from something that is stable, and when that happens the leave-taking is much more successful.

The previous individuation that was to have been evolving in adolescence is a prelude to what is now facing the family. This explains why many bulimics seem to first become symptomatic as they are being "launched" into the world or "leaving home." It is as if this becomes their "adolescence." This is true particularly with overprotective and perfect families. The differentiation that occurred during adolescence was a pseudo-individuation.

For example, an adolescent may get good grades, present no problems, and have an adequate circle of good friends. She is able to do this while continuing to remain emotionally tied in the family. Typically there is little evidence of rebellion. However, it is harder to remain emotionally tied to family expectations as a young adult, probably because social mores expect some version of physical separation and a demonstration of individual competence via rebellion and experimentation. Here again we see many instances of pseudo-differentiation, e.g., the young woman living away from home but in an apartment owned by her parents or working at a job in a company that a parent owns.

Again, the bulimia that presents itself now, in young adulthood (early twenties and on), has its roots in earlier stages and in earlier family life-cycle transitions that were not successfully negotiated. For example, Carla recalled that just as she was entering middle school, her parents divorced and her mother became seriously depressed and began to drink too much. Carla put aside all extracurricular activities and socialization for the next ten years. Essentially, Carla skipped adolescence. She became symptomatic at the time of her first serious dating when 23 years old. Failures at resolution left Carla poorly equipped to deal with the daily stressors of life. The denial of boundaries provided her with a poorly established sense of personal authority and autonomy.

Claudia, the youngest daughter in an overprotective family, had been her mother's co-dieter throughout childhood and adolescence. She had accepted that role and enjoyed the mutuality it afforded. Claudia began college with no history of eating disorder and maintained her role in the family by managing to be home every weekend. During her senior year, she began to seriously date for the first time and was coming home less frequently. Her recollection of her first binge/purge episode was a Thursday evening. She had called her mother to tell her she was not coming home. Her mother responded by telling her how much she had been counting on her being there, since she was so lonely and had been feeling depressed about how much time her husband was spending with a female associate. Claudia spent almost two hours on the phone with her mother that evening, listening to her cry and trying to offer suggestions. She even went so far as to call her father to the phone and tell him off. Claudia was also feeling increasingly upset about her physical appearance and was attributing this to her uncertainty about being sexually active with her boyfriend. She finally chose to not go home that weekend but overate that evening, panicked, and purged, with resultant feelings of relief. Over the next few months, she began to binge/purge daily.

Claudia's lack of boundaries with her mother and with her boyfriend, who was sometimes verbally abusive, was clearly evident. The family also had a long history of food-related concerns that provided a preexisting stress-reduction mechanism. The impending destabilization of the family system was interrupted, at least briefly. Claudia's mother separated from her father and moved into Claudia's apartment, with the result being a marked increase in bulimic symptoms that left her feeling completely out of control and eventually led to her seeking therapy.

Chaotic families appear different at this stage. Physically leaving home may have occurred much earlier, given familial expectations. We regularly see clients from these families as being forced in an accelerated fashion through these stages. This still makes for a pseudo-transition, even if the indicators of rites of passage, e.g., rebelliousness in adolescence, have occurred.

Lesbian and gay clients also have difficulties with launching. Part of successful launching includes formation of social relationships outside the family. The family and society fail to permit this, even more vigorously because of the meaning of gay relationships to the family. Heterosexual relationships can at least be tolerated. This serves to perpetuate these clients' stuckness in the launching phase.

Claudia and Laurie (see p. 71) provide graphic illustrations of how family life-cycle transitions involve the entire family. Parents are changing and possibly ending relationships at the same time the adolescents are doing the same. If the therapist simply looks at the family life-cycle as something that the child must move through and fails to be attuned to the parents' own development, many life-cycle issues will be missed.

Other variations in this simple, stage theory of family development are found in single-parent families or recombined families. A not too uncommon theme in single-parent families with a bulimic adolescent or young adult is for the mother and daughter to be developmentally parallel, e.g., dating, establishing intimate relationships. Here again, the possibilities for role reversal are endless, with the daughter "counseling my mom about her boyfriends. She made such dumb mistakes. You'd think she would have learned after 23 years of marriage."

Or, in a remarried family, the client may either get caught up in continuing warfare between her parents or she may feel prematurely excluded from the family as her parents start their own "new couple" phases and second families. We have been successful several times by removing the client from a central role between warring ex-spouses. For example, each of Tammy's parents confided in her about the other's misdeeds and regularly quizzed her about the other's activities. In the initial family session, both described their relationship as being at war with each other. The parents were asked to list the many issues that kept them "at war with each other." Their listing of reasons was extensive and impressive and we told them so. The war metaphor was very appropriate, since the father was a retired military officer. Yet in war, civilians get killed, and the father was asked about what the Geneva Accords had to say about killing civilians. This made the issue of Tammy's being in the middle very clear to both parties, but yet did not affect their behavior with each other, at least initially. For those first several sessions, the system was kept extremely intense by returning to the issue of what each was doing to "keep Tammy out of the line of fire." Tammy did her part to maintain the status quo by minimizing her parents' contributions and even reporting an increase in symptoms. Her behavior illustrates how all members of the system work together at this — it is too simplistic to call it a problem with parents' letting go.

In summary, life-cycle transitions must be negotiated by every family. The concept of life-cycle implies development, and it is useful to think about bulimics and their families getting stuck in their development, rather than one or the other being "sick." The most overt distress and stuckness seem to revolve around the gradual differentiation of the family as it grapples with adolescence and leaving home. However, as we have pointed out, the opportunities for stuckness are there at the beginning of system formation.

# PART III

# THE FAMILY
# TYPOLOGIES

# CHAPTER 7

# *Eating-Disordered Families: Current Literature*

THE FOLLOWING CHAPTERS introduce our conceptualization of the three family types that contribute to the development of bulimia: the *perfect* family, the *overprotective* family, and the *chaotic* family. Because there is little research specifically directed toward bulimic families, the differentiation that we present is derived from clinical experience and the eating disorders literature, which focuses primarily on anorexia nervosa.

The lack of literature on bulimic families is due to several factors. The primary reason is that bulimia has only been recognized as a disorder separate from anorexia nervosa since 1980. The two disorders are often not differentiated in terms of conceptualization of their development or in approaches to treatment. Two secondary reasons emerge to account for the lack of literature on bulimic families. The first is that treatment is often instigated when the bulimic individual is older, either because the onset of the bulimia is at a later age, as the individual is leaving home, or because it is a behavior that is concealed and acknowledged only when the individual is in her or his twenties or older. The second reason is related to the general lack of research on families due to the difficulties in conducting research on interactions as complex as those seen in families.

There has, however, been major work done in the field of the development of psychosomatic disorders, particularly anorexia, which will be briefly reviewed here. The earliest investigators of anorexia nervosa (Gull, 1874; Laseque, 1873) postulated that there were certain family interactions which were related to the development of the disorder. A number of clinicians and researchers have since suggested the use of family therapy in treatment of eating disorders (Bruch, 1973; Crisp, Harding, & McGuiness, 1974; Minuchin, 1974; Minuchin, et al., 1978), while others suggest family therapy if the client is younger than age 16 or as supplemental to other types of treatment (Garner, Garfinkel & Bemis, 1982).

Two theorists in particular, Salvador Minuchin (Minuchin et al., 1978) and Mara Selvini Palazzoli (1978) have offered conceptualizations of the development and maintenance of psychosomatic symptoms, including eating disorders, that focus on the dysfunctional family system. The eating-disordered behavior is seen as related to dysfunctional family patterns which allow the family to avoid conflict.

The family resists change, according to Selvini Palazzoli, because the symptomatic member provides homeostasis for the family. She theorizes that messages sent by family members are commonly rejected by others, resulting in little resolution of family conflict. The symptoms allow a "three-way matrimony" to exist in which the parents continue to interact by focusing on the symptomatic member or blaming each other for the symptomatic behavior. The anorectic behavior effectively masks the conflict in the parental relationship, making it impossible for the behavior to end until it no longer serves this purpose, which in the case of marital conflict could exist until one parent's death.

Minuchin (1974; Minuchin et al., 1978), a leader in the field of family therapy for eating-disordered behavior, has described a number of characteristics which typify psychosomatic families, including families of anorectics. Minuchin has characterized anorectic families as enmeshed, rigid, overprotective, and lacking in conflict resolution skills; he has also noted the involvement of the anorectic child in the marital conflict. He, like Selvini Palazzoli, sees the symptomatic child as included in the parental subsystem, through either triangulation, scapegoating, or parent-child coalitions. Anorexia is seen as a problem of family organization and functioning, and the goal of treatment is to change the patterns of interactions so that the behavior is no longer needed (Sargent, Liebman, & Silver, 1984).

While there has been research into conceptualization of factors and dynamics related to families of anorectics, there has been little attention devoted to families of bulimics. There have been scattered reports of case studies (Madanes, 1981; Saba, Barrett, & Schwartz, 1983; Schwartz, R., 1982), but with the exception of the recent family typologies suggested by Schwartz, Barrett, and Saba (1984), the literature on the families of bulimics has been sparse. Schwartz et al. (1984) report that the five characteristics that Minuchin describes are present in bulimic families and add three more: isolation, consciousness of appearance, and a special meaning attached to food and eating. We see these as operative, but also see individual differences among these families that make bulimic families quite heterogeneous. This heterogeneity needs to be appreciated both for assessment and for treatment purposes.

## THE DEVELOPMENT OF BULIMIA

There has been little offered in the research literature to explain why one psychosomatic behavior may develop rather than another. We endorse the view offered by others that bulimia is multidetermined (Garfinkel & Garner, 1982) and that a number of factors must converge in order for the symptom of bulimia to surface. Sociocultural pressures, victimization experiences (as a child or as an adult), individual factors such as body frame and set point, and family dynamics must be considered as vulnerability factors. We address ourselves here to the differences in families that influence the development of symptoms.

We believe that the development of anorexia nervosa is related to the difficulty that the family has in negotiating the passage of the child into adolescence, while bulimia represents a more advanced maturational state in which the adolescent and family have difficulty negotiating movement from adolescence into young adulthood and independence. This view has been suggested by Wooley and Kearney-Cooke (in press) and offers an explanation for the fact that, while anorectics often later develop bulimia, the reverse is seldom true. It also serves to explain age of onset of the symptoms. Anorexia is often developed in early adolescence, while bulimia most often occurs when the individual is around 18, a time of emancipation and launching.

Our concern is that because of the later onset for bulimia, many clinicians do not acknowledge the need for family therapy. Nevertheless, since bulimia may also be reflective of the family "stuckness," the most effective form of treatment is often family therapy.

In Chapters 8, 9, and 10, we describe three different family types in which a member is likely to develop the symptom of bulimia in order to maintain family homeostasis. The three types differ along important dimensions, although there are similarities across types. *All bulimic families have individual and subsystem boundary problems. Weight and appearance are important factors in all these families. And there is an inequitable distribution of power, which is reinforced by the cultural system.* The father usually holds the power in these families, and the bulimic individual is caught between her father and her powerless mother.

In most families described in the family therapy literature, the mother is portrayed as being overinvolved with her children to what appears to be a pathological degree. Little attention has been paid to the reason and accuracy of this portrayal, with the unspoken explanation being that this is somehow reflective of "bad mothering." While we do observe an overinvolvement on the part of many mothers of bulimics and a corresponding lack of involvement of fathers of bulimics, we suggest that this is not due to poor parenting; rather, it reflects the pathology of the cultural system and the difficulty negotiating the integration of masculine and feminine values, as described by Wooley and Kearney-Cooke (in press). Moreover, we do not observe maternal overinvolvement in all bulimic families, and certainly not in families in general. However, if it is part of the dysfunction of the family system, the task in therapy is to empower the mother and decrease the distance between the father and other members, a difficult task in the face of strong cultural pressures.

The family types will be described by the markers and signs that make them unique; familiar phrases and family messages will be offered as another way to recognize certain types of families. The way in which each family typically presents in therapy, as well as characteristics that distinguish the families, will be highlighted by the use of case examples. Since our approach is also developmental in nature, we will discuss the points at which each family gets stuck in the family life-cycle, with the bulimic behavior surfacing as a response to the "stuckness" of the family. Family-of-origin issues are discussed to emphasize the context within which the individual becomes vulnerable to developing symptoms in reaction to unresolved issues. Sometimes the symptoms reflect unresolved conflicts between the parents and grandparents, which is often the case when the problem persists in spite of therapeutic interventions with the individual. We highlight issues that must be addressed before the individual and the family are able to recover from the bulimia. Finally, the many systemic functions of the bulimic behavior are outlined for the reader.

While there are similiarities among the three family types, as well as similiarities between the family types offered here and those described in the eating disorders literature, the delineation of this typology provides the clinician with important information for conceptualization and treatment of bulimic individuals and their families. We do not suggest that every individual presenting with bulimia will fit neatly into one of the three family types. In our clinical experience, families often fit a combination of types. However, we do offer this typology as a framework within which to conceptualize salient issues, thereby facilitating both an understanding of the family's need for the symptom and treatment planning.

# CHAPTER 8

# *The Perfect Family*

*"A job worth doing is worth doing well."*

THE PERFECT FAMILY is similiar to many of the families of anorectics described in the popular literature (Cherry Boone O'Neil, Jane Fonda, Karen Carpenter). The family appears to be a success or "rags to riches" story; the symptomatic member is a "golden girl." Hallmarks of the perfect family include: an emphasis on *appearance*, *family reputation*, *family identity*, and *achievement*.

## THE PERFECT FAMILY INITIATES THERAPY

In the perfect family, either the parent or the child will make the initial contact for therapy, depending on the age of the client. If she is a teenager, typically the parent will call; if she is an adult, the call usually comes from the bulimic individual. The bulimic may present as intelligent, outgoing, physically attractive, and successful. If she has made the initial telephone call and is seen individually, she may strongly resist having the family involved. There may be a history of hiding the eating-disordered behavior from the family members and friends; in fact, the clinician may be the first and only person she has ever talked to about it. Hiding the behavior maintains the perfect veneer of the family. Common phrases heard during an initial interview include, "I feel like I'm living a lie," and "I'm living a double life."

The bulimia often began after a period of dieting or at the end of a relationship in which the bulimic was rejected. She may have attributed the failure of that relationship to shortcomings in her appearance. By the time a professional has been contacted, the bulimic has tried to end the bulimia by willpower (following family messages to solve problems on her own), reading self-help books, and promises of "never again." She feels frustrated and embarrassed that she cannot stop. The inability to stop on her own is used as evidence of a character flaw.

Like the bulimic individual, the parents "put on a happy face," even when faced with the fact that their daughter has an eating disorder. There is reinforcement for the very behavior that is a part of the bulimia — smiling when in pain, looking happy when distressed. Often members of this family type have "smiling depressions," a signal of the inability to resolve conflict in a realistic manner. Disappointment is just below the surface of the smile.

The family is concerned with finding "the perfect therapist" to help their daughter recover perfectly. The family sets up expectations so that the individual learns to hide her behavior extra carefully or tells the family that she has recovered when she has not. For example, there can be an expectation that the bulimic will constantly be making progress in therapy.

There is an intense family loyalty, to the exclusion of others, including the therapist. Emptiness and hollowness are salient features in this family. One client described her experience in her family by saying that it felt like they were all plastic robots. The perfect family becomes the perfect client in therapy — willing to come in when asked, reading books on bulimia, appearing concerned but not intrusive about the behavior. They overtly appear pleasant and cooperative. Joining with this family may appear to be easy on the surface, but the therapist may find that it is difficult to feel connected with family members. Members are resistant to the betrayal of perfection.

## ISSUES IN THE PERFECT FAMILY

### Boundaries

While the relationships in the perfect family have the overt appearance of clear boundaries, these boundaries often are rigid and impermeable. Yet there is enmeshment among all family members (most often mother and daughter), along with intense family loyalty that keeps family secrets and pain hidden. The enmeshment around feelings and behavior is evidenced as one family member completes a sentence for another or cries the tears of a third member. The pervasive explicit and implicit rules leave little room for differences. Often the parents are unable to detach and let their children learn from mistakes and life experiences.

### Identity and Self-image

Families expecting perfection can foster an unrealistic self-criticalness, as well as a search to do things "right" by the perceptions of others instead of one's own perceptions and feelings. The definition of self is based on externals (the scale, grades) and thus is subject to constant upheaval. Much energy is put into knowing the "right" answer, expression or opinion expected by the family, which leads the individual to be uncertain about how she really does feel. Repeated failure to control the bulimic behavior further contributes to a lack of self-esteem and a feeling of personal failure and disappointment.

Individuals from the perfect family lack a sense of identity apart from the family. The definition of self comes from what they achieve, their appearance, and the reactions of others. There is a "hurriedness" in these individuals, even when they are achieving. They are like a cup with a hole in the bottom — there is never enough to keep it full. The bulimic individual is exquisitely sensitive to the feelings of others toward her and constantly changes in order to please others.

## Expression of Feelings

Members of the perfect family are encouraged to see the positives in problem situations or to look for the silver lining in the clouds, making it difficult for them to express discouragement, depression, or unhappiness. Tears of happiness are okay to share, but tears of sadness are unacceptable. Smiling depression, as well as "empty happiness," is common. The therapist may see family members crying and smiling at the same time or a mother talking pleasantly about how difficult it has been for her to have a child with an eating disorder. Caring and love are expressed in this family, but with the underlying message that they are conditional upon appropriate behavior as defined by the family.

## Powerlessness

Power is distributed unevenly in the perfect family, with the men in the family holding most of the real power. Decision-making is supported as long as the correct decision is made in the eyes of the parents. This leads to a feeling of incompetency and indecisiveness in the bulimic member, who is afraid to make a wrong move. The family operates quickly and efficiently to give each member feedback on decisions — there is no mistake in the way that actions are viewed. This rigid feedback loop leads to submissiveness, passivity, and a lack of assertiveness. What appears to be autonomy is actually a pseudo-autonomy, since all actions require approval from others. This is often reflected in the relationships that the children in perfect families get into after leaving home.

*Grief and Loss*

There are often unresolved issues of grief and loss in the perfect family. There are usually rigid rules surrounding the appropriate time and manner of grieving for a loss, whether it is the loss of a parent or a sibling or a miscarriage. There are no other models for how to deal with loss or any indication that different members may grieve in different ways. The time and manner of grief are prescribed and all family members are expected to follow. Often, if there has been a loss, it may appear that the parents have handled it well, informing the children of what was happening and helping friends and others through the loss. This does not demonstrate resolution of the loss; rather, it is a reflection of the messages to give to others and not to express the pain and hurt experienced. The losses leave an emptiness and hollowness in the family, although this is not immediately evident to outsiders.

## FAMILY MESSAGES

Messages given in the perfect family stress appearances, positive feelings at the expense of not recognizing or dealing with emotions seen as negative, family unity, achievement, and overconcern for the feelings of others. Some of the messages are:

- United we stand, divided we fall.
- Don't rock the boat.
- What will people think?
- If you can't show a happy face, don't show your face at all.
- Listen quietly.
- Hear no evil, speak no evil, see no evil.
- A job worth doing is worth doing well.
- Be the best you can be.
- Make us proud of you.
- Be a good girl (boy).
- Think of others first.
- I am what I do.
- Don't hurt anyone's feelings.
- You have never caused us any problems (don't let us down now).
- She/he is not good enough for you.
- You are the perfect daughter (son).
- You can tell a man (woman) by her clothes.
- Go for what you really want.

The messages given, both overtly and covertly, can feel confusing to the children in the family because of the explicit injunctions to achieve and, at the same time, not hurt anyone's feelings. There is little emphasis on or recognition of internal qualities or attributes, and self is defined by who one marries or what one does or achieves. Messages can be incomplete. It is often the implied ending to the messages to which the symptomatic member responds.

## A PERSPECTIVE ON THE PERFECT FAMILY

The perfect family often looks "perfect" to outsiders. Upon closer inspection, it is a family in which there is an incredible number of very rigid rules and messages dictating behavior. Members must follow the rules in order to be included in the family. Inclusion comes at a high price.

This family type is characterized by special or high achievement by practically all family members. This can include achieving in work, sports, school, and/or appearance. However, not all members of this family type are professionals with advanced degrees, nor are members of the perfect family all doctors or white collar workers: The achievement is measured against family ideals and values. Thus, graduation from high school and getting a job in an area that the family values can be considered achieving in some perfect families. The essence of perfection rests in the rigidity of the rules and pressure to act, feel, achieve, and think right. Often, there is only one right way.

The family reputation is all-important; shame and failure for one family member are shame and failure for all. "What will other people think?" and variations on that theme are refrains in the perfect family. The dismay experienced upon learning that one of the children has developed an eating disorder may, in great part, be dismay at the thought of other people finding out about it and thinking less of the family. Often these other people, whose judgment is so important, are members of the family of origin. The parents can feel that somehow they have failed as parents in their own parents' eyes. There is a strong move to have the individual recover quickly and perfectly, while the problem is hidden from others (even other family members).

Because the family reputation is all-important, the development of an individual identity apart from the family identity is discouraged, especially when the individual identity conflicts with the norms or values set by the family rules. If a family member insists on being different, this insistence can lead to an almost matter-of-fact rejection by the family. Approval and acceptance by others are of utmost importance. Because the development of an individual identity is discouraged, there is a lack of a sense of self, leading to a feeling of hollowness and emptiness in the client. Family members often report feeling wounded by the actions of others in the family. The symptomatic member in this family is often the one who has the most options to do things differently from the other family members. But instead of encouraging this behavior, the family rigidly expects that, with the experience of the other siblings before her, she will be the one "to do it right."

Appearance is of paramount importance in the perfect family. The symptom threatens this veneer. "How could this be happening to us?" and feelings of embarrassment are often expressed to the bulimic member and to the therapist, creating a demand for a quick and happy cure. Parents are often overinvolved in the appearance of their children, commenting on or setting up rules concerning weight, hair, dress, and makeup. One patient commented,

> My dad used to have "inspections" before I was allowed to go out on a date. I'd have to get ready and then come downstairs and then he would tell me that I'd have to wear something different, or change my hair before I could go. I'd end up looking like what he wanted. Then I'd sneak upstairs and change before I went out.

Clearly, not all families that fit the description of the perfect family have a member who develops bulimia. We contend that it is this emphasis on appearance that is a major factor in the development of the symptom of bulimia, rather than a different symptom such as asthma. Bingeing and purging can be a way to look perfect, conform to family rules, and to rebel at the same time.

### Rules

The perfect family clearly depicts the discrepancy between overt and covert communication described in Chapter 4. For example, affection is expressed overtly, but covertly there are conditions. The rigid rules are more of the same. There are many overt and covert rules that members must follow in order to belong in the family. One rule is that family members are expected to behave in an age-appropriate manner. Leaving home, at least giving the appearance of separating, is done at the age-appropriate time. Dating, marriage, career choice and childbearing are also surrounded by strict rules about timing, leaving little room for individual development or difference.

Disturbing family rules creates an immediate demand by the family to restore harmony. If someone breaks the rules and refuses to conform under family pressure, he or she may be thrown out of the family in a quiet way (not speaking or visiting).

*Prior Anorexia*

In the perfect family, in contrast to overprotective and the chaotic families, there is often a history of anorexia in the bulimic individual. Usually she has "recovered" from the anorexia on her own or with a few sessions with a professional. The approval that she receives from this perfect recovery may further strengthen her desire not to let anyone in the family know about her bulimia, fearing disappointment. Because of the leverage that the family exerts on members to conform (use of silent treatment, overt rejection from the family), bulimia can be a silent rebellion during adolescence.

There are few obvious signs of chaos in this family type. There are few divorces; in fact, the parents may appear to have the perfect relationship. While there may be alcohol abuse, often in the father, it usually takes the form of "drinking to relax" after work and does not interfere with his on-the-job functioning. It can be hard to assess problems in the perfect family, since it is against the family rules to disclose weaknesses. However, the perfect family will most often tell the truth when questioned directly.

*Birth Order*

It is often the youngest daughter in the perfect family who develops bulimia. This is the last opportunity that the parents have to turn out the perfect child. Often viewed as "the good child," she may be expected to make up for the past imperfections in other siblings. Parents, when faced with the bulimia, may say, "I can't believe it, especially with this child—she has always been so good."

Females are more vulnerable than males in this family type to developing bulimia. This is due not only to societal expectations and pressures (supported by the family), but also to the struggle to balance confusing sex-role expectations. It is difficult for her to integrate behaving as a traditional female, especially in relationships, and achieving in school, sports, or a career. Bulimia can be both a reflection and a resolution of these contradictory expectations.

*Age of Onset*

Bulimia usually surfaces in late adolescence in the perfect family member. If the onset of the eating disorder is earlier, it is usually anorexia rather than bulimia. As demands by peers and in relationships to make decisions and to behave in ways counter to family rules increase, it becomes more difficult for the individual to balance family expectations and her feelings and desires. Bulimia can be a way to rebel and still appear perfect. Especially if the family reacted negatively to the earlier anorectic behavior by cutting off the individual, bulimia may be a way to continue the eating disorder secretly and still gain family approval. Given these factors, bulimia may surface as someone is just about ready to leave home or soon after leaving.

## FAMILY-OF-ORIGIN ISSUES

There is little history of psychological disturbances in the perfect family. However, one or both of the parents may be from a more distressed family, and their current behavior may reflect a flight from family-of-origin chaos. If there is a previous history of anorexia, and the bulimia has existed for several years, it is likely that the patterns of relationships and interactions are multigenerational.

There may also be a history of high academic or work achievement by one or both parents. The mother, due to the power imbalance in the parental relationship and the pressures from society, may have given up her achievement outside the home and channeled her energy into being the perfect mother. (The perfect mother has perfect children.) Part of being the perfect spouse may have meant having children and staying at home with them even if this was counter to her desires. In order to reinforce her decision, she may expect this same type of behavior from her daughters. As a result, the daughter may get a mixed message: Achieve outside the home, but not too much. Additionally, covert jealousy and competition may be experienced by her mother. The daughter may strive to be more like her father. She can join with him in academic or career achievement, and with her mother in traditionally female roles.

Looking at unresolved grief and loss and family disappointments can provide clues to the pressures on family members. One of the parents may have been the "disappointment" in her or his family, or older siblings of the bulimic may have disappointed the parents. Parental energies may be redoubled and redirected to the youngest, reinforced by a determination not to have her make the same mistakes as her siblings. Going to the right school, engaging in the right career (which is often a family business), or marrying the right man is of paramount importance. The individual's wishes are ignored if they are different from the wishes of the family. Her sense of self is not fostered when it is secondary to family expectations.

## THE FAMILY LIFE-CYCLE

If the parents in the perfect family have come from perfect families themselves, there were probably many expectations around finding the "right" partner and having children at the "right" time. As parents of young children, they placed many expectations on their children in terms of appearance and behavior. They may describe the bulimic individual as having been "the perfect baby" (although her behavior may simply have been a reflection of additional parenting skills learned through experience).

There are externally directed expectations regarding the expression of feelings, ways of reacting, and weight maintenance. This preoccupation with getting the child to feel and behave in the "right way" is a reflection of the lack of clear boundaries between parents and child. The parents' needs, not the child's, are being met. Belonging is contingent upon behavior, although autonomy is stressed. There is a lack of flexibility which goes with too many expectations. The inflexibility of rules and expectations make negotiating adolescence a difficult task, which is often not completed.

Anger is not allowed, and if it is expressed the person is told that it isn't reasonable to be angry or she is cut off (either emotionally or physically). Thus, this family gets stuck in the developmental task of adjusting to the adolescence of children.

Parental relationships on the surface appear stable and strong. However, underneath the appearance of an equal, strong relationship, there is a power imbalance, with the husband and males in the family holding the power. The last child to leave home will leave emptiness and discord between the parents or anger in the mother which is directed towards her husband.

In the perfect family, the eating disorder usually occurs at the beginning of adolescence, as the budding child is beginning the developmental task of separating and individuating from the family. While the actual physical launching from home does not appear to be delayed, since this would appear less than perfect, psychological launching is incomplete. If the child does psychologically separate and leave home, this forces the parents to rely on each other for meaning in their relationship. At this point depresssion is often seen in the mother, as she struggles to give her life meaning as her children need her less.

## THE FUNCTIONS OF THE BULIMIC BEHAVIOR

Bulimia in the perfect family serves a number of important functions, including rebellion, control, development of an individual identity, expression and suppression of feelings, and balancing traditional and nontraditional family expectations.

### The Perfect Rebellion

Bulimia can be one way that the individual can be less than perfect in a family that demands perfection in order to belong. It allows the bulimic to appear perfect (conforming to family rules) while covertly rebelling. The bulimic behavior can bring tremendous satisfaction in secretly breaking the rules (bingeing) and can also bring panic and the desire to belong (purging). The bulimia is often hidden from family — to share it would risk exclusion or "messing up" the perfect family.

### Individuation

One's identity in the perfect family is dictated by the family identity or defined by the company the individual keeps. Bulimia may become part of the individual's sense of self that is different from the family, thus making the bulimia very difficult to give up until she develops an identity that is separate from the family *and* from the bulimia.

### Anger

Both bingeing and purging can be ways to indirectly express the anger that is unacceptable in the perfect family. From an early age, the bulimic member may have repeatedly heard the message, "Of course you don't *really* feel that way," when she or a sibling expressed anger. Soon she learned to suppress angry feelings and later to not even recognize her anger. Bingeing and purging can serve to stuff angry feelings as well as to throw them up.

### Letting Go

The perfect family demonstrates extraordinary control over behavior and feelings. Bulimia provides a way to momentarily let go without anyone's knowing it. After the bulimia is discovered, parents may be aghast at the bulimic's lack of control.

### External vs. Internal Development

There is a lack of balance between external development, e.g., appearance and achievement, and internal development, e.g., fulfillment and emotional development. Bulimia is a natural response to this emphasis on externals and a way to attempt filling the internal emptiness.

### Reconciliation of Traditional Behavior and Nontraditional Expectations

In our society, females are expected to get to the top and at the same time to "be a lady about it." We know from classic studies (Broverman et al., 1970) that characteristics expected from women are not consistent with images of success. Bulimia, with the contradictory behaviors of bingeing and purging, is a way to act out against the system (bingeing) and then to conform to family and societal expectations (purging).

### Coping With Feelings

Most emotions in the perfect family carry a label of either "good" or "bad." Especially as one moves into adolescence and the development of relationships, many of the feelings that have been labeled "bad" are natural to experience. However, recognition and expression of pain, sadness, anger, guilt, and frustration (among others) are not allowed. Bulimia becomes a way to stuff down the feelings, to anesthesize oneself to feeling. Focusing on food directs attention away from feelings.

## THE HOWARDS: A PERFECT FAMILY

### Initial Contact

April, a 28-year-old woman married for two years, was bingeing and purging an average of seven times per day when her sister, Diane, who had heard of our group therapy program, referred her for an intake interview. She completed the time-limited group and was referred to one of the authors for ongoing therapy. Initially, April denied that her bulimia reflected anything other than her own approach-avoidance to food and spoke about her family members in a restrained fashion, casually commenting about their various accomplishments. She was beginning to have some discomfort about her role with her mother, who, she said, acted sometimes as a younger sister, but then she minimized the problem. By the end of group therapy, she was more aware of her family's dynamics but had not yet begun to establish control over her symptoms. In fact, she described the symptoms as worse.

She presented in a very poised, somewhat aloof manner, stating that her purpose was to "gather more information." She was college educated and verbally facile. She was currently working as a specialty chef and aspired to a serious art career. When informed that her husband was integral to future therapy, she initially stated that he would certainly avail himself if necessary, but she could not see how he was connected to the "problem," since she had been developing an eating disorder for the past 10 years.

### Family History

The genogram in Figure 2 identifies the primary players in this family's three-generational drama.

April is the older of two children born to a locally well-known and finan-

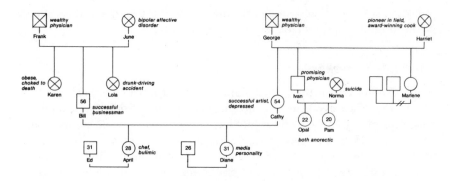

*Figure 2.* The Howard Family

cially successful businessman (Bill) and his wife (Cathy), who is a quite successful, regionally well-known artist. Her parents married after obtaining their college degrees, and she was born three years later. April's younger sister, Diane, is a locally well-known media personality. This pattern of success is replicated in many of the family members. Despite April's minimization of her accomplishments, she also is successful in her profession, as is her husband, Ed, a local businessman. Frank, the paternal grandfather, was a wealthy physician and landowner, as was George, the maternal grandfather. Harriet, the maternal grandmother, was one of the first women in her career at the time she graduated from college in the early 1920s, and her son, Ivan, April's uncle, is a prominent physician in another state. When Harriet gave up her career, she became an award-winning cook.

The remaining women in the Howard family were generally another story. June, April's maternal grandmother, had a long history of bipolar affective disorder and died in a psychiatric facility. Karen, April's father's sister, was morbidly obese, lived with her parents, and choked to death on food in her early thirties. Lola, his other sister, had initial success in business but was killed in a car accident that was a result of her driving while intoxicated. Marlene, April's mother's sister, was "anorectic-like" even currently, and Norma, Ivan's wife, committed suicide following a long history of depression. Ivan and Norma had two daughters, Opal and Pam, both with a history of anorexia, with Pam continuing to be symptomatic. This clearly suggested multigenerational patterning regarding eating disorders and being successful among the women in this family.

Bill was prematurely launched from his family due to his mother's illness, but distinguished himself early, being decorated in WWII. April was actually named after him, but she remembers that it was her mother to whom she felt closest. In fact, their closeness was clearly overinvolvement, as April was her mother's closest confidant. This was facilitated by Bill's working very long hours, including considerable extended travel. Cathy reported in a conjoint session that "April could pick up my every emotion, no matter how hard I tried to cover it. She is so much like me in that way — she feels everything so deeply and doubts herself continually." Diane was the child in the family who showed some adolescent rebellion, but both daughters were clearly successful when April entered therapy for bulimia. She had developed anorexia at 17, was hospitalized briefly at 19, and then stabilized her weight with bulimia, purging up to seven times per day when she began therapy at 28.

Several multigenerational themes seem to be operating in the Howard family. For example, each generation had its share of emotional cut-offs. Bill had nothing to do with his mother after leaving home and had never been able to get close to his father. The depth of this loss was reflected in his becoming tearful in an extended family session when discussing his parents. Cathy was unable to speak to her father, George, without extreme anxiety and had a conflicted relationship with her mother, Harriet, and her sister, Marlene. April and Diane were highly competitive, and although they were publicly civil, they distrusted each other and rarely spoke. In fact, Diane's method of informing April of the group was to send her a news clipping anonymously. April never felt heard by her father, Bill, yet displayed a level of hypersensitivity to her mother's feelings, even from a long distance, that was extremely eerie. Yet there was none of the delayed launching or overt inadequacy in this family that marks overprotective families with similar levels of enmeshment. Each of the four Howards and the two sons-in-law were proficient and successful.

A second theme pertains to food and physical appearance. The perfect veneer did not mask the operation of several processes germane to the development of a bulimic system. Food issues were evident with Harriet's cooking proficiency, which was handed down to April via many extended lessons with her grandmother. Karen's obesity and death by choking were graphic signs of the perils of overindulgence. As early as she could remember, April reported that her father insisted that his wife and daughters drink skim milk, while he got to drink whole milk. Physical appearance was extremely important, with all of the Howards being very athletic and extremely weight conscious. When the family got together on rare occasions, conversation revolved around everybody's latest running times.

Intimacy was not evident. Although Bill and Cathy had a "perfect" marriage and April initially reported that they never fought, April's parents' marriage was characterized by Bill's dominance and self-centeredness. He clearly seemed to view his wife primarily as someone who reflected his achievements. April had married Ed, a man who could not talk about his feelings, and Diane's relationship with her husband was characterized by numerous, mutual affairs. In contrast to the overprotective family, the members of the Howard family were generally reserved and aloof. Individuals went for months without contact, despite their living in the same town. The over-closeness of April and her mother seemed unusual given the other family relationships.

Depression was very prevalent in this family and reflective of the emotional cut-offs across several generations. Bill admitted to being petrified, first of April's anorexia and later of her bulimia. He was aware of April's bulimia but would never discuss this with her and worried outloud to his wife that April would meet the same fate as his mother, June. Cathy was also depressed and had been in therapy for several years. Her fears of her father were related to his tyrannical style with her and her mother, which was reflected partially by Bill in her current marriage. She had never felt heard by George, and after Harriet died she visited him only when family functions were scheduled and only with April. When George entered a nursing home, Cathy did not visit him once, although April did visit occasionally and then reported to Cathy what he had said.

## Systemic Functions of the Bulimia

An early therapy issue was April's emotional vulnerability to Bill and Cathy. She felt only partly whole when away from Cathy and felt personally violated by Bill whenever she was with him. She resented both of these positions but felt that she had to respond to her mother's every wish for support. This brought her into contact with her father. When these contacts occurred with both of them, April felt depleted and invaded simultaneously. She felt that her bulimia reduced her vulnerability to her parents, enabling her to be viewed as different and hence separate. She was removed from the parenting with her mother, and her mother would respond with greater solicitousness when April was overtly distressed. When the symptoms reduced in frequency and intensity, April was panicky about what excuse she now had not to "take care" of her mother.

Bulimia was also a vehicle for the expression of anger. As she began to separate from both of her parents, April's increasing competence forced her into a new position with her husband. Initially, April's increased assertiveness was met with avoidance by her husband, who in some ways was a younger version of Bill. Rather than confront him directly, April would purge and become depressed.

In sum, the perfect family is characterized by the overt appearance of appropriate coping responses. However, underneath the appearance of perfection, there are rigid expectations concerning achievement and appearance in order to be a part of the family. The family identity and reputation are of paramount importance; the development of the identity of the individual is allowed only if it fits with family expectations. Behaving in ways other than expected brings immediate demands to restore harmony. Bulimia reflects the individual's attempt to individuate, release "unacceptable feelings," and maintain the perfect veneer of this family.

# CHAPTER 9

# *The Overprotective Family*

*"All for one, and one for all."*

THE OVERPROTECTIVE FAMILY is similar to the bulimic families described in the treatment literature. They most closely parallel Minuchin's (1974) observations of psychosomatic families which are enmeshed and overprotective, lack conflict resolution skills, and involve children in marital conflict. In addition to these markers, the hallmarks of the overprotective family are the lack of confidence in the symptomatic member's competence, the lack of rules for age-appropriate behavior in the family, and the impact of unresolved family-of-origin issues, which are often related to victimization experiences in the mother.

## THE OVERPROTECTIVE FAMILY INITIATES THERAPY

Mother: I am calling to make an appointment for my daughter. She needs to see someone right away. She's throwing up her food and she could die. We're so worried.
Therapist: How old is your daughter?
Mother: 20 years old.
Therapist: Why are you calling, rather than your daughter?
Mother: (Pause, as though she doesn't understand the question) Because I'm her mother.

In this family type, the person most enmeshed with the symptomatic member (usually the mother) makes the initial telephone call to request therapy. She is extremely concerned with her daughter's behavior, asks many questions about the causes, treatment and prognosis, and usually wants to make the appointment for her daughter. She may say, when asked how she found out about the bulimia, that she "just knew." She may be eager to be involved in the therapy or express a wish to meet the professional. She may also have made a number of different contacts with professionals, searching for just the "right one." As the therapist listens, she may be surprised upon finding out the client's age; often, from the parental description, the bulimic individual sounds much younger than she actually is.

Some of the phrases that the therapist is likely to hear include:

- "How could this be happening to us?"
- "I just knew something was wrong — but I couldn't talk about it."
- "She's too scared to call so I told her I would do it."
- "I've been so depressed ever since I found out about it."
- "This is hurting us all so much."

When the family comes for the first therapy appointment, the parents or siblings may help the bulimic fill out the necessary forms or fill them out for her. The bulimic individual often looks and acts younger than her age.

One or both of the parents may be in their "element" in the discovery of the bulimia. The fact that their child has a problem and needs their support may energize them out of a depression and into action, as the bulimic child provides them with a reason to act married (hence Palazzoli's term, "three-way matrimony").

The parent(s) may also be able to describe the symptom in great detail. For example,

It seems like a lot of times the bingeing starts in the early afternoon, especially if there are potato chips or other certain foods around. I know when she is doing it and I've tried to get her to stop. I can hear her when she's in the bathroom running the shower and trying to throw up. I am worried because it seems to take her so long and I don't know what she's doing to her body.

## ISSUES IN THE OVERPROTECTIVE FAMILY

### Boundaries

Attention to boundary issues is particularly important because the bulimic symptoms function to establish boundaries in this family. Separateness is difficult to achieve in the overprotective family because of the enmeshment, particularly between mother and daughter and husband and wife. Hallmarks of the lack of boundaries include parents' talking in terms of "we" when speaking about their daughter, a description of "mental telepathy" between mother and daughter, or one family member's crying for another. Either or both parents will talk for the daughter when she is perfectly capable of speaking for herself. Parents will speak of their daughter's emotions or experiences as if they were their own. There is an intrusive quality to interactions between family members, with members exchanging clothes without asking, reading each other's mail, etc.

Therapist: Jill, how old are you?
(Jill starts to answer but is interrupted.)
Mother: 17
Therapist: How long have you considered your bulimia a problem?
(Jill looks at her mother.)
Mother: Three years
Therapist: Hmm. Jill, is your mother always so helpful?
Jill: Mom just cares a lot and tries to help. I know that my bulimia hurts her.
(Mother's face starts to turn pink and tears well up in her eyes. Jill starts
        to cry.)

Often the overprotection of the child has come out of unresolved experiences of one of the parents. The mother may try to live her life through the daughter and thus vicariously experience what she missed when she was growing up. One client described her feelings:

> When I was in high school, my mother pushed me to try out for the cheerleading team. I don't think that I was really very interested, but it seemed so important to her. She would practice the cheers with me every day after school. I think that she was more disappointed than I was when I did not make the team.

### Identity

The lack of boundaries in the overprotective family inhibits the development of individual identities of the family members. Since family members are permeable to the feelings of other members, separateness is difficult to achieve. The individual is unable to describe who she is in terms other than weight and appearance and words her parents have used to describe her.

### Autonomy

The smothering of the youngest child by the parents leads to a lack of autonomous functioning on her part. Decision-making is usually done for the child; thus, she is not allowed to develop skills needed in this area to function independently from her parents. Actions that lead to separation are discouraged, and family members are given conflicting messages about achievment and independence.

## Expressions of Feelings

Feelings of sadness and anger are not allowed expression in the overprotective family. Because of the lack of separateness in family members, "negative" or painful emotions are viewed as hurting the entire family. Family members have little experience with successful resolution of conflict and avoid it. Love and affection are freely expressed and are age-inappropriate and smothering. Conflict is rarely effectively resolved and members often report feeling guilty about creating conflict or expressing feelings other than love and affection.

## Grief and Loss

Unresolved issues of grief and loss are a salient feature of the overprotective family. If the parents have divorced, the child may take on parental depression, sadness, or loneliness. If one of the children in the family has died or if the mother has had miscarriages (events often seen in these families), the surviving child may become the focus of parental love and overprotection.

## FAMILY MESSAGES

Listed below are some of the messages that are given in the overprotective family. Their themes include the importance of cohesiveness, a lack of trust of anyone outside the family, and the idea that the parents know what is best for their children.

- All for one, one for all.
- No one is good enough for my daughter/son.
- You know we will always be there for you, no matter what you do.
- There's no place like home.
- He's only after your . . . (body, money, etc.).
- Don't hurt anyone's feelings.
- What am I going to do when you are gone?
- Find a nice man to take care of you.
- You can't trust anyone outside of the family.
- No one will treat you the way we do.
- The boogie man will get you if you don't watch out.

These messages are confusing and contradictory. For instance, the message to "find a nice man to take care of you" conflicts with the message, "no one is good enough for you," and, "no one outside the family is to be trusted."

## A PERSPECTIVE ON THE OVERPROTECTIVE FAMILY

The overprotective family is marked by its lack of recognition and encouragement of their child's competence and need for independence, especially as she reaches the teen years. This family overtly provides a very safe, secure environment during the early years of growing up because of the parents' sensitivity to their children's needs. However, this sensitivity becomes smothering and age-incongruent in the teen and young adult years, when less involvement is appropriate. It becomes clear that this family has a difficult time allowing children, in particular the youngest child, to grow up or leave home.

There is a lack of opportunity for children to make decisions, as the parents make these in "the best interests" of the children. This makes it difficult for the child to leave home successfully when the time comes because the parents' sheltering and protection have robbed the child of the necessary opportunities to take risks and make choices. There has been little trial-and-error learning and the world is painted as a scary place.

The overprotective family is cohesive by guilt ("It hurts me to hear you say that . . . "). A good child is one who doesn't hurt one's parents (or who protects her parents from anger, disappointment, etc.). Families are described by others as caring, sensitive, and considerate. Members of this family type often report feeling smothered by love and affection; food is often the symbol of affection. Anger is viewed as a hurtful emotion so that, instead of being expressed directly, it is often expressed in passive-aggressive actions or statements. Consequently, it is difficult for the adolescent to be rebellious. Her rebellion is bound to result in a parent's becoming depressed.

## FAMILY-OF-ORIGIN ISSUES

Unresolved multigenerational issues that surface in the overprotective family include: a reaction to victimization experiences of the mother during her childhood; parental difficulty leaving home; unresolved relationships in the parents' family of origin; parents' being faced with being a couple again; and lack of individuation of the family members.

If the mother was molested or abused as a child, she may feel the need to guard her children closely. Often the molestation has not been addressed; in fact, it may be disclosed for the first time in the family therapy. As Mrs. M. shares:

> I was determined that nothing would happen to Kathy like what happened to me. When I was six or seven, my father first started it. He would come into my room at night, to make sure that I was okay, or so he said. He gave me backrubs to get to sleep, although I remember that they weren't the kind of backrubs he or my mother gave me at other times. He kept on going . . . and I was scared to death. Even now, I have trouble going to sleep without a light on or the door open. I have made sure that no one has ever bothered Kathy like that.

The "protection" that this mother gave to her daughter was protection for both of them. In making sure that her daughter was not molested, she did not allow her to experience her growing-up years independently. The daughter had difficulty in having close relationships with men, including her father and brothers.

Another issue that often surfaces in this family type is one or both parents' difficulty in leaving home. In one family, the parents had spent their first four years after being married living with the wife's parents. They had two of their children before having a chance to live on their own as a couple. Consequently, the couple had little chance to create its own family identity. Although they since had moved to a town about 30 miles away from her parents, they visited weekly and were unable, until the entire extended family came to therapy, to separate. With no adult models for leaving home, the children in this family had no idea how to leave home in an effective manner.

Parents are faced with the task of becoming a couple again after the children leave. If they were not able to accomplish this task before the children were born, or if the parents have centered their relationship around their children, this task will be difficult. The grandparents in this system may not have yet established a couple relationship and may still be overinvolved in the lives of their grown children or wedded to a parent in the previous generation. And so the pattern is repeated in the next generation.

If these issues are not resolved, the person with the eating disorder is likely to choose a partner with a similar lack of individuation who continues the overprotection. The partner reinforces the lack of competence and decision-making skills. Thus, the eating disorder continues to be supported even after the individual leaves home.

## THE FAMILY-LIFE CYCLE

As discussed above, often the bulimia begins when the individual is making decisions to leave home. Carol vividly describes her experience:

> Everything seemed to be fine as I grew up. Mom and I have always been close — she was always there for me when I needed her. But it seems like things

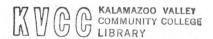

started to change when I became a teenager. My body was changing and I
was beginning to look more like a woman and my mom just freaked out. She
had some friends that had a kid that was rebellious — drinking and staying out
all night. She was determined that this was not going to happen in her family and kept a tight rein on everything I did. My friends were too wild or not
good enough for me. I had to tell her everything I did, everyone I talked to,
and every move I made. I went away to school for one year — it was the best
year of my life.

    Then my parents decided that they couldn't afford college anymore and
wanted me to come home and attend junior college. I remember that time
feeling in sort of a fog. I decided that if I moved back home, I would never
be able to leave. I decided to drop out of school and get a job so that I could
afford my own apartment.

    At first, my mother pleaded with me to move home. When I said no, she
said that I was on my own. "You've made your bed and now you have to lie
in it." If anything happened, she said I had to take care of it on my own. I
felt so cut off and scared. But there was a part of me that knew, for my own
survival, that I couldn't go back home. But I moved back to the same town
and got my own apartment. The bulimia was terrible. I spent every spare
minute bingeing and throwing up. I felt like I had lost my best friend.

Carol was able to make a physical break from her parents, although she
did move back to the same town. Emotional launching of the young adult
did not occur. Leaving home became an intense struggle for survival and
the penalty was emotional cut-off.

As children leave home, the task of the parents is to allow them to leave
and to readjust to being a couple again. When the marital relationship is
poor, the child may feel herself pulled to stay home. The bulimia becomes
an issue around which the marital pair can be involved. It can also become
a weapon for blame between parents and thus keep them involved with each
other.

### Birth Order

In this family type, it is most often the youngest daughter who develops
the symptom of bulimia, for several different reasons. In Western cultures,
females are often viewed as being weak and dependent. This socialization
process begins very early and both overt and covert messages are transmitted
by the peers and the family, as in Jill's experience:

    When I was in eighth grade, I decided that I wanted to be on the track
team in junior high. I did really well — I could even beat some of the boys my
age. Then my friends started to tease me, saying that I was getting muscles
and that boys didn't want a girlfriend who could beat them up. I stopped running as well as I had been and eventually dropped the team.

Until adolescence the youngest female in the family is usually the weakest and smallest. She is also the last child to leave home. It is likely that other siblings have also had difficulty leaving home. If they have moved out, often this has been accomplished only after a major blow-up, which gave them the emotional distance to leave. The youngest has been left with the "wreckage" and has seen the depression and sadness in the parents after her sibling(s) has left. As Kay explains:

> My older sister moved out about two years ago. She had been dating some-one my parents didn't like and my father had given her an ultimatum: "Either stop seeing Mark, or you can't live here anymore." She went behind their back, but she was pretty daring about it — almost as though she wanted them to find out. My dad caught them making out in Mark's car and threw her out. My mother cried for days. She said that I was the only reason she was able to go on . . .

### Age of Onset

In the overprotective family, the bulimic behavior usually begins as the child is starting the process of leaving home. Struggles around independence and autonomy, often centered on food and weight, may begin when she reaches the teenage years. The bulimia may either begin or worsen significantly as decisions to attend college or move out into her own apartment are made.

## FUNCTIONS OF THE BULIMIC BEHAVIOR

Bulimia, in the overprotective family, enables the bulimic individual to stay young and dependent; at the same time, it is a way to passively rebel and create personal space. The eating disorder supports the parents' worry that their daughter needs their protection and can be used against the daughter as evidence that she is not ready to leave home. Further, it is a way to shut down feelings that are unacceptable in the family.

### Creation of Personal Space/Boundaries

"The bathroom has the only door in our house that it is okay to have shut." Bulimia is a way to create boundaries where there are none. The enmeshment in the family relationships, particularly between mother and daughter, can feel suffocating and overwhelming to the bulimic individual. Bulimia can be a way to individuate and to distance between the bulimic individual and other family members.

### Expression of Anger

Bulimia becomes a way to express anger in an indirect manner and to passively rebel. Unless the dysfunctional pattern of communication is changed,
the symptom of bulimia is one of the few ways in which the individual is
able to express her frustration and anger.

### Involvement of the Marital Pair

The father in the overprotective family is often the scapegoat and the child
may feel guilty about leaving her mother all alone. Often, the parents have
stayed together "for the sake of the children"; when the time comes for the
children to leave, the spouses find that they have little in common. Late
divorces are often seen in this family type, which can add to the guilt of the
children in leaving their parents. Bulimia becomes an issue around which
the marital pair can stay involved. As Kari shares:

> My parents hardly talk to each other anymore. They have probably com-
> municated more with each other since they found out about my bulimia. They
> try not to leave me alone at home since they are afraid that I'll binge. I think
> they take turns watching me—eating, going to the bathroom, or when I am
> just sitting around.

### Homeostatic Function Around Leaving Home

Bulimia can be used as evidence that "the child" is not yet ready to leave
home and be on her own in a world that is scary and dangerous. The family works together in a familiar way—parents reinforcing the family messages
and the child bingeing and purging—with the result that the daughter
becomes less and less able to leave home.

### Shutting Down Feelings

Many feelings, especially those of anger, sadness, rebelliousness, and independence, are not acceptable in the overprotective family. Since these feelings are a natural and reasonable response to situations that one encounters
in life, the individual must find a way to either express them or not feel them.
Bingeing becomes a way to stuff down unacceptable feelings and purging
can be the result of the inability to keep herself totally shut down.

Bulimia can be a mask for other problems in the family, such as depression, parental ineffectiveness, alcohol or prescription drug abuse in a parent.
Thus, the bulimia serves many important functions in the overprotective
family; these must be addressed before the individual is able to recover.

## THE HOLMES: AN OVERPROTECTIVE FAMILY

### Initial Contact

Lisa, age 19, was a freshman at the state university, living in a sorority. Her mother, Valerie, age 50, called one of the authors who was working at the university counseling center to request therapy for her daughter's bulimia. Valerie had been called by two of Lisa's friends, who were concerned about Lisa's bulimic behavior. They told her that they had tried to talk to Lisa about it, but she refused to acknowledge it, saying that she was sick to her stomach because of the flu, not because she was trying to lose weight.

Valerie sounded panicked and scared about her daughter's behavior and had made a number of telephone calls in order to find "the right person to treat my daughter." When told that her daughter would need to call to request an appointment, she replied that Lisa was too upset to call and that she refused to acknowledge that anything was wrong.

Lisa did call several days later, after going home and being confronted by her mother, who demanded that she call, saying that her behavior was hurting the entire family and harming the reputation of the sorority. The mother dialed the telephone for Lisa and stood by while she talked. After I talked with Lisa, Valerie asked to speak to me and asked whether I felt that Lisa should leave the sorority and come back home to live until "her eating problem cleared up." I advised the mother not to have Lisa immediately move home, and encouraged her to attend family therapy if this were indicated.

An initial consultation and assessment were conducted with Lisa individually since only students were seen at the student counseling center. There were several signals during the initial telephone contact that this was an overprotective family: the mother's making the initial contact although her daughter was not living at home; the mother's speaking for her daughter on the telephone; the remarks about hurting the entire family; the mother's anxious suggestion that Lisa move home immediately; the bulimia beginning at the time of leaving home; and the mother's report that Lisa's boyfriend, of whom she did not approve, was the cause of her bulimia.

Lisa, while smiling throughout the consultation, was clearly angry at being "forced" into the appointment. She did not feel that she had a problem, saying that she only vomited in order to lose a few pounds and that she could stop at any time. Her weight was within normal limits, although she was about 10 pounds over her ideal body weight. In the consultation, I provided some information about bulimia, referred her to a physician due to the physical symptoms she reported, and suggested that she test her statement that she could stop at any time by setting some limits to her bingeing and purging. I offered some predictions about the behavior if she was unable to control it and did not seek treatment. She clearly was not ready for therapy, but did see a physician. It was suggested that the family seek consultation with Lisa involved, which she resisted.

The next contact with the Holmes was approximately one year later, when Valerie called again to request therapy for Lisa. She had quit school and returned home to live the same month that her older sister had gotten married and moved out of state. Valerie had been faithfully attending a local support group for family members of people with eating disorders, although Lisa and the rest of the family refused to participate. At the time of the second call, Lisa had lost 17 pounds and Valerie expressed concern about her physical state. Lisa was still reluctant to be in treatment, but was willing to do so since her mother had set that as a condition for her living at home. At this point, the entire family was seen.

*Family History*

Lisa's father, Joe, 51, and Valerie met in grade school in a small town where their families knew each other well. They dated throughout high school and college and married one year after finishing school. Valerie lived with her parents, as did Joe, until they were married. They waited for five years to have children, until their financial situation was stable. Cari, the oldest girl, was described as the perfect baby and Valerie reported that she put a great deal of energy into being a good mother. She constantly called her mother to check when Cari had a cold or fever and to see if her mother felt that she should take her to a doctor. Three years later, Lisa was born. The parents reported that she was a fussy baby and that she was more difficult to get close to than Cari. Four years later, to their delight, John was born. Valerie said that she had hoped for "a boy for Joe since I had the two girls." The early years of the family were described as very happy and secure, with many family activities and outings.

When Lisa was 15, her sister graduated from high school and went to college several hours away from home. Her launching was extremely difficult for Valerie, who felt close to Cari. Lisa described seeing a drastic change in her mother when Cari left. Valerie had been actively involved in the PTA, volunteer work, attending the children's activities — which ceased when Cari left home. That summer Valerie was diagnosed with a heart problem and "took to her bed" per doctor's orders. Cari came home often to check on her mother, and Lisa negotiated adolescence by alternating between staying at home with her mother and acting-out by staying out late and seeing friends whom her mother disliked. Joe threw himself into his job and detached more from his daughters and wife, spending more time with John, fishing and playing sports.

Food issues were salient for all members of the Holmes family. Valerie began to gain weight at the time of Cari's leaving home, which greatly disturbed Lisa. Joe reported that he frequently binged and had "spells" when he threw up chunks of foods which he had not chewed enough, John was on a weight gain program for his sports activities, and Cari was dieting frequently.

## Family of Origin

The genogram in Figure 3 illustrates the characters in this family. Valerie, the younger of two daughters, described her older sister Lillian as bossy and parental towards her. Her relationship with her mother was extremely close. She was not close to her father, who died of a heart attack when Valerie was 40, with his obesity being a contributing factor to the stress on his heart. He "didn't know what to do with two girls," as Valerie described it. There was no history of alcohol abuse or psychological disturbances.

Joe was the youngest of three boys in his family and grew up on a farm that "was my dad's life." His oldest brother married and moved out of state; the middle brother had a long history of alcohol abuse. His mother also had alcohol problems as well as depression. When his parents lost their farm due

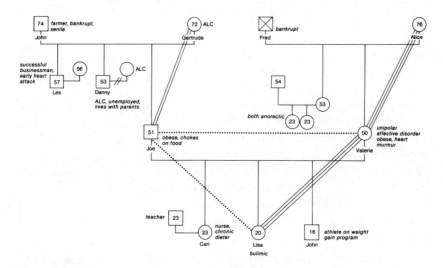

*Figure 3.* The Holmes Family

to financial setbacks, they blamed Joe for the loss, since he had not stayed on the farm to work. Joe's alcoholic brother Danny was the child favored by his mother, and at age 53 he still lives at home with his parents, who support his alcoholism by giving him money. They even provided him with a car after his was wrecked and he was cited for drunk driving. Joe felt guilty about not being a good son, a theme constantly reinforced by his mother. He said that he did not know how to relate to his daughters since he had no sisters, using almost the same words that Valerie had used to describe her father.

Cari and Lisa reenacted the relationship between Valerie and Lillian to the point that they were given the nicknames Val (Lisa) and Lil (Cari). The fusion of Valerie and Lil and Valerie's lack of individuation from her mother were repeated in Lisa's difficulty separating from her family. The scapegoating of Joe in his family was repeated by his being scapegoated for his lack of involvement with Valerie and his daughters.

### The Function of the Bulimia

The parents blamed Lisa's boyfriend for her bulimia, saying that his rejection of her and the abusiveness of the relationship were the sole factors in Lisa's development of her bulimia. Lisa's understanding of her bulimia centered around her desire to be thin to attract a boyfriend and to get attention from her father. It was clear from the consultation with the family that part of the function of the bulimia was to create personal space and to construct boundaries between Lisa and her mother, who was very intrusive (reading her mail, balancing her checkbook, reading her diary, intercepting her telephone calls). It was also a way to stay young and remain home. Leaving home would mean the abandonment of her mother, who would no longer have a friend and confidant. Lisa described her mother as her closest friend and worried that her mother would no longer have a reason to get dressed or to get out of bed in the morning if Lisa left.

Her bulimia served to energize the system, to increase her father's involvement, and to keep her mother from being depressed. The bulimia kept Lisa from feeling and expressing her anger, and from getting into positive relationships with men (who are never there for you, anyway, according to the beliefs of the women in the family). It also served to keep her parents from dealing with their marital relationship, as Joe's alcoholic brother's behavior had done in his family.

### Goals of Therapy

The initial goal of therapy was to decrease Valerie's involvement in Lisa's symptoms and to help the parents work together as a unit. Constructing appropriate boundaries between Valerie and Lisa and decreasing the distance between Joe and Lisa were major goals throughout the therapy. As the parents began to work together more, family-of-origin issues were brought into focus as they related to the scapegoating of Joe and the wedding of Valerie to her mother. Finally, the marital issues were addressed through couples therapy, with Lisa being seen individually and in a group in order to strengthen the separation and work on relationships with men. The couple was taught to shut their door, to take vacations together without the children, and to cope with depression. The therapy took many forms over the two years of treatment: family therapy, group and individual therapy for Lisa, education, and couples therapy for Joe and Valerie.

The overprotective family is easily identified by the markers of age-inappropriate overprotection of family members, particularly the females. This can be due to a flight from the chaos in one of the parent's family of origin, reflecting multigenerational issues. Bulimia becomes a way to balance distance and fusion of members of the family; it can create momentary boundaries against the intrusiveness of others. Both the case presentation of the Holmes family here and the description of the treatment of the Longs in Chapter 19 illustrate the enmeshment, overprotection, and lack of age-appropriate rules for the symptomatic member.

# CHAPTER 10

# *The Chaotic Family*

*"The only one you can really count on is yourself."*

WHILE MANY THEORISTS and researchers have described eating-disordered families similar to the perfect family and the overprotective family (Bruch, 1978; Minuchin et al., 1978; Schwartz et al., 1984), the chaotic family type frequently observed in bulimia has not been described in the literature on eating disorders. Instead, chaotic families, not often seen as the context for anorexia nervosa, resemble substance-abusing families as described by Stanton and Todd (1982). The experiences of children growing up in alcoholic families are similar to those of bulimics from chaotic families: They learn not to talk, trust, or feel (Black, 1981).

While enmeshment and lack of conflict resolution skills exist in the chaotic family, as in the other two family types, many of the markers and signs of this family's patterns are distinct from the overprotective and the perfect family. For example, while the perfect and overprotective family types are hallmarked by their rigid rules, the chaotic family is hallmarked by the inconsistency of its rules. Other hallmarks of the chaotic family type are: unavailability of one or both parents, victimization experiences of the family member (or members), frequent expression of anger, and substance abuse.

## THE CHAOTIC FAMILY INITIATES THERAPY

Client: (Timidly) I wanted to get some information.
Therapist: Is this for yourself?
Client: (Pause) Yes. (Pause) If I'm bothering you I can call back at a better time.

112

Therapist: I have time now. What kind of information are you looking for?

Client: (Hesitantly) Well, I don't know for sure. You see, I started getting rid of my food when I'd eat and I lost a lot of weight and my parents got suspicious that I was doing something bad because I was eating a lot. And then my best friend told my mom what I was doing. She told my dad and now they're really disgusted with me. They're not talking to me. They told me I had to stop, but I can't. So that's what I want help with.

Therapist: (Wondering whether she wants help with her eating or her parents) You've probably tried to stop by yourself. One could feel pretty stuck with such pressure. How old are you?

Client: Fifteen.

It is not unusual for the bulimic individual in the chaotic family to make the initial therapy contact. The contact is usually made in the midst of a crisis or immediately after a crisis. The precociousness and resourcefulness of these clients become evident early on; often they have persistently searched for help, even after initially coming up with little information. Contact may also be made with the professional by a family friend who recognizes her distress, by in-laws, or by the parents. When the parents make the contact for therapy, their motivations may vary widely. For example, it may be that they have decided to be "a parent for the day" (as one client expressed it), or that they are in crisis, or that they wish to relinquish total responsibility to the therapist.

Despite their resourcefulness and persistence, clients or families may make a number of contacts before actually making an appointment. There is also a greater probability than with other bulimic families that they will not show up at a scheduled appointment. These difficulties arise because of the individual's fear of being disloyal to her family, fear of asking for family resources to go towards her treatment, or difficulty believing anyone can help the situation. Also, it may be that the crisis which precipitated the phone call has abated.

Few others in the bulimic's environment are aware of the eating-disordered behavior. This can be due to the individual's not wanting to burden parents further when there are already many problems in the family. More typically, the behavior is obvious but the parents are so exhausted physically or emotionally that the behavior is ignored, unless it becomes very extreme or additional symptoms become apparent in the bulimic, such as suicide gestures. The emotional unavailability of parents for their child is characteristic of the chaotic family. This pattern of unavailability leads many clients to question the usefulness of family therapy. They are more used to "doing it on their own."

Often, there are few financial resources available in the chaotic family. Perhaps this is why these clients and their families are more likely to be seen in community mental health centers or other public agencies. The facts that these families do not fit the common stereotype of the "perfect family" from which the person with the eating disorder develops, that they tend to leave treatment prematurely, and that they are seen in public agencies (with little money designated for research) may explain why chaotic families have not been described in the literature on eating disorders.

## ISSUES IN THE CHAOTIC FAMILY

The chaotic family is a multiproblem family. The issues are not difficult to see, as this family type is less able (perhaps because of less emotional energy) to consistently cover up dysfunctional patterns. The salient issues associated with the chaotic family include: lack of boundaries, difficulty individuating, pseudo-autonomy, powerlessness, uncontrolled expression of anger, depression, inability to express love and affection, and unresolved grief and loss.

### Boundaries

Boundaries alternate between being too permeable or impermeable. Individuals seldom experience a healthy balance between these two for any extended period of time.

The lack of well developed and appropriate boundaries in the bulimic individual signals a lack of emotional boundaries with one of the parents (usually the mother). A lack of boundaries is also attributed to experiences of physical victimization. Repeated boundary violations by family members' physical and emotional intrusiveness neglect the individual's need for privacy. These intrusions further contribute to the individual's sense of powerlessness over herself or the environment.

The development of impermeable boundaries serves to ward off attacks, intrusion, and invasion, which are frequently part of the bulimic's developmental experience through physical victimization, psychological abuse or intimidation. Her experiences contribute to a style of protecting herself from further intrusion or abuse by hypervigilance, avoidance of relationships, or dissocation. (Nash and Baker (1984) have identified an increased degree of dissociation in individuals who have been physically or sexually abused.) These experiences and ways of relating result in an individual who can be perceived as superficially appropriate, but who forms intimate, trusting relations very slowly.

Boundaries between the parents' subsystem and the children's subsystem are also often lacking. Enmeshment seems to be facilitated between certain family members as a result of their shared victimization experiences. The enmeshment most typically occurs between mother and daughter; they subsequently form an ambivalent alliance against the father. Often the bulimic has served in a parental role and fluidly shifts back and forth between being part of the children's subsystem and part of the parents' subsystem. This experience contributes to a feeling of "not belonging." These experiences further compromise the extent of emotional connection the bulimic develops in other relationships. She is practicing an approach-avoidance relational system, which will contribute to her difficulty establishing relationships outside of the family.

## Identity

When you consider the rapidly fluctuating alliances and inconsistent relational patterns, it makes sense that there is considerable difficulty in developing either a family identity or an individual identity within the chaotic family. The development of a self-identity is impaired because of a failure in the "holding environment" parents can provide (Kegan, 1982). This connection with parents is essential to the development of a sense of belonging, integration, and its converse, differentiation.

The bulimic and other family members may go to great lengths to obtain a pseudo-identity that hides the pervasive family dysfunction and individual confusion. This identity, however, is poorly developed, easily threatened, and easily lost. The bulimic's personality, opinions, and feelings may change as often as the clothes she wears.

## Autonomy

Autonomy — or, rather, pseudo-autonomy — is thrust upon the individual when she is very young. For example, a six-year-old may be cooking breakfast for her younger brother and sisters; an 11-year-old may be given custody of her drunken father as the police put them in a taxicab because no one else is available; or a 15-year-old is kicked out of her mother's home to find somewhere else to live because she does not get along with her mother's current boyfriend. In all of these examples (which are not unusual for chaotic families), the child is unprepared for the responsibility, but feels that she has little choice. Once again, the child experiences powerlessness while surviving by focusing on her pseudo-autonomy.

The precociousness required of this child creates confusion. Not only is she unsure of her personal limits but she also has few effective models for functioning in an autonomous manner. It is here that compulsivity gets established as an initially adaptive mechanism to cope with the anxiety generated by her required autonomy. She may attempt to establish rituals and to adhere to implicit or explicit rules in order to give herself guidelines within which to function. Food rituals may emerge, particularly if the family has a pattern of problems related to food.

### Powerlessness

A major issue in the chaotic family is the lack of power and control felt by family members. This seems paradoxical when one considers the precocious emergence of autonomy. However, the victimization experienced by family members can lead to a feeling of resignation and lack of perceived control over self, destiny, and the environment. Unfortunately, but predictably, the bulimic individual frequently gets into relationships which reinforce familiar feelings of powerlessness and victimization. The intrusion and powerlessness experienced provide further motivation for the individual to develop compulsive behaviors and routines in order to numb these feelings or to feel a sense of pseudo-mastery over her environment. This allows her to feel a superficial sense of control of the world through compulsivity around food. Often, the bulimia emerges as a means towards establishing power. Crystal, a 24-year-old client, heard her mother criticize bulimics, and began to try this behavior, although secretly. Her mother came into therapy with her, and responded to Crystal's disclosure of her bulimia with, "You always had to do something to get me going."

### Expression of Feelings

The three major feelings that are unexpressed or expressed inappropriately in this family type are anger, love, and sadness. *Anger* is pervasive, explosive, and unpredictable. Angry feelings can be conveyed in eruptions of violence or denied and stifled. The explosiveness of anger may be related to rules about expressing anger which require members to stifle it. When people reach their limit they explode. Alcohol can also contribute to the explosiveness and unpredictability of the way in which anger is handled. Alternatively, anger may be stifled because of family rules to provide a "civilized appearance" or because of fear that "once it starts it will never stop."

*Love and affection* are shown inconsistently and conditionally. Unlike the perfect and the overprotective families, the chaotic family has conditions for love and approval that change for reasons that are not always apparent or reasonable, especially to small children. There are few ways of behaving that one can count on to get affection and approval. The individual can be running on empty for a long time.

*Sadness* is seldom differentiated from depression. It goes unrecognized and, if expressed, is shown as depression. It is not surprising that there is so much substance abuse and depression in chaotic families. The substance abuse often numbs the depression. The sadness and depression that are apparent serve many generations. Because anger, love, and sadness are seldom expressed effectively in this family type, bulimic behavior can become a way to feel and then not feel these feelings.

### Grief and Loss

The chaotic family has usually sustained many losses, including: separation, multiple divorces, severe illness, unavailability of parents, suicide, molestation, depression, death, and abuse. The depression and sadness inherent in the losses are feelings to avoid — family rules make sure of this. For example, grieving or depression may be labeled a sign of weakness. Grieving is not facilitated or accepted in family members, so that new losses remind them of past unresolved losses. Because of the pervasive enmeshment of family members, the bulimic may go to great lengths to hide her grief and depression, so as not to bring these feelings up for other members. People in the family may be cut off with little warning, creating additional losses, which again are unresolved. Therapy in the chaotic family needs to address these losses and to facilitate the grieving process.

### FAMILY MESSAGES

Messages in the chaotic family carry themes of emotional cut-offs, disengagement, mistrust, coercion, and isolation. Common messages include:

- Don't ask questions.
- You can't trust anyone.
- Spare the rod, spoil the child.
- Every person for herself/himself.
- Don't do as I do; do as you are told.
- Children should be seen and not heard.
- The only person you can count on is yourself.
- I wouldn't yell at you if I didn't love you.
- When the going gets tough, the tough get going.
- You're asking for it if you upset your father/mother.

These messages contribute to the patterns of cut-off in the chaotic family. For example, the messages, "Children should be seen and not heard," "The only person you can count on is yourself," and "You can't trust anyone," support the detachment and isolation of family members. The messages in the chaotic family also tend to be inconsistent, and consequently, confusing. For example, "Don't do as I do; do as I say," leaves children without a role model or punished at times for following the role model their parent supplies. "I wouldn't yell at you if I didn't love you," can contribute to difficult relationships. The intensity of conflict in the family can become family members' measure of association and connectedness. Because parents may not have the capacity for love or attachment their children need, the children may settle for the intensity of their anger, as this may be the emotion that allows them the most connection to their parent.

## PERSPECTIVE ON THE CHAOTIC FAMILY

The chaotic bulimic family appears similar to centrifugal (Stierlin, 1973) or addictive (Elkin, 1984; Stanton & Todd, 1982) families described elsewhere in the family therapy literature. A cardinal feature is the lack of consistent rules and organization. Rules in this family type change constantly and are enforced inconsistently. Role and status changes among the members are frequent. Because of the lack of rules and organization, there are few guidelines or models for effective decision-making. Consequently, long-range planning and financial stability are not that common.

The expression of emotions is also unpredictable. Family members are not certain who is available to them for emotional support and help. Indeed, parents may be emotionally and/or physically unavailable for the children. Depression, suicide, divorce, physical illness, and/or alcohol and drug abuse are commonly observed in the parents of chaotic family. The expression of love and positive feelings is unpredictable. Children grow up feeling unsure of their worth and lacking trust in relationships.

There is a paucity of appropriate models for conflict resolution. Resolution can be forced and take on the essence of "pseudo-resolution," as physical force and/or psychological intimidation are used to resolve conflict. This is unfortunate, because there is a tremendous amount of anger, which is often expressed inappropriately, explosively, and unpredictably. The members that are powerless (usually mother and daughter who are enmeshed) express their anger passive-aggressively. Anger (emotional or physical) can be lethal in these families. Family members consequently vacillate between being hardened to the anger and walking on eggshells. Habituation and tolerance for anger also compromise the individual's judgments about physical safety. Problems tend to be resolved through inappropriate physical acting-out, use of alcohol or drugs, or withdrawal through depression.

Usually, chaotic family members become symptomatic when they have difficulty negotiating change in their life-cycle. Each stage with which they have difficulty sets them up to have further difficulty negotiating the next stage, unless they truly do learn how to make the necessary changes for vertical movement in the family life-cycle. There can be a pattern of psychological disturbances in family members, as well as a history of suicide attempts and successful suicides. Since sadness and grief are unexpressed and unrecognized, unresolved grief and loss are pervasive. The bulimic individual is unlikely to be the first symptomatic member. One of the parents is likely to have had ongoing symptoms, or parents may have taken turns being symptomatic. For example, in a 16-year-old's family, her mother's depression lifted when her father became unemployed. When he was employed again, her mother started drinking. After the mother got treatment for her alcoholism (which the 16-year-old initiated at age 14), the father sustained back injuries which kept him from going back to work.

Expectations are inconsistent and age-inappropriate. This reflects the cross-generational violations common in this family type. At times, children are treated as older and expected to behave as adults or as the parents' parents. Some of the competence the client demonstrates on initial contact is a function of this "training." At other times, they are treated much younger than their age. As Sandi shares,

> I always felt different from other kids my age. My mom drank alot and she would pass out on the couch or, some days, never got out of bed. Dad worked all the time so I could pretty much do as I wanted. But he wouldn't let me date until I was 17, even though in reality I had guys over to the house when I was 13. Mom didn't care as long as I didn't bother her.

In the chaotic family, too much autonomony is given to the young child. As Mahler and colleagues would describe it, the child is "prematurely hatched" (Mahler, Pine, & Bergman, 1975). This can lead to a reduced level of parent-child attachment and result in feelings of abandonment. This is another loss for the child to have to work through. Often the bulimic individual will speak of feeling different from her peers, reflecting the lack of belonging she experiences in the family. A common metaphor used in working with individuals with this pattern of "incomplete parenting" is "learning how to feed themselves appropriately."

## Birth Order

It is often the oldest female in the chaotic family who develops bulimia. As the oldest, she precociously gives up her childhood in order to take on the responsibility of holding the family together. This often replicates her mother's role in her family of origin. At an early age she may take on the task of cooking and cleaning or may go to work outside the home in order to help pay bills. This is similar to Elkin's (1984) description of the role of "mother's assistant," which often falls to the oldest girl in alcoholic families. Her role is that of the family organizer and smoother of conflict. She may attempt to get her mother out of an abusive relationship or to divert the abuse away from her mother or younger siblings and towards herself, feeling that she is stronger or more able to survive it. In extreme cases, the bulimic may resort to shoplifting to get food for the family or presents for others.

Her caretaking, while providing an essential, otherwise absent role in the family, simultaneously provides her with a sense of importance and specialness which is lacking. Unfortunately, because much of what she accomplishes is precociously required of her, she takes on tasks without knowing her limits. It becomes difficult for her to ask for help because she may fear sharing or giving up her special role as her mother's "savior" or father's "best girl."

### Age of Onset

In the chaotic family, the bulimic individual often develops the symptoms of bulimia at an earlier age than in the other two family types. Sometimes there is a mixed picture of previous history of anorexia or obesity, both of which may have also been attempts to establish boundaries and separateness within the family.

## FAMILY-OF-ORIGIN ISSUES

In the chaotic family, salient family-of-origin issues include: repetitive patterns of physical and sexual abuse, lack of close relationships, grief and loss, and patterns of using alcohol or drugs to deal with emotions.

There can be a pattern of molestation, battering, and abuse across several generations, which contributes to the chronic powerlessness most often experienced by women and girls in the family. Parental relationships are often abusive, either physically or emotionally. the tenuousness and instability of their relationship with each other leave them unavailable to provide adequate parenting for their children. Pregnancies can be unplanned, unwanted, or the result of sexual abuse. Pregnancy can also be a way for the mother to escape her frequently abusive, chaotic family of origin.

Relationships are marked by a lack of trust and attachment. Emotional cut-offs are common and alliances between family members change quickly, without warning. The individual is not encouraged to be close to another individual. The difficulty establishing close relationships is further compounded by the inadequate attachment and bonding between parent and child (Bowlby, 1979), either because the parent lacks this capacity or because she is unavailable. Bulimia is reflective of the disengagement of the family members and is a way to isolate the individual from close relationships.

There is almost always a history of unresolved grief and loss throughout the generations of the chaotic family. As mentioned earlier, this feature is shared in other chaotic families (Stanton & Todd, 1982). Death through violent acts, suicide, and accident is common. Yet the deceased is rarely talked about and the grief is poorly resolved. As Sherri recounts,

> Grandmother died of an overdose when I was 13. I wasn't told, although as I look back I realize that there was something funny about it. My mom didn't tell me how she died and she would cry whenever I mentioned her. I'd ask her what was wrong, but she wouldn't say anything. When I was 20 and helping my mom move, I found the death certificate, which said "death by overdose." My mom still refuses to talk about it.

A recent loss in the family inevitably reactivates earlier unresolved losses and seems to make family members even less available. Consequently, leaving home becomes a difficult task, especially for the oldest daughter, who has performed a valuable "cohesion-enhancing" role in the family. The bulimic client from the chaotic family tends to have a difficult time with therapist absences. Discussing her feelings and reactions to the therapist's vacations provides a useful avenue to addressing a history of losses.

Repeated patterns of alcohol and drug abuse are seen across the generations. Chemicals are used to cope with unresolved feelings and regulate emotional closeness and distance. The bulimic individual may have vowed never to abuse alcohol or drugs. Yet her abuse of food is similar to other family members' abuse of drugs or alcohol. One client's disclosure illustrates this point well:

> One day I had this awful realization. My mother—I promised myself I would never be like her—used to pass out from drinking and then have a hangover the next day. I go to sleep after bingeing and purging and feel like I have a "sugar hangover" the next morning.

## THE FAMILY LIFE-CYCLE

There are several places where the chaotic family fails to successfully negotiate life-cycle stages. This seems to lead to the person's developing a greater vulnerability to having an eating disorder. When individuals who have a number of problems marry, they may lack sufficient emotional stability to provide a cohesive safe environment in which to raise children. People who are at similar stages in emotional and psychological development often choose one another as mates. Thus, it is not unlikely that both parents in a chaotic family have chaotic backgrounds. The implication is that they will not be well equipped to deal with their own conflicts constructively or to parent their children.

If the person's emotional resources are exhausted, this can lead to stress, both in the marital relationship and in the establishment of family relationships. The addition of children to an already burdened, stressed relationship overwhelms the parents, who lack the flexibility to deal with this task. Often, in chaotic families there is personal boundary violation in the form of spouse abuse. This seems to foster a mother-child coalition in the newly developing family.

Because insufficient attention is given to the children, which reflects the depleted marital relationship, parent-child attachment is impaired. The child has little sense of belonging. This inhibits the development of a sense of self and an individual identity in family members. This is a poor balance of belonging and autonomy, with too much autonomy given to the children. In fact, the demonstration of autonomy or toughness may be a way for the client to receive special acknowledgment from a parent. This lack of resolution at the stage of the birth and early years of growing up leads to problems later on when it is time to differentiate.

As a young adult, the person prepares herself to invest in an independent and separate life. A secondary goal is to maintain some connectedness with the family. In the chaotic family, departures at the launching stage can be sudden and violent, which can leave the individual feeling emotionally cut off from the family. As one client describes leaving home,

> At the end of my senior year in high school, my mother announced that she was leaving my father and moving in with her boyfriend. They moved to a town about 30 miles away, to a one-bedroom apartment. I wanted to graduate from my high school and anyway there was no place for me with them. My father started to drink more and more, and would yell at me, saying I'd be a whore like my mom. I couldn't take it so I moved in with a friend and finished the last month of school, working full-time as a waitress. I haven't had a home since then.

There is no supportive home base or surety of love and caring to serve as a foundation from which to launch. The adolescent is set adrift, often abruptly, to find her own way in the world — and frequently to repeat the patterns of the chaotic family.

## FUNCTIONS OF THE BULIMIC BEHAVIOR

For the individual from the chaotic family, bulimia serves to provide the individual with the affection and nurturance lacking in the family, becomes a safe way to express anger, numbs her to her rage and pain, and is a way to get emotional distance from the intrusion of others.

## Affection and Nurturance

In the chaotic family, parents are unavailable as a source of support, caring, and love. Bulimia is a symbol and a symptom of the individual's search for this affection; at the same time it convinces her that she is unlovable because of the behavior. Bulimia may be described as "a friend who is always there when I need it." The emptiness experienced after purging is reminiscent of the emptiness of the family relationships.

## Anger

Bulimia serves as a vehicle by which the individual can express her rage and anger at an abusive family member in a secret and safe manner. It enables her to feel the anger and then to stuff the feelings back down. The cycle is reinforcing, as she feels and then stops feeling.

## Creation of Emotional Distance

The physical and emotional intrusion that is experienced in the chaotic family is reflected in the bulimic behavior. Bingeing and purging create boundaries and space for the bulimic individual.

## Self-Abuse

The bulimic behavior is a way to continue the cycle of abuse, as well as to reinforce to the individual that she is not worthy of affection and caring. The abusiveness apparent in bingeing to the point of being uncomfortable and the intense violence of the purging recreate the familiar feelings of powerlessness and abuse experienced in the family.

## Dissociation From Reality

The bulimic behavior is a way to help the individual separate herself from reality, creating a fog. Especially in families in which there is a history of physical abuse and molestation, dissociating from reality is a way for the individual to cope with those experiences.

## Relinquishing Responsibility

As the parent figure in the chaotic family, the oldest female has taken on responsibility for other siblings and her parents. She cooks, shops, baby-sits, smooths conflict, diverts anger, and cares for others. Bulimia can be a way to let go of her responsibilities for others and focus on herself. With a lack of models for taking care of oneself and no one to do so if she gives it up, bulimia is a way to let go.

*Predictability*

In a chaotic environment, one is unable to predict the behavior of others. There is no sure way to predict the mood of the parents or their availability. A parent may come out of a depression, or decide to quit drinking, and be a "parent for a day." With such constantly changing rules, quickly shifting emotions, and unstable family members, bulimia serves as one predictable behavior. It can be a stabilizing force for the individual, the only way she feels control. Rituals become important and the bulimic individual alternates between being rigidly in control and totally out of control.

*A Way to Catastrophize*

The professional treating the chaotic family may find that the bulimic behavior consistently gets worse when the family environment becomes stable. This can be an attempt to return the family to prior functioning or a way for the individual to remind herself that all is not well and that the family could erupt into chaos at any time. Clients feel apprehensive when things go smoothly, anticipating that at any moment this will change.

*A Way to Stay Young and Solicit Support*

Bulimia reflects the individual's need to stay young in the family. She often feels older and different from others her age. The eating disorder can be a way to let her family know that she is not ready to be on her own or to take on the responsibility for others.

## THE PALMERS: A CHAOTIC FAMILY

*Initial Contact*

Andrea moved to Seattle "to get away from my family." Her mother and siblings were living over 900 miles away in another state. She had obtained a job in a restaurant and was experiencing considerable difficulty with bingeing and purging. She heard of our group treatment program (described in Chapter 15) and began therapy. The group was time-limited, and since she was pleased that she had made some progress controlling her bingeing, Andrea asked for a referral to continue therapy and began to see one of the authors in therapy. At the time Andrea entered group therapy, she was completely ignorant of the functions of her bulimia and its role in her family. She felt guilty about leaving her mother and guilty over the relief she felt when not living with her. This lack of understanding at the time Andrea entered therapy accurately reflected the degree to which she remained enmeshed with her mother and was unable to "step outside" and view the family more objectively.

Her manner of presentation was as a very young teenager. She dressed as if younger than her age of 22 and maintained a smiling, happy demeanor at all times. She was also a client who was impossible to reach by telephone. For example, in trying to reach her to set up a referral for individual therapy, the therapist had to resort to a letter. Andrea later informed us that she stayed away from home most the time and kept her phone unplugged when she was there.

*Family History*

Let's turn to the genogram in Figure 4, which identifies the primary players in this family's four-generational drama. Andrea, age 22, is the youngest of five children born to an alcoholic dentist, Bob, and his wife, Carol, who was 17 at the time they got married. Andrea's oldest brother,

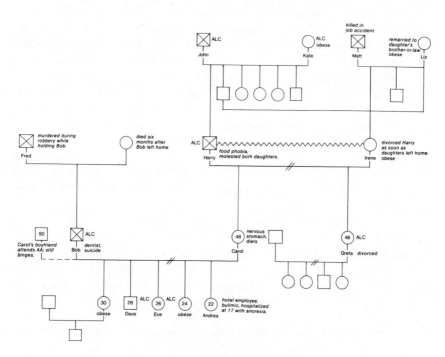

*Figure 4.* The Palmer Family

Dave, and one older sister, Eve, are alcoholic, with Dave being alcoholic since the age of 13. Bob committed suicide one year after his divorce from Carol, when Andrea was three years old. Andrea was first informed of the suicide in a family-of-origin session with her mother when she was 21.

Bob's father, Fred, was murdered during the Depression while holding Bob, then four years old, in his arms. He operated a small business and was killed during a robbery. Andrea's mother, Carol, and her younger sister, Greta, were born to Harry and Irene, who fought throughout their marriage and divorced as soon as both daughters left home. Carol described their relationship as highly and overtly conflictual, with numerous instances of physical fighting. Harry was also alcoholic and died, friendless and without family, the same year Andrea became anorectic. It is very interesting that both Harry and Carol had "food phobias" and had severely restrictive diets, and Carol reported a long history of a nervous stomach and vomiting when anxious.

Harry, Andrea's grandfather, was born to John and Kate, both of whom had alcohol problems. According to Carol, both John and Kate had run away from their own families of origin prior to age 15. Irene, Andrea's grandmother, was born to Liz and Matt. Matt died from a tragic industrial accident, and Liz promptly married her daughter's brother-in-law. This graphically illustrates the incestuous nature of the family. Carol and Greta reported being molested by Harry, their father. Liz and Irene were described as always at odds with each other, to the point of physical violence. Carol reported that she was still extremely fearful of her own mother and on occasion asked Andrea to visit Irene in her place. Andrea essentially was her mother's ambassador to Irene and kept their relationship going, bearing messages back and forth between the two.

When Bob killed himself, Carol moved to Australia with her children, even though she had no family or friends there. This reflected a long-term pattern of "running" from one's problems and the absence of any emotional support from one's family. The Palmer family remained there for the next ten years.

Several multigenerational themes seem to be operating. The first is a long history of premature departure from the family, e.g., John, Kate, Irene, Carol, Eve, Dave, Andrea, a feature common in centrifugal families. Despite this premature physical departure, at the time of therapy Dave and Eve were living with Carol, and Andrea was in daily phone contact with her mother. The second is the pervasive substance abuse, with alcoholics on both sides of Andrea's family. Two of her siblings are alcoholic, and Carol's current boyfriend attends AA, but still binges several times each year. Andrea is afraid to drink because, she reports, "I like it too much."

A third theme is problematic marital relationships, with not a single marital relationship in this family being reported as satisfactory. Carol has been divorced for 20 years and has not had any interest in remarrying, feeling that marriages are restrictive and hazardous to one's health. Andrea keeps her relationships brief and superficial, ending them when the male shows interest. Or she pursues older, unattainable men who are both alcoholic and depressed.

A fourth theme is the blurring of generational boundaries. Bob became the surrogate husband after his father, Fred, was killed. His mother died six months after Bob left home, for no apparent physical reason. Liz married the brother-in-law of her daughter, and Andrea and Carol report a relationship that is akin to being sisters, with each being remarkably tuned in to the other's emotions. Andrea does for Carol what she cannot do, visit her own mother, Irene.

The fifth theme is related to diet and weight. Kate, Liz, and Irene were described as extremely overweight. Carol and Greta were chronically on diets and two of Andrea's three sisters were considerably overweight and had been so for many years. Andrea's dieting reflected her identification with her mother.

A sixth theme has to do with violent deaths and sudden losses, none of which seemed to be resolved. Fred's death by shooting was paralleled by Bob's shooting himself, and Andrea never hearing the truth about it until much later. Matt, who was one of the few nonalcoholic males in the family, died suddenly and tragically, with Liz responding to it by almost immediately getting married. This theme has numerous implications for depression and incomplete mourning in the family. Andrea recounted numerous instances of incredible sibling fights that occurred when her mother was at work. These episodes seemed to be the flip side of the loss and incomplete mourning. In addition to yelling and screaming, physical attacks with fists and knives were not uncommon. Her brother was once rushed to the emergency room after being stabbed by Eve. Andrea said that "as soon as we heard mom pull up outside, it stopped and we pretended nothing had happened."

Andrea became anorectic in early adolescence. This persisted for several years, resulting in her hospitalization at the age of 17. She was in individual therapy for almost one year after that. She left home with a boyfriend and traveled before high school graduation, moving to the Seattle area by herself when she was 19. She began to gradually gain weight within the year, but began to use bingeing and purging as a weight control mechanism. The origins of Andrea's anorexia in early adolescence, coupled with substance abuse disorders beginning in her siblings at similar developmental periods, strongly suggests that this family had problems with moving into adolescence. Andrea prided herself on looking asexual and boyish and was unable to pronounce the words "woman" or "breasts" without stuttering until she was 20 years old. A premature and false launching occurred when Andrea "left home" with a boyfriend prior to completing high school. The presence of a boyfriend would imply sexual development, but Andrea was actually almost asexual and described herself as "sworn off of men," with all men being "jerks".

### Systemic Functions of the Bulimia

What systemic functions did the bulimia serve the Palmer family? From Andrea's perspective, bulimia was the only constant in her life. She scheduled her binges at the end of the day and felt she needed them in order to "stop racing." She also began to recognize that she would binge/purge in response to stress at work or tension with men she was dating. Her eating disorder, along with alcoholism in two of three other siblings, effectively interrupted the movement of this family into a new life-cycle phase, launching. This "nondevelopment" effectively staved off, for several years, the loss of Andrea to the family. She was regularly begged by one or another family member to move home. Yet she felt that if she moved home, her symptoms would worsen and it would only enable Eve or Dave to "get out." In a family whose history was replete with tragic, unresolved loss, further loss was avoided at considerable cost. The initial dieting reflected an overidentification with the mother, as did the later adoption of purging. When Andrea entered therapy, all siblings, except her oldest sister, were either living with their mother or checking in with her on the phone. Andrea gradually became aware of how much her mom "needed" her children when Carol commented, "I don't know what I would do without all of you to worry about."

Goals established for Andrea's therapy involved dealing with family-of-origin issues, as well as controlling the bulimia. In addition, despite Andrea's premature introduction to heterosexual relationships, she was extremely avoidant of males and found the prospect of a semi-committed relationship panic-arousing. Andrea began to learn how the bulimia served as a "boundary" for her in relationships and also provided a chance for sameness and stability, in sharp contrast to the chaos she experienced in her family.

The chaotic family is identified by the unavailabilty of one or both parents, the victimization experiences of the family members, the chaotic organization and rules, and the inappropriate and often violent expression of anger. Bulimia becomes a response of the individual to the chaos and abuse. The clinician working with individuals and families of this type must be willing to address these issues, as will be illustrated in Chapter 20, a case example of the treatment of a chaotic family.

# PART IV

# THE TREATMENT OF BULIMIA

# CHAPTER 11

# *Assessment*

A CAREFUL ASSESSMENT allows the therapist to tailor treatment to the client. This chapter is intended to help the clinician with assessment by pointing out important areas of inquiry, organizing data, and facilitating innovative and integrative thinking. It is divided into two broad sections. In tune with our systemic focus, the first covers family assessment. The second is concerned with individual assessment of the bulimic client (within a family focus). We provide a framework which the therapist can use to generate hypotheses about the individual and the family and to determine who should be involved and when. We also introduce the Bulimia and Related Eating Disorders Screen, an instrument that can be utilized to obtain important clinical information. Important questions to attend to during the assessment include: What are the family patterns and how are those related to treatment consideration? Who should be involved? What is the client and family's readiness for therapy? Are there medical issues that also demand treatment?

## FAMILY ASSESSMENT

Nichols (1984) recently wrote that family therapists pay too little attention to assessment. He states that all too often therapists display a tendency to treat all families the same. This seems to be particularly true of therapists with powerful techniques but limited conceptual schemes.

Our assessment of numerous bulimic families has made us aware of their heterogeneity and prompted increasing flexibility in our treatment approach. Consequently, we believe that families should be assessed in the same systematic way that individual clients are assessed. In fact, we would rather know the interpersonal world of the client than any other single variable. Ob-

taining a sense of this necessitates assessing significant relationships, boundaries, the family's rules, hierarchical structure, and flexibility and motivation for change. What we do in this section is describe our approach to
assessment — what we look for and how we do this — specifically with bulimic
families.

First, however, we would like to provide a brief sketch of what it is that
different theoretical schools of family therapy propose that therapists assess.
The various schools of family therapy differ widely in their emphasis on
assessment and in the methods used to make assessments. The school's theoretical formulations about family functioning guide where their adherents
look for problems and what they see. "Some look at the whole family (structural, Bowenian); some look at individuals and dyads (psychoanalytic, experiential); and some focus narrowly on sequences that maintain symptoms
(strategic, behavioral)" (Nichols, 1984, p. 555).

Our theoretical perspectives subsume the structural, strategic, and Bowen
schools, and we will briefly discuss the assessment process of each. Structural family therapists observe family members interacting among themselves, frequently directing families in an enactment of an interaction. Patterns of enmeshment and disengagement, central themes in the bulimic's
family, are observed. For example, if the therapist enacts a discussion between the parents who are then frequently interrupted by the child, the
assumption is that the parents are disengaged and the child is enmeshed.
This would suggest directing energies into strengthening the boundary between parents and child and enhancing parental involvement. Naturalisti-
cally, the family also exhibits structures, oftentimes with regards to who sits
where and who speaks to whom. This naturally occurring data also direct
the therapist's course. For example, the structural family therapist would
expect to see indicators of enmeshment in bulimic families, e.g., mother
speaks for daughter.

Strategic family therapists may begin by asking about the presenting
symptom and then listen to determine how the family maintains the problem through attempts at solutions. The family's current stuckness is seen as
the direct result of "solutions that have become the problem" (Watzlawick,
Weakland, & Fisch, 1974). For example, the adolescent's increasing efforts
at autonomy, when viewed by the family as pathological, may activate
"solutions" of restrictions and limit-setting, which lead to further autonomy-
reducing behavior and an increasingly rigid view of the adolescent as de-
viant and in need of help. Strategic therapists will also use directives and
reframings early in their contact with the family; the family's response will
provide information about the relative compliance of the family.

Bowen therapists are devoted history-takers and are very interested in
both the past and the present. Bowen therapists assess the presence of emo-

tional cut-offs from the extended family system and the subsequent level of family member differentiation that invites triangulation. Frequently, three-generational genograms, recording important figures and dates, are developed to provide a panoramic view of the entire family and its individual members. The genograms presented throughout this book reflect our interest in and appreciation of the influence of multigenerational issues in the development of bulimia.

## Specific Family Assessment Techniques

Our discussion here is limited to clinical observations. Although we use questionnaires as part of our ongoing research, e.g., Family Environment Scale (Moos & Moos, 1981), those are not discussed, since we are focusing on bulimic-specific family issues. Our method of family assessment combines direct questioning with observation of family patterns; we also use assignments and enactments as more active assessment techniques.

## Boundaries

The range of possibilities includes rigidly impermeable to highly permeable boundaries. Family data that illuminate the nature of boundaries emerge at the first contact. If the mother is there in part because, "I was reading her diary and I know I am not supposed to, but a mother has certain rights," that is certainly a very overt indicator of permeable mother-daughter boundaries, as are facts about co-dieting and wearing each other's clothes. Family members' interrupting and speaking for other family members are other indicators of permeability. Directly asking the family how the current distress is being manifested may bring to light the fact that the identified patient has been sleeping with the mother lately — a further indicator of boundaries that are too permeable. A history of incest documents a particularly toxic boundary permeability that has long-term implications for family and individual treatment.

While boundaries in bulimic families are often too permeable, the opposite extreme also occurs. For example, fathers who are difficult to enlist in therapy or who sit in the chair furthermost from the rest of the family members are probably emotionally outside the family. Difficulty in having access to a parent can constitute impermeability. Such is the case where a mother becomes ill whenever her daughter starts to move emotionally closer to her father. This effectively cuts off the promise of a second relationship that could titrate the intensity of the mother-daughter relationship.

However, these quite obvious indicators are most frequently seen in overprotective families or between dyads in chaotic families. Evidence of enmeshment in perfect families is more subtle. For example, a woman from a perfect family whose parents were medical professionals reported, "The only decision I ever made that was different from my family's expectations was not becoming a doctor." During several extended family interviews, few overt signs of boundary violation were evidenced, i.e., no interruptions or speaking for each other. Instead, statements of respect for each other's feelings were observed. Yet this was a family where the daughter reported feeling "sucked dry" whenever she was with her mother or "violated" when with her father. The clearest indicators of these problems came via enactment, when father and daughter recreated a discussion several months' previous, in which the daughter was informing her father of her decision to leave graduate school. After several attempts at creating the enactment, what was clear was markedly increased anxiety in both mother and daughter and a seemingly total inability of the father to hear what his daughter was saying. He clearly had expectations of her that were very rigid. However, this was difficult to see in the family until the enactment.

A particularly useful method of assessing boundaries in the family is to determine who knows what about the bulimic symptoms. In early sessions, it is important to elicit the family members' perceptions of the symptoms. Entirely different pictures emerge from a family where the mother is intimately familiar with every episode, versus a family where the daughter only is bulimic when at her mother's house (and this fact is studiously avoided by the mother), versus a family where no one is aware of the symptom. What this would suggest about the first family is that extreme enmeshment characterizes the mother-daughter relationship — it is overt and in some ways a more straightforward treatment issue, because overt symptoms of this sort are more amenable to interventions, e.g., reframings, symptom prescription, and boundary clarification by restricting the intrusion.

The second family's pattern of awareness — daughter bulimic only at her mother's house and mother "unaware" — is suggestive of a conflicted, estranged mother-daughter relationship, and in this case role reversal, where the daughter was a "parental figure" to her mother and was much more closely aligned with the father. The mother defended her lack of awareness of her daughter's symptoms with the statement, "I have always worked hard to instill a sense of personal authority and privacy for each of my children. She knows that she can come to me with her concerns, but she is older now and needs to make the moves. I made the moves when she was younger." This type of rejoinder is difficult to argue with, since it is exactly what we like to see parents able to say. The naive therapist might accept the mother's words at face value, but we chose to have the mother and daughter enact a scene where the daughter was informing her mother about her bulimia and asking her mother for some concrete manifestations of support. The intensity that was created in this simple exercise pulled in the father, who began to yell at his wife; his tirade ended only when the identified patient burst into tears.

In the final family, where everyone reported ignorance about the symptoms, the emotional cut-offs among family members were very clear. This last family was quite chaotic in style, whereas the first was more overprotective in nature and the second was primarily a perfect family.

Chaotic families can be illusory with regards to no boundaries. The increased incidence of various types of aggression and abuse would certainly suggest boundary problems, but the lack of consistent, ongoing relationships implies a "you live your life, I live mine" attitude. However, consider Andrea, described in Chapter 10, who, despite the geographic distance, routinely found herself "counseling" her mother over the phone and then bingeing and purging after each telephone call. She described the experience as "being four years old again." Minuchin (1974) has stated that all families at the extremes of engagement/disengagement leave their offspring ill-prepared for emotionally successful adulthood. Bulimic families occupy these extremes; careful assessment allows for tailoring interventions that interrupt the sequences or alter the structures of the family.

Questions that we ask families to illuminate boundaries include the following:

- What do you know about your sister/daughter's symptoms?
- Who do you talk to about this?
- Who would it be hardest to talk to?
- What have you tried to do to help your daughter/sister?
- Do you think your father and mother talk to each other about this?
- What do they say to each other? Who ends the conversation first?
- What kinds of eating problems have you had?
- Who talks to whom in this family?
- Who does not talk?
- Who is most distressed by the bulimia?

### Conflict Resolution

Many bulimic families have an extremely difficult time resolving conflict, often because of poor boundaries between members. If you have the perception that everybody knows everything about you anyway, you devote little time to more overt, direct communication. Phenomena related to these boundary problems are triangulation and conflict-detouring. Most often, triangulation in bulimic families forces the daughter into the role of parent or, less frequently, scapegoat. Manifestations of a family with a parentified daughter include speaking on behalf of one of the parents in the session, protecting parents from information "that just might kill them," the presence of a parent who is a physical invalid and has been so over much of the daughter's life, a son who covers for his parents' inadequacies, and a daughter who still remains the confidant of parent and sibling alike. During one family interview, for example, it came out that the identified patient was the only other family member aware that her father had remortgaged the house and was concerned about a dark spot found during x-rays of his lungs. This particular woman did not live in the family home but was in daily phone contact with her parents, mediating their various conflicts with each other.

Enactments are an excellent way of assessing how the family resolves conflict. The ensuing information is used to activate the family towards change. An 18-year-old bulimic client, Diane, and her family, with whom she was living, came in for their second session after having been given an assignment to think about what Diane's behavior might be telling the family. Halfway through the session, the father tentatively suggested that Diane might be responding to the fact that "we sometimes get a little upset with each other." The mother demurred about this and said, "Not only can I not remember when we last argued, but I'm sure we did it out of earshot." The therapist asked the parents to talk about something they regularly disagreed about. After some preliminary assurances that each "had learned to live with it and it was no longer a problem," the two began an increasingly strained discussion about overdue house repairs. Not only did Diane become visibly distressed, but she ran from the room yelling, "Stop it! Stop it!" This enactment clearly marked the triangulation in the parental relationship and how this had prevented appropriate conflict resolution between them. This intervention, which shifted the focus from Diane's bulimia to the parents' marriage, illustrates how often assessment and intervention are complementary.

With the overprotective family, the therapist often has to be very alert for indications of problems with conflict resolution. The mother of one adult client steadfastly denied that her husband's binge drinking upset her. She stated several times, in a variety of ways, "It is something I'm used to," "At least he's a good provider," and "There's nothing I can do about it, so I just don't get involved." Since this father refused to come to the sessions, we asked the mother in the session to convince her daughter of this. This activated a sequence of behavior where the mother began to cry, the daughter comforted her, and then both minimized the tears. It underscored the fusion between the daughter and mother and demonstrated how the client "sponged up" her mother's emotional distress.

We have also found circular questioning to be a useful technique in assessing conflictual issues. This is a technique from the Milan group (Selvini Palazzoli, Boscolo, Cecchin, & Prata, 1978) that was developed with the belief that the pattern of questioning may "release" information into the system, enabling it to change on its own. Once the therapist has a hypothesis about the problem presented by the family, she may interview the family in a circular rather than a linear fashion. A common type of circular question is a "difference" question, e.g., asking about differences between relationships ("Is father closer to Diane or to Bob?"). A difference always reflects a relationship that is reciprocal and hence circular. Other examples of circular questions pertain to behavioral effects, e.g., "When does Sally usually refuse to eat?" "What does mother do when she doesn't eat?" "What does father do when mother yells?" (Tomm, 1984, p. 260). This type of questioning frequently allows for greater openness and disclosure and begins to teach the family about the systemic nature of the symptoms.

Assessing how the family deals with conflict provides valuable information about the link between bulimic episodes and lack of conflict resolution. Teresa, a 15-year-old bulimic client, began several years earlier to have more contact with her mother and stepfather, something that bitterly hurt her father, who had custody of her. This animosity, long dormant, was now more overt, and yet nobody was able to communicate about it very clearly. The parents denied discussing each other in front of her, but we know from family communications theory that nonverbal communication of affect may be even more potent. The importance of this issue was underscored when we were able to bring the parents together for a series of successful sessions and Teresa's symptoms began to diminish.

With chaotic families, conflict may appear to be much more freely expressed and the naive therapist may equate that with conflict resolution. We have found that *the expression of conflict does not necessarily equal the resolution of conflict*, and in chaotic families the expression of conflict frequently leaves the recipient feeling violated. (In fact, assessing for battering should be done routinely and specifically in these families.) The emotional distance characteristic of chaotic families does not make for resolution.

Questions we have found to be very useful in evaluating a family's ability to resolve conflict include:

- What does this family do with angry feelings?
- Who gets hurt the most when mom is angry?
- When does dad's Mr. Nice Guy image disappear?
- Who knows when you are angry?
- Does anybody get beat up in this family?

*Family Protection*

Assessing unresolved multigenerational issues can provide a variety of avenues for intervention. When we ask parents who the bulimic client most closely resembles of various family members on both maternal and paternal sides, sometimes we get responses such as, "She is her own person, she doesn't remind us of anyone," but more often than not, with persistent questioning, the family identifies an individual whose role illuminates some of the projection operating in the family. For example, a firstborn daughter may be the focus of projection because, as the first child, she is a convenient object for the parents' ambivalence about their marriage, the grandparents' displeasure in their marriage, and each parent's feelings about self, either as a female or as a male relating to a female.

Questioning of the family regarding what was happening at the time of the child's birth can identify the existence of unresolved losses, conflicts, disengagement, etc., that have affected the child's place in the family vis-à-vis her parents. Stanton and Landau-Stanton (1984) have also mentioned the importance of assessing whether the parents received "permission" to get married, as well as "permission" to have children, from their own parents. Failure to receive "permission" can severely affect the parents' marriage and relationship with the grandparents, thus creating more opportunities for emotional cut-offs from the family of origin. Another line of questioning assesses the mother's and father's expectations for this daughter and how those differ from expectations for various other children in the family. Particularly when the presenting dynamics of the family offer few intervention angles, as is sometimes the case with perfect families, assessing the family by way of family-of-origin projections opens cracks in the family's veneer.

Questions that we have found to be very useful in evaluating a family's projections include:

- Is there anybody in the family you grew up in whom your daughter reminds you of?
- What significant things were happening when this daughter was born?
- What did your parents say about your marrying your wife?
- What would they say now?
- When your daughter was born, how did you want her to be different from your son?

*Likelihood of Change*

Watzlawick et al. (1974) have provided the therapist with the very useful understanding that persistence and change need to be considered together, despite seeming to be opposite in nature. Thinking about change in this way reminds therapists that any system's expressed desire to change is counter-balanced by a similar desire to persist. Not every family that begins therapy is going to make a second-order change where the system itself changes. Some families will not even go through the motions of first-order change or change where the system itself remains the same. Yet the therapist must be able to assess whether this family will embark on a difficult task together.

If we plan to do family therapy, we need to involve the key players in the system. A first step in assessing likelihood of change is seeing whether these players are available for therapy. A client who urges you not to invite in her father "because of his heart" is giving an indication that therapy can-not proceed as necessary. On the other hand, perfect and overprotective families often readily show up, either because of their need to maintain ap-pearances or because of their sense of family unity. This is not necessarily correlated with likelihood of change, however, because these are rigid family systems that seemingly resist change.

Another useful indicator is the degree of distress or crisis that is apparent. For a family with a long history of stability, acting-out in an adolescent may be enough of a crisis to accelerate the parents into adopting new roles and permitting greater autonomy for the adolescent. That is not likely in bulimic families. Conflict and crises are detoured or absorbed at a remarkable rate, and it is necessary for the system to be in a considerable state of flux for change to occur. If the family does not seem "uncomfortable" about the symptoms, intensification of the distress must occur. For example, a fami-ly that has already seen one or two therapists for prolonged periods of time with no apparent change is definitely a family where the therapist must help to build intensity. Since life-cycle transformations activate systems, it is useful to assess the family along this dimension as well.

Some therapists speak of "probes" that essentially are tests to determine whether the family is motivated to change. These may take a variety of forms, including assignments that test for willingness to cooperate with the change process and reframing symptoms in a way that is bound to alter the family's comfort level. However, overprotective families in particular will cooperate with what the therapist asks, yet continue to be very slow to change. It is ironic, but in these situations the family therapist may be frustrated by the presence of the family. It has come to represent an over-turned pot of glue that persists in not changing. Here again, the therapist can be misled and find herself working "too hard" with a family that in many ways is not "ready" to change.

In summary, assessment should be the first step in family therapy. To know the patterns, sequences, and projections is to have a guide to how the family got stuck on its evolutionary path, what needs to happen to get it unstuck, and whether therapy has a chance of being successful at this time. Let us turn now to assessing the individual client.

## INDIVIDUAL ASSESSMENT

While the concept of individual assessment may seem alien to family therapists who insist on either seeing the entire family or seeing no one at all, we believe there are several instances in which an individual session is warranted, even if the bulimic individual is currently living at home.

There are several systems-related questions that the therapist working with bulimic families needs to consider when making a decision about whether to involve the entire family from the outset or to see the individual for an initial evaluation. Since assessment is sometimes synonymous with intervention, we might ask:

- How might an individual session help the establishment of boundaries in the family?
- Would granting an individual session facilitate joining with the family or the individual?
- Is there the possibility of abuse in the family which needs to be assessed individually?

### Establishment of Boundaries

One of the hallmarks of the bulimic families is poor boundary definition between family members and family subsystems. Individual autonomy in the perfect and overprotective family is severely inhibited, and enmeshment and invasiveness characterize family interactions. Often there is an extreme lack of privacy, a necessary component in the development of separateness and individuation. Parents may be overinvolved in the behavior and may be able to recount the number of times their daughter threw up or binged. While these issues certainly need to be addressed in the family therapy, individual sessions can be used at the beginning of therapy to provide necessary differentiation between members, to acknowledge the need for space and privacy, and to facilitate the beginning of the establishment of clearer boundaries. The risk is that the individual session will confirm the family's belief in the "special needs" of the identified patient. However, we feel that the individual session frees us to act more assertively with the family because of the "special" insights that we now have. For example, without violating confidentiality, if that has been guaranteed, the therapist may say, "I have been wondering, especially since my session with Kimberly, about . . . "

### Joining

A second reason for conducting an individual session during the initial assessment is to facilitate joining with the bulimic individual. If the client is using bulimia to establish personal space and boundaries, she may see therapy as a further invasion by the family, especially if she is forced to participate. It would be appropriate for the bulimic client to act rebellious regarding treatment. Granting an individual interview is one technique that the therapist can use to join with the resistant member, encouraging her to speak up, acknowledging her anger or reticence to proceed facilitating a therapeutic alliance. If the person is from a chaotic family, there can be a lack of trust and suspiciousness due to the history of abuse, invasiveness, and parental unavailability. The individual session can facilitate the establishment of a trusting relationship, which can help the therapist function as a change agent in the family.

In a rather curious way, individual sessions enable joining with the family. Family members see the identified patient as sick, and our affording some respect to that position goes a long way towards connecting with the dominant members of the family. The therapist does not have to fight the family on every front from the very beginning. As long as you are clear about a rationale for your decision to see someone individually, do so. However, to act without a clear rationale is to invite and encourage obstacles to treatment.

### Possibility of Abuse

Perhaps the most important reason to conduct an individual interview is to investigate victimization experiences in the bulimic's life, extrafamilial or intrafamilial. While we strongly advocate family treatment of bulimia and realize that seeing a client individually may support dysfunctional dynamics present in the family system, we feel that it is a lesser error to see the client individually if there is any suspicion of abuse than to conduct family or couples therapy with the secret hidden and not discussed. In a recent study, it was found that over 66% of 172 bulimic women had had a victimization experience (rape, molestation, and physical abuse). The therapist must be sensitive to the signs and signals that abuse may be present in the family. These signals include the family's "walking on eggshells," a history of alcohol or drug abuse, suicidal behavior, or fright at the thought of having a certain family member included in the sessions. The therapist must have sufficient experience to be able to separate resistance from signs of abuse. The assessment should begin at the first telephone contact between the individual and the therapist and can be facilitated by the use of a screening instrument such as the Bulimia and Related Eating Disorders Screen.

### Bulimia and Related Eating Disorders Screen

The Bulimia and Related Eating Disorders Screen (BREDS) (Root & Fallon, 1983b) is an instrument developed for both research and clinical assessment. We ask that clients complete this questionnaire and return it

before the initial consultation session. It can be completed in approximately 20 minutes and can be used as a semistructured clinical interview. During the session, this information is discussed, with the therapist asking for
additional information and confirming or disconfirming data.

The BREDS is divided into seven sections, which provide information on
demographics, family history, psychological and psychiatric history, eating
disorders history, current eating attitudes and behavior, habits, and medical
history (see Table 4).

DEMOGRAPHIC. This section asks for information relating to marital status,
family size, and educational level. We pay special attention to level of education and educational plans, since the client's disclosure can provide information about personal/familial beliefs about achievement, so important in
the perfect family. Information on birth order and living arrangements can
also provide useful information. We have learned that the oldest females
who are bulimic have a greater likelihood of being from chaotic families,
with youngest females signaling overprotective families with difficulty letting go. Living at home or by oneself is useful diagnostically. We find that
social isolation increases directly with the chronicity of the symptom.

FAMILY HISTORY. This section compiles information on family history in
terms of past history of eating disorders, drug and alcohol abuse, depression, and psychological disturbances. Typically in the chaotic family many
family members will have a history of disturbance in several of these areas.
Thus, one can already begin to make hypotheses about family typology and
the availability of family members for therapy. A "checkerboard" response
in this section (where numerous indicators are checked) is an indication that
an individual session should be considered to check for abuse. The presence
of a mother or other sibling with bulimia or anorexia is further evidence of
family rigidity.

PSYCHOLOGICAL AND PSYCHIATRIC HISTORY. In this section, information on
past treatment, suicide threats and attempts, and victimization experiences
is obtained. Particular attention should be paid to the section on victimization experiences. This is the most difficult section for many clients to complete and sometimes is left unchecked. Clients will report that they "missed
it" when filling out the screen. This is often a clue that there has been some
victimization experience which she may not have acknowledged or labeled
as physical abuse (e.g., date rape, sexual molestation that occurred one time
or did not involve intercourse). Even if this section is checked "no," it is important to go over the questions in the interview. Questions should be stated
in a way that allows the client to share information. "Molestation (abuse,

## TABLE 4

Name: _____ Date: _/_/_  Identification:$_{1-3}$ _____ (Card 1)
Age:$_{7,8}$ _____
Birthdate:$_{9-14}$ _____

## BULIMIA & RELATED EATING DISORDERS SCREEN

This questionnaire is a comprehensive screening tool. Please answer every question honestly. Some of the questions may not apply to you. Many questions require that you indicate the answer that best describes you most of the time. The information that you provide is strictly confidential.

## I. BACKGROUND INFORMATION

1. Marital Status:$_{15}$ __$_1$Single __$_2$Married __$_3$Divorced __$_4$Widowed

2. Number of sisters:$_{16}$ ____   Number of brothers:$_{17}$____

3. Birth order in your family:$_{18}$ __$_1$Oldest __$_2$Middle (#___) __$_3$Youngest __$_0$Only

4. Education:$_{19}$ ___$_1$Elementary School    ___$_5$Vocational or Business Certificate or Training

   ___$_2$GED    ___$_6$Four Year College Degree

   ___$_3$High School Diploma    ___$_7$Master's Degree

   ___$_4$Two Year College Degree    ___$_8$Ph.D. or Professional Degree

5. Occupation:$_{20}$ _____

6. Income per year$_{21}$(combined household if in long-term relationship):

   ___$_1$Less than $7,500    ___$_5$$20,000 to $25,000

   ___$_2$$7,500 to $12,000    ___$_6$$25,000 to $30,000

   ___$_3$$12,000 to $16,000    ___$_7$$30,000 to $40,000

   ___$_4$$16,000 to $20,000    ___$_8$Over $40,000 annually

7. Living arrangement:$_{22}$

   ___$_1$Parents    ___$_4$Alone

   ___$_2$Spouse or Partner    ___$_5$Sorority

   ___$_3$Roommate    ___$_6$Dorm

## II. FAMILY HISTORY

1. Parents' Marital Status:$_{23}$ __$_1$Single __$_2$Married __$_3$Divorced __$_4$Widowed

2. Parents' Education: Indicate highest grade completed. F-father$_{24}$, M-mother$_{25}$.

   ___$_1$Elementary School    ___$_5$Vocational or Business Certificate or Training

   ___$_2$GED    ___$_6$Four Year College Degree

   ___$_3$High School Diploma    ___$_7$Master's Degree

   ___$_4$Two Year College Degree    ___$_8$Ph.D. or Professional Degree (M.D., J.D.)

3. Father's Occupation:$_{26}$    Mother's Occupation:$_{27}$

_____    _____

Please indicate Family members who have been:

| | Mother | Father | Sister | Brother | Grandparents | Aunts, Uncles, Cousins |
|---|---|---|---|---|---|---|
| 4. Obese . . . . . . . . . . . . . . . | 28___ | 36___ | 44___ | 52___ | 60___ | 68___ |
| 5. Anorexic . . . . . . . . . . . . . | 29___ | 37___ | 45___ | 53___ | 61___ | 69___ |
| 6. Bulimic . . . . . . . . . . . . . | 30___ | 38___ | 46___ | 54___ | 62___ | 70___ |
| 7. Treated for drug abuse. . . . . . . . | 31___ | 39___ | 47___ | 55___ | 63___ | 71___ |
| 8. Treated for alcohol abuse . . . . . . | 32___ | 40___ | 48___ | 56___ | 64___ | 72___ |
| 9. Treated for depression or mood disorder | 33___ | 41___ | 49___ | 57___ | 65___ | 73___ |
| 10. Hospitalized for psychiatric reasons. . | 34___ | 42___ | 50___ | 58___ | 66___ | 74___ |
| 11. Threatened suicide or attempted suicide | 35___ | 43___ | 51___ | 59___ | 67___ | 75___ |

## III. PSYCHOLOGICAL AND PSYCHIATRIC HISTORY

Card 2

1. Sexual identification:[7]
   ____[1]Exclusively heterosexual    ____[4]Mostly homosexual
   ____[2]Mostly heterosexual    ____[5]Exclusively homosexual
   ____[3]Bisexual

2. Age at first intercourse?[8,9]____ years

|  | Yes[1] | No[0] |
|---|---|---|
| 3. Have you ever been in therapy? | | |
| If yes, was it for an eating disorder? [10]___ | ___ | |
| Did your therapist know that you had an eating disorder? [11]___ | ___ | |
| Name of therapist _____ [12] ___ | ___ | |

4. Are you currently in therapy? [13]___ ___
   If yes, is it for an eating disorder? [14]___ ___
   Does your therapist know that you have an eating disorder? [15]___ ___
   Name of therapist _____

5. Have you ever been prescribed psychiatric medication? [16]___ ___
   Present medication:[17] _____   Past medication:[18] _____
   Reason:[19] _____   Reason:[20] _____

6. Have you ever been hospitalized for psychiatric reasons? [21]___ ___
   When:[22,23] _____ Reason:[24] _____

7. Have you ever threatened suicide? [25]___ ___
   Age at last threat:[26,27]____ years

8. Have you ever attempted suicide? [28]___ ___
   Age at last attempt:[29,30]____ years

9. Please check if you have ever been a victim of:

| | | Yes | No |
|---|---|---|---|
| | Rape | [31]___ | ___ |
| | Sexual molestation | [32]___ | ___ |
| | Physical abuse as a child | [33]___ | ___ |
| | Physical abuse by partner | [3c]___ | ___ |

## IV. EATING DISORDERS HISTORY

1. Height:[35,36]_____

2. Current weight:[37-39]_____   Lowest weight:[40-42]_____   Date:[43,44]_____
   Desired weight:[45-47]_____   Highest weight:[48-50]_____   Date:[51,52]_____

3. How do you see yourself?[53]    4. How do others see you?[54]

   _____[1] Very overweight [1]_____
   _____[2] Overweight [2]_____
   _____[3] Just right [3]_____
   _____[4] Underweight [4]_____
   _____[5] Very underweight [5]_____

5. Age you first felt too fat:[55,56]____ years

6. Age you first dieted:[57,58]____ years

7. How often do you diet?[59]____ [4]All the time   ____[3]Once a week   ____[2]Once a month
   ____[1]A few times a year   ____[0]Never

8. Please check if you have ever had:(place an H if you have been hospitalized)

| | Younger than 13 | Adolescence | Adulthood (18+) |
|---|---|---|---|
| a. Anorexia Nervosa | [60]_____ | [63]_____ [69]H | [66]_____ [72]H |
| b. Obesity | [61]_____ | [64]_____ [70]H | [67]_____ [73]H |
| c. Bulimia | [62]_____ | [65]_____ [71]H | [68]_____ [74]H |

## V. EATING ATTITUDES AND BEHAVIORS

Card 3   A. Binge-eating

|  | Yes[1] | No[0] |
|---|---|---|
| 1. Do you feel that you have a problem binge-eating? | [7]___ | ___ |
| If your answer is no, skip to section B. | | |

2. Do you:

| | Never[0] | Sometimes[1] | Usually[2] | Always[3] |
|---|---|---|---|---|
| a. Find yourself preoccupied with thoughts of food and eating? | [8]___ | ___ | ___ | ___ |
| b. Eat a large quantity of food in a short time? | [9]___ | ___ | ___ | ___ |
| c. Feel that you cannot stop eating during a binge? | [10]___ | ___ | ___ | ___ |
| d. Feel depressed and anxious after a binge? | [11]___ | ___ | ___ | ___ |
| e. Worry that someone will find out about your binging behavior? | [12]___ | ___ | ___ | ___ |
| f. End a binge by inducing vomiting? | [13]___ | ___ | ___ | ___ |
| g. End a binge by using laxatives? | [14]___ | ___ | ___ | ___ |

3. How old were you when you first considered binge-eating a problem?$_{15,16}$____ years

4. How long have you been binge-eating as part of a pattern (habit)? $_{17,18}$____ years

5. What is the longest period of time that you have been able to go without binging?$_{19,20}$____ days$_{21,22}$____ weeks$_{23,24}$____ months$_{25,26}$____ years

6. How often do you binge?$_{27}$
   ____$_{7}$More than once a day: ____ times        ____$_{4}$Once a week
   ____$_{6}$Every day                               ____$_{3}$A few times a month
   ____$_{5}$A few times a week:   ____ times        ____$_{2}$Once a month

7. How long does a binge typically last?$_{28}$
   ____$_{1}$Under 30 minutes  ____$_{2}$30 to 60 minutes  ____$_{3}$1 to 2 hours  ____$_{4}$Over 2 hours

8. What time of the day are you most likely to binge?$_{29}$
   ____$_{1}$Morning ____$_{2}$Afternoon ____$_{3}$Evening ____$_{4}$Night ____$_{5}$Middle of the night

9. On the average, how much do you spend on a binge?$_{30,31}$_____ dollars.

## B. Vomiting

1. Do you induce yourself to vomit to control your weight? $_{35}$____$_{1}$Yes ____$_{0}$No
   If your answer is no, skip to Section C.

2. Do you:

|  | Never$_0$ | Sometimes$_1$ | Usually$_2$ | Always$_3$ |
|---|---|---|---|---|
| a. Vomit only after binging? . . . . . . . $_{36}$____ | __ | __ | __ |
| b. Vomit after every meal? . . . . . . . . . $_{37}$____ | __ | __ | __ |
| c. Vomit without necessarily having binged? $_{38}$____ | __ | __ | __ |
| d. Binge eat in order to vomit?. . . . . . $_{39}$____ | __ | __ | __ |

3. How old were you when you first used vomiting to control your weight?$_{40,41}$____ years

4. How long have you been vomiting as part of a pattern (habit)?    $_{42,43}$____ years

5. What is the longest period of time you have been able to go without vomiting?
   $_{44,45}$____ days$_{46,47}$____ weeks$_{48,49}$____ months$_{50,51}$_____ years

6. How often do you vomit?$_{52}$
   ____$_{7}$More than once a day: ____ times        ____$_{4}$Once a week
   ____$_{6}$Every day                               ____$_{3}$A few times a month
   ____$_{5}$A few times a week:   ____ times        ____$_{2}$Once a month
                                                     ____$_{1}$Less than once a month

7. What time of day are you most likely to vomit?$_{53}$
   ____$_{1}$Morning ____$_{2}$Afternoon ____$_{3}$Evening ____$_{4}$Night ____$_{5}$Middle of the night

## C. Laxative Use

1. **Do you use laxatives for weight control?**            $_{57}$____$_{1}$Yes ____$_{0}$No
   **If your answer is no, skip to Section D.**

2. Do you:

|  | Never$_0$ | Sometimes$_1$ | Usually$_2$ | Always$_3$ |
|---|---|---|---|---|
| a. Use laxatives only after binging?. . . $_{58}$____ | __ | __ | __ |
| b. Use laxatives after every meal? . . . $_{59}$____ | __ | __ | __ |
| c. Use laxatives without necessarily having binged? . . . . . . . . . . . . $_{60}$____ | __ | __ | __ |
| d. Use laxatives routinely, regardless of what you eat?. . . . . . . . . . . . $_{61}$____ | __ | __ | __ |

3. How old were you when you first used laxatives to control your weight?$_{62,63}$____ years

4. How long have you been using laxatives as part of a pattern (habit)? $_{64,65}$____ years

5. What is the longest amount of time that you have been able to go without using them?
   $_{66,67}$____ days$_{68,69}$____ weeks$_{70,71}$____ months$_{72,73}$____ years

6. How often do you use laxatives?$_{74}$
   ____$_{7}$More than once a day: ____ times        ____$_{4}$Once a week
   ____$_{6}$Every day                               ____$_{3}$A few times a month
   ____$_{5}$A few times a week:   ____ times        ____$_{2}$Once a month
                                                     ____$_{1}$Less than once a month

7. How many laxatives do you typically take at a time? $_{75\,76}$_____

8. What time of day are you most likely to take them? $_{77}$
   ____$_{1}$ Morning ____$_{2}$ Afternoon ____$_{3}$ Evening ____$_{4}$ Night ____$_{5}$ Middle of the night

9. How do you determine how many you take at a time? -_____

  **D.** Rank order your control over the following behaviors (1=most control; 3=least control)
   $_{78}$____ Binge-eating    $_{79}$____ Vomiting    $_{80}$____ Laxative use

**Card 4 E. Fasting**
1. Do you fast to control your weight?     $_{5}$____$_{1}$ Yes ____$_{0}$ No
2. Do you fast to compensate for overeating?    $_{4}$____$_{1}$ Yes ____$_{0}$ No

## VI. HABITS

1. Please indicate the frequency with which you use:

|  | More than$_{6}$ once/day | Daily$_{5}$ | Weekly$_{4}$ | Monthly$_{3}$ | Less than$_{2}$ monthly | Used to$_{1}$ | Never$_{0}$ |
|---|---|---|---|---|---|---|---|
| a. Cigarettes. . | $_{7}$____ | ____ | ____ | ____ | ____ | ____ | ____ |
| b. Coffee. . . . | $_{8}$____ | ____ | ____ | ____ | ____ | ____ | ____ |
| c. Alcohol . . . | $_{9}$____ | ____ | ____ | ____ | ____ | ____ | ____ |
| d. Marijuana . . | $_{10}$____ | ____ | ____ | ____ | ____ | ____ | ____ |
| e. Tranquilizers | $_{11}$____ | ____ | ____ | ____ | ____ | ____ | ____ |
| f. Barbiturates. | $_{12}$____ | ____ | ____ | ____ | ____ | ____ | ____ |
| g. Cocaine . . . | $_{13}$____ | ____ | ____ | ____ | ____ | ____ | ____ |
| h. Amphetamines. | $_{14}$____ | ____ | ____ | ____ | ____ | ____ | ____ |
| i. Hallucinogens | $_{15}$____ | ____ | ____ | ____ | ____ | ____ | ____ |
| j. Heroin. . . . | $_{16}$____ | ____ | ____ | ____ | ____ | ____ | ____ |
| k. Other: ____ | $_{17}$____ | ____ | ____ | ____ | ____ | ____ | ____ |

                                                Yes$_{1}$    No$_{0}$

2. Have you been in treatment for alcohol abuse?
   Date $_{1920}$_____ Were you hospitalized?   $_{18}$____ ____

3. Have you been in treatment for drug abuse?
   Date $_{22\,23}$_____ Were you hospitalized?   $_{21}$____ ____

4. How often do you exercise? $_{24}$ ____$_{1}$ Monthly ____$_{2}$ Weekly ____$_{3}$ A few times a week
   ____$_{4}$ Daily ____$_{5}$ Several times/day ____$_{0}$ Never

5. How much time do you spend exercising each time? $_{25}$ ____$_{1}$ Less than 30 minutes
   ____$_{2}$ 30 minutes to 1 hour ____$_{3}$ 1 to 2 hours ____$_{4}$ 2 to 3 hours ____$_{5}$ More

6. What types of exercise do you commonly do? $_{26}$_____ , $_{27}$_____

|  | Adolescent Yes$_{1}$   No$_{0}$ |  | Adult (18+) Yes$_{1}$   No$_{0}$ |  |
|---|---|---|---|---|

7. Have you ever shoplifted:
   Cosmetics? . . . . . . . . . . . . . . . . . $_{28}$____ ____    $_{33}$____ ____
   Clothes? . . . . . . . . . . . . . . . . . . $_{29}$____ ____    $_{34}$____ ____
   Food?. . . . . . . . . . . . . . . . . . . . $_{30}$____ ____    $_{35}$____ ____
   Jewelry? . . . . . . . . . . . . . . . . . . $_{31}$____ ____    $_{36}$____ ____
   Other: _____ $_{32}$____ ____    $_{37}$____ ____

8. Have you ever been arrested for shoplifting? $_{38}$____$_{1}$ Yes ____$_{0}$ No Date $_{39\,40}$_____

## VII. MEDICAL HISTORY

1. Do you have any chronic illnesses? $_{41}$____$_{1}$ Yes ____$_{0}$ No
   If yes, please describe: _____

2. Age of first menstrual period: $_{42\,43}$____ years.

3. Do you have a regular cycle? $_{44}$____$_{1}$ Yes ____$_{0}$ No

4. Is there any time other than pregnancy during which you have stopped menstruating?
   ____$_{1}$ Yes ____$_{0}$ No If yes, for how long? $_{46\,47}$____ Months $_{48\,49}$____ Years

5. Date of last physical: $_{50\,51}$_____

6. Are you currently using any of the following forms of birth control? $_{52}$
   ____$_{1}$ Birth control pills ____$_{2}$ Diaphragm ____$_{3}$ IUD ____$_{4}$ Condom ____$_{5}$ Other

7. Please mark the following symptoms that you experience frequently:
   $_{53}$____ Swollen glands    $_{60}$____ Muscle weakness    $_{65}$____ Dry skin
   $_{54}$____ Excess gas    $_{61}$____ Tingling    $_{66}$____ Hair breakage
   $_{55}$____ Rectal bleeding    $_{62}$____ Muscle spasms    $_{67}$____ Brittle nails
   $_{56}$____ Easily cold    $_{63}$____ Muscle cramps    $_{68}$____ Frequent thirst
   $_{57}$____ Amenorrhea    $_{64}$____ Poor circulation    $_{69}$____ Dizziness
   $_{58}$____ Difficulty                                $_{70}$____ Fainting
           concentrating                           $_{71}$____ Fluid retention
   $_{59}$____ Dental problems
   Please estimate the cost of your dental care in the last two years $_{72\text{-}74}$_____

8. Have you noticed any changes in your physical health since you have been
   binging and purging? $_{75}$____ Yes ____ No If yes, please describe: _____
   _____
   _____

rape) are common experiences, especially in women who develop bulimia. Has anything like that happened to you?" Even if she says "no," a further question, such as, "Have you felt confused about the touches of father (brother, strangers)?" may be illuminating. Date rapes can be explored by asking if the first intercourse experience was by choice or forced.

Recently, a client was referred to one of the therapists by a clinician who had been working with the entire family, including the remarried spouses. Therapy was going slowly and he felt that perhaps group therapy would be a better treatment modality. During the pretreatment interview with one of the authors, the client shared that there was an incident, about six years ago, when the stepfather had come into her room late at night and fondled her. She had not shared this with anyone, and we were convinced that this was certainly part of the reason that the family therapy was at a standstill. While we do not suggest that the therapist automatically assume that the client has been victimized, we feel that often this is an area that is not talked about or investigated in enough depth.

EATING DISORDERS HISTORY. This section assesses client perceptions around body-image and weight. The therapist can use the information provided to ask additional questions surrounding the circumstances of weight gain or loss, as well as to talk with the client about whether her desired weight is a reasonable goal. The question on how she sees herself and how others see her can provide important diagnostic distinctions between anorectic and bulimic clients. For example, it can give information on whether the client is dissatisfied with her weight or body but is able to assess it realistically, or whether there is a distortion in her assessment of her current weight and body image. The anorectic sees herself as overweight (or just right at a very low weight) and thinks others see her similarly. In contrast, the bulimic often has a more accurate perception of her body-image and can more easily distinguish between *seeing* herself as "fat" and *feeling* "fat." The therapist can also obtain important information on hospitalization experiences and reactions to previous treatments.

EATING ATTITUDES AND BEHAVIORS. This section is subdivided into sections on bingeing, vomiting, laxative use, and fasting. This can be a less threatening way to get this information, although the therapist should inquire into accuracy of the responses of the client. The questions correspond to the DSM-III (APA, 1980) criteria for bulimia and also ask the client to begin to think about times when she is more vulnerable to binge-eating, purging, or abuse of laxatives. One subsection here asks the client to rank order her control over the bingeing, vomiting, and laxative abuse. This is valuable in several ways. The question asks her to think about which of the behaviors may be the easiest to control and helps her to realize that she does have some control over some of the bulimic behavior. The anorectic client will typically have more difficulty controlling the purging behavior, while the bulimic client will usually report more difficulty controlling the bingeing behavior, especially when pressed to make a distinction between bingeing and vomiting.

HABITS. This section is designed to elicit information on the past and present use of alcohol and drugs, exercise behavior, and shoplifting. The questions on drug and alcohol use should be carefully investigated in order to assess the possibility of these problems in addition to the bulimia. The therapist should note the use of alcohol in order to see if this has been a problem in the past or present. We frequently ask, "Have you ever felt, or has anyone told you, that you drink too much?" "Have you ever blacked out or been unable to remember periods of time during which you had been drinking?" We have found that as the individual is working to recover from the bulimia, she may increase her use of alcohol to compensate for a decrease in the release that she previously found with bulimia. Or a bulimic recently treated for alcoholism is likely to show an increase in bulimic symptomatology. Use of marijuana should be explored to determine if the individual's use of marijuana is contributing to her urges to binge more frequently. If there are any doubts about a substance abuse dependency or addiction, we recommend that the individual be referred for evaluation by a specialist such as a certified alcohol counselor.

While a history of shoplifting behavior is occasionally observed in non-eating-disordered adolescents, shoplifting is often observed in bulimic clients of all ages and has increasingly become a precipitating event for the initiation of court-mandated treatment. It is our experience that clients may have difficulty answering these questions truthfully if they fear or sense disapproval on the part of the therapist, lack trust in the therapist, or deny substance abuse problems.

MEDICAL HISTORY. This section seeks information about physiological effects of the bingeing and purging behavior, major illnesses, and menstruation history. A list of symptoms for the client to check can give the therapist a ready reference on the physical effects of the bulimia. Symptoms are geared towards detecting dehydration and electrolyte imbalances. We strongly suggest that any client presenting with bulimia be seen by a physician experienced with eating disorders in order to assess her physical symptoms.

## Using the BREDS

The BREDS is a unique instrument that the treating professional can use to compile information in a quick and thorough manner. Significant aspects include questions which can help the therapist make a decision on whether an individual session may be indicated, distinguish in a preliminary manner whether it is likely that the individual is anorectic or bulimic in behavior or cognition, and open up discussion of victimization experiences. Many of the questions require the client to begin to think about the relationship of life events and family stresses to weight, dieting, and bulimic behavior and to look at patterns of responses to these stresses.

With the BREDS in hand, the therapist can begin to hypothesize about the family type, as well as the appropriateness of having the family in at the beginning of therapy. Clients from perfect families often show patterns of high achievement in parental occupations, little history of psychiatric disturbance in the family, and relatively less incidence of impulsive behavior. Individuals from overprotective families are usually youngest girls, may be living at home at an older age, and report a history of maternal depression and obesity. Individuals from chaotic families are usually oldest girls in the family, report that parents are divorced, dead, or never married, have a "checkerboard" pattern of responses on the family history section, reveal a history of abuse, and exhibit many types of impulsive behavior, including drug and alcohol abuse as well as shoplifting.

Thus, the BREDS can be used to develop hypotheses about family structure and functioning, to provide the therapist with information which may take many interviews to elicit, and to gather information on the medical consequences of bulimia. Whether it is used as the basis for an individual interview or as a way to collect information before seeing the family for an initial interview, the information is essential for the therapist to have as she or he begins treatment.

# CHAPTER 12

# The Role of Consultation

CONSULTATION, AS AN INTERVENTION technique with bulimic families, differs from therapy in several ways. A consultation is a brief, time-limited contract (usually one session, rarely more than three sessions), which is clearly stated from the outset of the consultation. During the consultation, the therapist assesses the family system; while he or she may make some interventions, they are limited. Because the therapist sees consultation as a more tolerable intervention than therapy for some families and individuals, he or she must clearly set goals for themselves and the family and resist the urge to intervene or offer more than the family can tolerate.

Three different types of consultation situations are discussed here: 1) the family is seeking help for the first time for the symptomatic member; 2) the therapist invites the family for a consultation while the bulimic member is in individual or group treatment; and 3) another professional who is currently working with the family initiates the consultation. We offer guidelines for conducting this type of session and excerpts from a consultation conducted with a family who sought help for their bulimic daughter.

## THE FAMILY SEEKS CONSULTATION

The first appointment with a family is usually conducted as a consultation. A consultation format can be less threatening to parents, who may feel that the eating disorder is their fault and fear that they will be blamed for the development of the bulimia. In a sense, the consultation can "whet the family's appetite for therapy" offered in a supportive, nonthreatening manner. For psychologically unsophisticated families, perfect families, or families from certain cultural backgrounds that do not comprehend therapy, a consultation can be used to dispel myths about therapy and to overcome

150

family messages and injunctions around seeking help from an outsider.

This approach has several advantages. First of all, it allows the therapist to assess the therapist-family fit for therapy. The style of the family, the language used, and the personality of members and the therapist should be evaluated to determine ways of joining with the family members. When the first session is conducted in this way, no one is committed to continuing the therapy. It allows the therapist to consider how much energy treatment of this family will demand (taking into account the other clients and families on her or his caseload), and to assess how this family may generate family-of-origin issues in the therapist's own family. A consultation format allows a graceful out for the therapist who may, after seeing the family, feel that another therapist would be more appropriate for the family.

Second, a consultation helps the therapist to assess how available the family members are for family therapy and to assess whether the family system can tolerate open-ended therapy. If the symptomatic member is totally opposed to treatment, the therapist's using the consultation to offer predictions about the behavior and to connect the symptoms to the family dynamics, rather than to an individual problem, may help her to be more open to treatment.

For some families, particularly chaotic ones, a consultation or a series of consultations may be all that the family can tolerate. Attempting to involve the family in an open-ended type of family therapy could repeat old patterns of family or parental unavailability.

Sometimes the family seeking help has a history of numerous contacts with other health-care professionals. This type of history usually indicates a family that is difficult to treat because they do not have adequate motivation to change, have had difficulty locating an appropriate therapist, or have run into obstacles in the mental health care delivery system. The consultation session can be used to explore the reasons for a complex treatment history.

## CONSULTATION INITIATED BY THE THERAPIST

The second type of consultation is initiated by the therapist after working with the bulimic client in individual or in group therapy. The family may not have been directly involved in the therapy for several reasons: The client needed individual or group therapy to strengthen her for the family or couples therapy; the family is geographically unavailable except on a consultation basis; or a consultation was all that the family was able to tolerate.

The therapist-initiated consultation may be similar to the one initiated by the family. Regardless of the reason that the consultation is suggested, the therapist should carefully consider whether the client should be the one to ask in the family or whether the therapist should take this responsibility.

For some clients, part of the work of therapy may be asking the family in, acknowledging that she needs their support to recover. For other families, especially if there is a possibility that the family may refuse to come in, the therapist may decide to call. It is important for the client to understand why the family is invited at this time.

For clients from unpredictable chaotic families, it can be helpful to talk about the goals of the consultation — what might be realistically accomplished and what may happen during the session — in order to provide some predictability.

## CONSULTATION REQUESTED BY ANOTHER PROFESSIONAL

A consultation may be requested by another treating professional, such as an alcohol counselor, a therapist, a physician, or nutritionist. Consultation may also be initiated by court order. It is essential that the therapist take time to talk to the referring professional about the reason for the request. Possible reasons include:

- Assessment of the eating disorder (the diagnosis has not yet been made).
- The professional wants the consultant to reinforce interpretations that have been made to the family.
- The family or the therapist is stuck and wants a second opinion.
- A magic cure is desired on the part of the professional.
- The professional wants confirmation or disconfirmation of a hypothesis.
- The professional wants to discontinue treatment and a consultation is a way to end therapy.

Depending upon the reason for the request, the consultant must decide whether it will be honored. A psychologist recently requested that one of the authors see a family that she had been working with for several months. Talking with the psychologist revealed that she was engaged in a power struggle with the family and that the purpose of the consultation was to engage the therapist on her side. She wanted to limit the interpretations and control the session so that her view of the bulimia was supported. The consultant declined to do the consultation on these terms.

## THE GOALS OF THE CONSULTATION

There are four primary goals in conducting a consultation with a family. They include: joining with the family members, assessing the family system, linking the symptoms to the family, and providing education.

*Joining*

Joining is essential to the consultation process; if the therapist does not join with the family members, it is unlikely that they will be able to hear or use the information provided by the therapist. Joining begins with the first telephone call; the therapist must be willing to take time to talk with the caller and listen to his or her concerns. Families quickly decide whether or not the therapist will hear and respond to their concerns. This may mean that the therapist needs to initially accept the family's view of the problem before introducing new ways of understanding the bulimia. These cautions also apply to joining with the professional initiating the consultation.

With a rebellious adolescent, joining may be facilitated by respecting that she does not want to talk or to be involved in the session. By allowing her not to talk, the therapist can, in fact, encourage her participation. Joining with parents can involve responding to their fears and concerns around the bulimia and emphasizing that the eating disorder is not their fault. Often, parents come to therapy expecting to be blamed for causing the bulimia, and subsequently are threatened by hypotheses about the family's involvement in the bulimia if the therapist offers these too early in the session.

The therapist must respect the family rules and organization in order to be able to join with the family. Ignoring the rules will sabotage the consultation. For example, while we like to hear what each member would like out of the consultation, we may turn to the father or mother and ask to hear him/her first. If the therapist is successful in joining with the family, it increases the likelihood that the family will be willing to participate in therapy.

*Assessment of the Family System*

Assessment of the family system is an essential part of the consultation. As discussed in the preceding chapter on assessment, this involves assessing: interpersonal boundaries, family type, family history, unresolved multigenerational issues, communication patterns, availability of members for therapy, and the systemic function of the bulimia. The therapist can determine who is the most distressed by the bulimia. The consultation can also be used to generate and test hypotheses about the family functioning.

*Shifting From an Individual Focus*
*to a Family Focus*

Accepting the family's reality is central to joining and then allows the therapist leverage for proposing variations on this reality. In this way, the therapist can guide the family from seeing the bulimia as the problem of the individual to a view that incorporates the family. Often, it is the bulimic individual who is most resistant to enlarging the view to include the family.

*Education*

We often use a consultation session to provide information to the family and to the symptomatic member about the process of recovery from bulimia. With the increased media attention to bulimia, families often come in with misinformation about what bulimia is and the physical effects of bingeing and purging. We also offer information about the process of therapy and what family members can expect if they do decide to participate in therapy.

While the interventions made in a consultation are limited, we often do set up some guidelines around the bingeing and purging behavior. If it is possible, we suggest that the bulimic individual contract to replace binge food within 24 hours of eating it. We also direct the individual to be responsible for cleaning up the bathroom and kitchen after a bulimic episode. These two interventions make the bulimic individual responsible for her behavior and can relieve some of the tension around the behavior. These interventions also have the effect of letting the family know that she will not be able to stop the bulimic behavior immediately, while facilitating joining with the parents by directly addressing and intervening in the bulimic behavior. The therapist does need to evaluate whether these interventions are realistic and whether the family can follow through with these directives.

We have found it useful in working with families to offer handouts to reinforce the ideas presented in the consultation. We typically offer a handout to the family with suggestions for avoiding power struggles around the bulimic behavior, discouraging dieting, and setting limits. We do not suggest that the family attempt to follow all of the suggestions. We do stress making her responsible for her behavior, staying out of power struggles around food, and developing ways of interacting other than around food. This handout is provided in Table 5.


## A CONSULTATION SESSION

The following is an excerpt from a consultation conducted by one of the authors. The family, a working-class family from a small town referred by their physician, requested a consultation for their daughter Terri, a 17-year-old who had been bingeing and purging for one year. We use the excerpts to highlight the joining process and to illustrate the way in which the therapist moved from an individual view of the problem to a view which included the family. Kathy and Steve are the parents. Mary, the 21-year-old daughter, was away at school and not present for the session.

*Joining and Setting Goals of the Consultation*

Therapist: Terri, your family has asked for this consultation with me. Everyone is worried about you, and maybe we could start out by having you fill me in on what everyone is so worried about.

Terri: Yeah. (Angrily, looking out the window) I think you know about why everyone is worried.

Therapist: I want to know from you. That's part of why I am doing this consultation. So I would be really interested in why you think everyone is so concerned or if they have any reason to be concerned, but I think it could feel like a real invasion of your privacy to be coming in and talking about your bulimia with a perfect stranger. So I'll let you get a sense of me. I'll talk with your parents for a while. Steve and Kathy, what would you like to get out of the consultation today?

Kathy: Well, I'd like to find out more about this bulimia, because I don't know much about it, you know. And Terri said that the last couple of days she has been more in control of herself, she hasn't vomited, so that's encouraging. But I really don't know much about it and what to do. I can't really do anything because she is responsible for herself. It is a big worry for us. We don't see her eating what she should be eating and she goes in the bathroom and gets rid of it. It's just a lot of stress.

Therapist: So you would like some information about what this is all about and how one gets better, how one gets over this?

Kathy: Right.

Therapist: Maybe it is also hard to know what is the right thing to do as parents—how you should be acting towards Terri.

Kathy: It is hard to know what to do because when we talk about it, she gets upset and leaves the room.

Terri: Mom! (pause) It just gets old after a while. And I don't know how to explain it to them.

Therapist: So for you Terri, you would like to be able to understand more of why this is happening. Maybe I can help you and your parents understand this a little better. (Terri nods.) Steve, what would you like from today?

Steve: I would just like to know why Terri has to be like this, you know, why she is so mixed up. Why she doesn't eat like the rest of us, why she goes to the bathroom after she eats and eats and eats . . .

Therapist: Like why she is having to throw it away like that.

Steve: It worries me, for her to keep throwing up all the time after she eats.

Therapist: What do you worry about, Steve?

Table 5

Guidelines for Family Members Who Want to Help a Family Member
Recover From an Eating Disorder

There are no quick or easy solutions for recovery from an eating disorder. Therapists, physicians, and other "experts" have no magic that can cure your loved one. Be wary if someone offers guarantees or quick cures. If she is to recover, she will need to make some changes in her attitudes and behaviors. You cannot make them for her. You and the other members of the family may also need to make some changes to accommodate her growth. Hopefully, all of you will take advantage of professional help to make the rough spots a little smoother.

Allow yourself not to know all the answers about how to help the person you love. This does not make you any less of a parent, partner, or sibling. Admitting your lack of understanding of the problem demonstrates that you are human. There are resources for help with this problem. You do not have to be the expert.

If your child is younger than 18 (legal adulthood), GET HER INTO THERAPY IMMEDIATELY. Do not hesitate out of fear that she will hate you or become increasingly ill. If she is over 18, you need to admit that you have no control over her. She can choose to be helped, or not. You do, however, have control over how much you will let her take advantage of you. You do not have to continue living with behavior you find unacceptable. You do not have to provide her with opportunities to abuse your love and generosity. To protect yourself, you may have to set limits on the amenities you provide her which reinforce her eating behavior.

In any close relationship, you need to set limits on how much you can give of yourself. If you can do this, you not only model taking care of yourself, but remove some of the debt the person you love may feel she owes you. You need to set limits on how much you can do.

Once your child/spouse/sibling is in therapy, avoid getting involved in discussions or arguments over weight and food behaviors. If you become concerned about weight loss, dehydration, or other signs of medical jeopardy, call the therapist, physician, or both.

Cooperate with the therapist in devising and sticking to a plan that will encourage your loved one to become mature, self-loving and responsible.

If your child/spouse/sibling is food shopping or cooking for the family, realize that she may be using this nurturing role to deny her own need for food by feeding others.

LEARN TO TAKE CARE OF YOURSELF! Do not become a martyr. Do not sacrifice yourself for your loved one. You will accomplish nothing, and you will end up feeling exhausted and resentful. Do not let family life or your relationship revolve around the eating disorder. Make sure you and the other members of the family make time for satisfying activities and fun. Do not neglect fulfilling relationships. Do not spend all of your time with the person with the eating disorder; you will only encourage her to be more dependent on you. She needs to be making friends and contacts outside the family circle and your relationship.

Do not allow her to run the family. Her eating habits and food choices should not dominate your kitchen, your refrigerator, your meals, or your schedule. She should not be responsible for what the family eats, which restaurants you patronize,

TABLE 5
(*Continued*)

or where you go on outings and vacations. Remember, other family members are entitled to have input into these kinds of decisions.

Give your daughter/spouse/sister responsibility for the consequences of her words, actions, decisions, and behaviors. She needs to learn how to deal with disappointment, frustration, and anger. Do not protect her by giving her the power to avoid all situations she finds distressing. Give her the responsibility to replace what she has eaten on a binge or to clean the bathroom after she purges. This responsibility is aimed to help her deal with reality rather than punish her behavior. However, realize in that many instances the person with an eating disorder is not financially able to replace what she has eaten.

Verbally and physically express honest love and affection for her. Do not tie your caring to sermons about eating or demands to gain weight.

Admit you sometimes feel angry, frustrated, helpless, afraid, powerless, and enraged. Showing these emotions does not take away from your love for her. By sharing your feelings, you are providing the most direct permission for her to feel and express her feelings. Your feelings may be different from hers.

Participate in family therapy or a parent/spouse support group to work through these feelings and get support from others. Don't become isolated with your problem. Keeping it a secret does not necessarily help anyone.

Develop ways of sharing and socializing that do not involve food. This does not mean that you need to exclude socializing that centers around food. Develop dialogues with her about issues other than food, weight and diets. Discuss current affairs, feelings, the arts, sports or any other good topics.

Sometimes when discussing issues and feelings, you can hear things the way you want to. This also goes for the person with the eating disorder. Check to make sure that you are accurately hearing what is being said to you. It is equally important for you to make sure that you have been heard accurately.

Practice good sense. Do not go on diets. It's hard to explain why it's OK for you to diet but not for the person with the eating disorder. Take an honest look at your reasons for dieting and exercise. Are you giving your appearance priority over your health? Are these activities primarily for weight loss? It is hard for the individual with an eating disorder to try to change her thinking about weight loss and the importance of her appearance when significant others around her are reinforcing the importance of weight loss and thinness.

Recognize your daughter, sister, or partner for qualities that are independent of her appearance or achievements. Sharing with her what you appreciate about her or are attracted to can support her development of a sense of self that is secure, unique, and definitely less subject to the changing fancies of fads and fashion. Of course, such observations and sharing are helpful only when spontaneous and sincere.

Avoid power struggles with your loved one over gaining weight or stopping the bingeing and purging. She will always win. Avoid power struggles of any kind for the same reason.

Do not try to manipulate her with statements like "If you won't change for yourself do it for me (or us)," "You are ruining the whole family," or "Why are you do-

*continued*

TABLE 5
(*Continued*)

ing this to me?" She will feel guilty and responsible for the welfare of the rest of the family, something she most likely already feels. These feelings will not help her to change her behavior. You need to take care of your own welfare. Do not make her responsible for your happiness.

Avoid making requests such as, "What can I do to help you?" and "Help me to help you." She does not know what she needs; if she did she would probably seek it.

Let her know that you are available for emotional and psychological support. You may even ask, "What kind of support could you use at this time?" or "How can I support you?" These questions are different from the questions, "Help me to help you," or "How can I help you?"

Do not ask, "Are you better?" This is a loaded question and pulls for the response, "Yes, of course." Judge progress for yourself. For example: Is she more aware of her feelings? Is she thinking more realistically some of the time? Is she being less critical of herself? Look for broader definitions of recovery than just changes in eating behavior or weight.

Realize that at best your child/spouse/sibling is probably ambivalent about wanting to get well. At times she may want to recover; at others she will retreat into what she perceives as the relative safety and security of her rituals and other relationships with food.

Realize you are trying to do what is right and best in an extremely difficult situation. Recovery takes time, patience, and professional help. Allow yourself to seek the resources you need during this time.

Adapted from the ANRED ALERT by Dr. Jean Rubel.

Steve: Well, it could damage her brain or kill her like Karen Carpenter.
Therapist: Kathy and Steve, you would like to understand what is happening to Terri and how you can help her to recover. Also, Steve, you said that you would like some information about the physical effects of the bulimia. Terri, you would like to be able to talk to your parents about the bulimia and understand it more. Have I heard each of you? (Therapist looks at each person in turn as they nod.)

So what I'll do is ask for information from each of you. I think that some of what I can offer you will come from my questioning about things in the family. If I didn't need to ask about the family, I would have asked only Terri to come in. But I do need some information about the family, I need each of your perspectives, thinking that you could have three different views of what goes on, what happens. That will help me to understand why Terri needs her bulimia. This will also help me to make some recommendations as to what needs to take place to help Terri to recover.

The therapist subsequently asked for information about the bulimia, attending to the needs of the family for some understanding of the behavior. The consultation would have failed if the therapist had not been sensitive to the need of the parents to at least initially talk about the bulimia and their worry about the physical effects of the behavior. Acknowledging their concern facilitated joining with the family members and increased the likelihood that they would be able to connect the symptom to the family later in the consultation.

### Linking the Symptoms to the Family

The next step in the consultation was to link the symptom to the family issues. The therapist accomplished this by asking each member to offer ideas about the purpose of the bulimia.

Steve: I don't understand! Terri, you know you look okay, you are skinny enough. Why do you keep doing this? You don't need to . . .

Therapist: So why do you think that Terri does this, if it has nothing to do with her weight or has to do with issues other than her weight? Why does she need to do this?

Kathy: I asked her if it had anything to do with us, and she said no.

Therapist: If it did have to do with the family, how do you think it is connected?

Steve: It's probably me. I'm the bad guy. (Parents look at each other and laugh.) I'd like her to tell me what throwing up has to do with me. Do you know that this is dangerous if you do it all the time?

Therapist: Steve, what does being the bad guy have to do with Terri's throwing up?

Kathy: He's just kidding. (Therapist motions her to stop talking.)

Therapist: Steve?

Steve: I don't know. Maybe she's mad at me or doesn't like me. Maybe she thinks I'm too mean.

Therapist: I think it could be related.

Kathy: Oh, Steve, you're not so mean. (Turning to Terri) Right, Terri? Tell him. (Therapist motions Terri not to answer.)

Therapist: Kathy, Steve really took a chance saying Terri's throwing up might be because she's mad at him or he's too mean (therapist will follow up on theme of potential abuse later after she feels that she has joined with Terri). Kathy, how do you think Terri's bulimia is connected with the family?

Kathy: I don't know. I never thought about it like that. (Pause) I just love her and want her to get better. (Pause) Maybe she's jealous of her sister.

(Pause) Do you really think it has something to do with the family?

Therapist: There are certain reasons that Terri does this and part of what you wanted from the consultation was to understand the reasons for her bulimia. Terri, without knowing it, I think that some of what you are trying to do is to help your parents get ready for you to leave home when you grow up. Because, if you were to leave home now, or in the next year, and things were just the way they are, I think you would be really worried about your mom. (Mom tears up.)

Terri: Yeah. She's lonely a lot and dad gets so mad sometimes. She and dad hardly talk at all, except when one of them is mad at me for eating all the food.

Therapist: I think that you would be really worried and guilty about leaving your mom alone, and you are giving your mom and dad some practice to get used to worrying together and being more of a team. I don't think that you planned it that way, but that's some of what is happening. (Turning to parents) So I think she is giving you some practice, to see how you will handle it.

The session continued to focus on Terri's concerns for her parents and the linking of her bulimia to the issues in the family. Terri expressed concern about her father's increased drinking and leaving her mother alone. It was important for the therapist to limit what could be accomplished in the session, and to resist trying to address all of the issues in the consultation. The issue of Steve's meanness was addressed again—directly with the family. Steve was given direct suggestions about what to do if he felt like hitting Terri. (It was assessed that he was likely to use these suggestions.) Terri was given instructions as to what to do for her safety if she felt her father's anger was reaching an explosive point. The session ended with a discussion of recovery and the issues that the family would probably need to address if they chose to participate in therapy. Each member was given some information on ways that to help Terri towards recovery. The referring physician was also alerted to the possibility of physical abuse.

Ironically, Kathy later called for therapy to ask if the depression she had been experiencing could be related to Terri's bulimia, her growing up, and Kathy's fear of "losing her baby." If the therapist had pushed for family therapy during the consultation, it is likely that they would not have been amenable to treatment. By allowing the family the space and the time to choose therapy, the likelihood of a successful treatment outcome was increased.

# CHAPTER 13

# *Individual Systemic Therapy*

MOST THERAPISTS AGREE that family issues are salient in the development and maintenance of an individual's bulimia. Nevertheless, most therapists facilitate an individual's recovery from bulimia through nonsystemic individual therapy. While some of our clients have recovered without physically bringing their families into the therapist's office, all of our clients in individual therapy have completed some family-of-origin work.

We believe that individual therapy for bulimia can be successful if it is conceptually systemic. This may initially seem like a misnomer, but the therapeutic assumptions in individual systemic therapy are radically different from those in psychodynamically based individual therapy. For example, therapists with the latter approach believe that the origins of bulimia are intrapsychic in nature, whereas the systemic therapist believes that bulimia arises from and is maintained by the client's interactions with the various members of her system. This disagreement about the "site" of the problem is manifested in differences in approach to treatment, e.g., a focus on insight with the psychodynamic therapist, and a focus on ongoing interaction patterns with the systemic therapist.

As the individual responds differently to interaction patterns, she changes and thereby changes patterns in the family. Although these changes are small, they set into motion changes within the system that reverberate and activate other pattern changes in the family. The systemic therapist has an appreciation for the system's homeostatic responses to these changes, and aids the client in anticipating the system's moves to right itself.

This chapter examines the purpose and process of systemic individual therapy. What we provide by considering the individual modality of treatment is flexibility in working with clients, appreciation of the importance

161

and appropriateness of individual therapy for some clients, and acknowledgment of individual differences among clients. We outline indications and contraindications for individual therapy, explore the client-therapist relationship as it relates to individuals from each of the three family types, and offer some guidelines for facilitating symptom control and for beginning and ending therapy.

## INDICATIONS FOR INDIVIDUAL THERAPY

There are certain times when individual therapy is the most appropriate form of treatment. Individual therapy can be a safe place in which to work through victimization experiences, establish physical boundaries from extremely enmeshed and/or intrusive families, support individuation and separation from family of origin, strengthen the individual so that she can tolerate family therapy, and teach tools for symptom control. Each of these situations is briefly outlined below.

We routinely ask ourselves two of the simplest but often overlooked questions to determine the appropriateness of individual therapy at a given point in time: 1) What is the work this individual needs to do first and can this be done in individual therapy? and 2) What are the limitations to individual therapy? These two questions enable us to conduct individual therapy even though there is also family or couple work to be done. If family or couples therapy is more appropriate for what is currently going on with the individual, we do not do individual therapy. When we do offer individual therapy, we inform the client of the limitations of individual therapy, pointing out that it may be one phase of treatment in the recovery process. At a later date couples therapy or family therapy may be more appropriate and helpful.

### Teaching Symptom Control

Some elementary tools can be taught to the bulimic to help her understand some of the purposes of her symptoms, to take responsibility for as much of her behavior as she can, and to become more conscious of her choices to binge and or purge, so that she owns her bulimia. Without this ownership, as indicated by the individual's language (e.g., "my bulimia," "I" instead of "it"), she will not have control over her symptoms. The therapist needs to assess the amount of control the client can realistically be expected to take, given the role of the symptom in the larger network. We offer a more in-depth discussion of symptom control later in this chapter.

*Working Through Victimization Experiences*

The majority of bulimics with whom we work have histories of physical victimization (rape, sexual molestation, physical abuse) occurring before as well as during their bulimia. Furthermore, many of these individuals have not been able to speak to anyone about these experiences. The family rules about distress, blame, communication, and responsibility may restrain the individual from disclosing information in a family session — even if the perpetrator of the violence is not a family member. The therapist must be sensitive to cues that signal such experiences — both past and current. Questions such as the following facilitate disclosure (Root & Fallon, 1985):

1) Have you ever been forced into sexual acts as a child or adult?
2) As a child had you ever been physically punished in a way that left bruises or was more extreme than your friends experienced?
3) Have you ever been hit, spanked, slapped, or shoved by a parent (or partner)?
4) When you were a child, did anyone ever touch your breasts or genitals, or ask you to touch them in ways that made you feel uncomfortable, "dirty," or scared?
5) Have you ever felt scared for your physical safety if you said no to sex?
6) Was your first experience with sexual intercourse by choice or were you forced?
7) In any sexual relationship have you ever felt that you did not have the option to say no to sexual activities without physically being endangered?
8) Have you ever had to dress in a certain way to hide the fact that you and your partner had a fight?
9) As a child or teenager did teachers ever question you about bruises or marks you received from an adult?

We find that providing clients with information about the prevalence of such experiences among women with eating disorders and connecting these experiences to subsequent feelings of powerlessness and depression facilitate disclosure.

Individual therapy helps to validate the woman's experience and memory of these traumatic events. If a woman or teenager has been victimized by a family member, eventually she will need to challenge the dysfunctional rules in the family and talk about her experiences with family members. With the chaotic family, it may be difficult for the woman to determine whom she should or can tell about her experience(s): Parents have not been available or trustworthy in the past and may be no more available at the present time.

### Strengthening for Family Therapy

Some families can be too difficult to live with (much less to treat). Individual therapy can help the bulimic clarify and validate her experiences in the family. It can also prepare her for the anticipated stress of family therapy. Subsequently she can feel more powerful as she enters into that phase of treatment.

### Establishment of Boundaries

An initial assessment or consultation with the family can provide information about family members' respect for individual psychological and physical space. Individual therapy can be a structural intervention to create separate psychological and physical space for the bulimic. This was part of the reason for shifting from family therapy to individual therapy with the Weisfields (see Chapter 20). A similar shift can be made with a couple in which the "nonsymptomatic" person is extremely intrusive and "helpful."

### Supporting the Developmental Process of Separation and Individuation

The process of recovery reflects the leaving home or launching of adolescents (or young adults) from the family. Shifting from family therapy to individual therapy can mirror a parallel process in the family. This was the reason for shifting from family therapy to individual therapy at the end of treatment with the Long family (see Chapter 19).

### The Family is Geographically Unavailable

When the family is geographically unavailable, the therapist needs to determine during the consultation if there is a portion of recovery that can be accomplished in individual therapy during the consultation. Family therapy can be conducted in a series of consultations during vacations or visits. However, to proceed with individual therapy if it is contraindicated under these circumstances will contribute to treatment failure.

## CONTRAINDICATIONS FOR INDIVIDUAL THERAPY

There are several contraindications for individual therapy: when a client is being coerced into therapy; when the individual is repeating a dysfunctional pattern of protecting family members; when therapy is at an impasse because the family is sabotaging therapy; when the client does not feel ready for therapy but feels it is the right thing to do to appease worried people; or when the family is geographically unavailable, though needed, for therapy.

### The Individual Is Coerced Into Therapy

Initiating therapy under these conditions is more likely to occur overtly with the chaotic family and covertly with the perfect family. Obviously, this is a terrible condition under which to establish trust and a working rapport with an individual. If someone is not ready or has reasons to reject help, then even the best help will be useless; premature termination is most likely to be the outcome of such therapy. When therapy is initiated with such coercion, the individual is likely to feel powerless. To go ahead with the therapy reinforces the individual's feelings of being powerless and/or victimized by the family.

The coercive family is often looking for a professional to do substitute parenting, as well as to keep the individual in the symptomatic role. The parents can then point to the bulimic as having failed "even with the best help," so this confirms her role as "the problem" which once again diverts attention away from the real problems of communication, dysfunctional distribution of power, and dysfunctional relationships. This experience reinforces her symptomatic role in the family as "the one who cannot follow through" or "the one who is beyond help." To avoid these pitfalls, some therapists will even ask not just the parents, but also the grandparents, to come in for the initial interview, especially when the symptom has been persistent (Selvini Palazzoli, 1978).

### Dysfunctional Protection of the Family

Many persons enter therapy and acknowledge that family members are affected by or affect their symptoms. Nevertheless, they insist that family members do not need to be included in therapy. This usually occurs with chaotic and overprotective families. In contrast, individuals from perfect families may let you know that the family could not possibly be involved in their symptoms because the family is loving, caring, and perfect. Often, persons from the perfect or overprotective families keep their bulimia a secret for fear of hurting other people's feelings or making their parents feel guilty.

We seldom make the decision to see an adolescent without her family, although many adolescents request that their families not be involved. Doing individual therapy with an adolescent when the whole family needs to be there can feel like conducting therapy with a room full of empty chairs. Some families drop their teenager off with the therapist as they drop a younger child off with the babysitter. They absolve themselves of responsibility and involvement, which may be a major aspect of the family's dysfunction.

The adolescent or young adult who wants to keep the family out of therapy may have various reasons, ranging from protection of the family to acceptance of the blame for the symptoms or family dysfunction. A consultation helps the therapist to assess the basis for the bulimic's (or family's) request. Sometimes, for reasons mentioned previously, it is appropriate to work individually with the adolescent from a chaotic family, the partner in an abusive relationship, or the physically victimized individual.

## Significant Others Are Sabotaging Therapy

If the bulimic in individual therapy gets stuck inexplicably, it is likely that someone in the family is invested in keeping the individual symptomatic. Put simply, it is likely that the family is sabotaging therapy or the individual's efforts at change. An example comes to mind of a mother who initially wanted her daughter in treatment; as therapy progressed, the daughter became more appropriately separate from her mother. As this change occurred, the mother started to sabotage treatment by telling the client how she had not seen any progress, doubting the competence of the therapist, and generally portraying herself as a victim of the therapist, a role she had played with the client's father. Subsequently, the client relapsed, became the focus of her parents' conflict, and enabled the parents once again to avoid directly addressing their marital conflict.

Other examples of family sabotage can take the form of placing unreasonable expectations or responsibilities on the bulimic, such as asking her to cook or do the grocery shopping. A partner may be subtly sabotaging the work by arranging more activities around food (for example, a husband takes his wife out for dinner more frequently so as to relieve her of the stress of meal preparation or cleanup). Such interactions should alert the therapist that the family does not intend to let go of the symptomatic individual easily.

Often at the outset of individual therapy we ask the partner or the family to come in for a consultation and inform them that they will need to be included in the therapy at some point in time. We explain that individual change usually is best supported by fine-tuning important relationships. In the course of recovery, the individual is learning to become cognizant of her critical needs, and to actively seek to fulfill them; her relationships will inevitably need to change. There are no exceptions to this.

## THE THERAPIST-CLIENT RELATIONSHIP

The degree to which the therapist will be able to facilitate family work at a distance is related to the therapist's awareness of the subtle ways in which signals of dysfunctional family patterns surface in the therapist-client relationship. The bulimic client will repeat patterns of dysfunctional cognitive, communication, and relationship patterns learned in her family with the therapist. Assessment of the client's family type during the initial interviews allows the therapist to anticipate common dysfunctional patterns.

### The Perfect Therapist-Client Relationship

The client from the perfect family is used to aiming to please and is likely to repeat this pattern with the therapist. She may try to make changes too fast or prevent herself from talking about her fear, anxiety or uncertainty for fear of appearing weak. The therapist and client may collude to uphold the perfect therapist-client relationship. For example, if the perfect client falters or is not making progress, the therapist feels embarrassed or works extra hard to get her on the right track. Or, it may be difficult for the therapist in this type of relationship to prescribe a relapse to the client.

### The Overprotective Therapist-Client Relationship

Clients from overprotective families have had lots of practice taking care of others and avoiding hurting family members, especially mother and father. Therefore, these clients may not let the therapist know when things are difficult, worrying that this information could hurt or offend their therapist. Clients can get sidetracked by working towards recovery for the therapist, for the family, but not for themselves. We have also seen the situation in which the client's attempts to take care of the therapist have been an indirect pull for the therapist to take care of the client. This is not surprising, given the level of ambivalence about dependency in these families.

*The Chaotic Therapist-Client Relationship*

Trust is the most salient therapist-client issue with clients from chaotic families. This client is used to feeling that the only one she can count on is herself (even though she does not even trust herself). Therefore, she will have a difficult time asking for help, may need to take breaks from therapy for fear of getting too close or developing a dependence on the therapist or therapy, or may act in ways to test the limits of the therapist's "caring" for her. Testing the limits may occur in breaking treatment contracts, coming late to sessions, or missing sessions. The therapist can be overprotective of the chaotic client because of her often sad and traumatic history. While the client may want this protection, this degree of caring scares her away from therapy.

## PREMATURE TERMINATION

All bulimics entering therapy are ambivalent about giving up their bulimia. This ambivalence can be reflected in the client's history of premature terminations from therapy and "therapist shopping." It is important for the therapist to note that the bulimic's "therapist shopping" can be legitimate, given a history of bad experiences with therapists. Shopping may reflect these experiences rather than ambivalence about therapy or fear of commitment. The likelihood of premature termination can be significantly decreased if the therapist is aware of the client's past patterns in relationships, previous therapy experiences, and readiness for therapy.

In a study by one of the authors (Root, 1983), factors related to premature termination from time-limited group therapy were explored. These factors appear to be relevant for clients who prematurely terminate from individual treatment as well. The clients who dropped out of treatment were younger, less isolated, and bulimic for shorter time. Additionally, these clients perceived themselves to be heavier and had more frequent episodes of bulimia per month. In summary, it appeared that those clients who dropped out of treatment were the most ambivalent about giving up their eating disorders. They had not reached the chronic stages of bulimia; i.e., they still had many friends and received much reinforcement for any weight loss.

*It is important to conduct a consultation to assess the bulimic's readiness for therapy.* This consultation can address several questions:

1) Is the individual willing to risk gaining weight in order to recover?
2) Has she told anyone about her bulimia?
3) Is she aware that her bulimia is more than a food or weight problem?
4) Is she willing to involve significant others in her therapy if necessary (e.g., partner or family members)?

Affirmative answers to these questions indicate her readiness for therapy.

During the consultation the therapist should evaluate the client's treatment history. How and why did the previous therapy end? This is important information that the therapist can use to help the client become aware of the patterns that characterized her earlier termination(s). The therapist can discuss with her what those are, how the two of them would recognize them if they emerged again, and even contract to discuss these patterns as they emerge in this new therapy relationship. The therapist can also provide information to support the client's right to terminate at any time, with some guidelines on how to do it (e.g., taking two sessions to terminate).

Because of the difficulty bulimic families experience in resolving conflict, expressing feelings, or dealing with loss, the bulimic has rarely had positive experiences or practice in ending relationships. Taking a history of separations and endings (e.g., leaving home, going away to college, getting married) provides information useful for anticipating likely times for her wanting to leave therapy. The therapist can talk about the risks the client might have to take in therapy, e.g., looking at family relationships and past experiences, and the reasons the therapist anticipates that the client might terminate early.

Clients from perfect families may terminate therapy after they have developed some tools and started to manage their bulimia because of the family rule, "You should be able to solve your own problems; going to therapy is a sign of weakness." Additionally, they may feel they are taking too long to recover. Being in therapy is uncomfortable for bulimic clients because it is a reminder that they are not perfect. It is important for the therapist to avoid a perfect recovery process with these clients.

Clients from overprotective families may terminate because they feel they are failing the therapist and perhaps wasting his or her time (protecting the therapist). If the therapist is reenacting dysfunctional family relationship patterns, she or he may insist that these clients stay in therapy, making the decision for them or rescuing them from themselves. If these relationship possibilities are talked about at the beginning of therapy, they are much more likely to be recognized early on, thus avoiding premature termination.

Clients from chaotic families may not be used to so much attention and caring and run from therapy for fear of closeness. They may also run for fear of rejection (better to leave than to get kicked out). Premature termination can be avoided by anticipating client's tolerance for therapy and planning breaks which respect those tolerance limits.

In general, premature termination can be avoided by assessing the client's readiness and tolerance for therapy. Providing realistic information about recovery, encouraging the client not to make a perfect recovery, and maintaining a clear sense of the therapist-client relationship will facilitate therapy.

## DETERMINING WHERE TO BEGIN

Treatment planning begins with a thorough assessment (see Chapter 11). Once the client has started therapy, a simple technique to determine a starting point is to have the individual write about the purpose of her bulimia. This technique is also an intervention, as it often helps the client become clearer about the purposes of her symptoms beyond "weight control." It can be used repeatedly throughout therapy as part of ongoing assessment, as well as to determine readiness for new phases in recovery or therapy as illustrated in the examples below.

This first example is from a young woman who was in therapy for the first time. The excerpt below was written after the second session and provides glimmers of understanding of the purpose of her symptom as it involves her interactions with significant others and herself.

> It helps me not gain weight. I don't want to gain weight and be fat. The world doesn't like fat people. I like having the pretty clothes and getting the attention I didn't used to get when I was fat. It also makes me mad that I have to do this to get all this approval. It satisfies my craving to be filled up. It also relieves my panic and anxiety after I've binged. It's like erasing my mistake and starting all over again.

The next example is by a teenager after five months of therapy. Her writing captures the intensity of her confusion and anger, her need for privacy, and her need to experience control and power in her life.

> I need something that is *mine* which no one can take away. Bulimia takes the place of being close to people because I don't trust friends to stay. Being able to eat bizarre amounts of food and still be thin gives me a feeling of power. I need that feeling because of things that happened over which I had no control, like being raped and years of being a misdirected parcel between my parents' homes.
>
> There are so many feelings within me that I am afraid to let out because there isn't a safe place for them to go. Purging is a way of feeling that something is getting out of me. I wish there was a way to empty myself out completely so there is nothing inside. However, I don't always want to be empty because if I was I would need to binge. That's part of what is so changeable about bulimia.
>
> Sometimes I need to binge in order to give myself something that is mine. Food is there when I feel lonely or depressed. Bingeing is also a counterreaction to how little I eat the rest of the time. I don't know how to eat normally anymore.

The last example is from a 19-year-old woman who has struggled with depression and bulimia. As she describes the vicious cycle she experiences and the purpose it serves her, her understanding is clearly more complex than that of the previous two women.

Bulimia helps me to not think about my problems. I can block out reality and hide from the outside world. I plan out the best time for binges — this makes me feel like I have a friend and it gives me a way to block out all of my thoughts for a while. It's like getting drunk or high — but when I'm all done I feel worse, and even more worthless and out of control because I lost it again. By being bulimic I don't take risks so that I can't get hurt. The overprotection of my bulimia then turns into other problems, and that's where my depression arises from. The conflict turns into a matter of control, or moreover, a lack of control.

This lack of control is only known to me though. Others around me see me as a person who really knows what she wants. Only I know that that isn't true. My bulimia covers up the vulnerability that I am afraid to express.

The examples above, from different individuals at different points in therapy, are marked by a decreasing dissociation from their symptoms. The woman who had just started therapy demonstrates by her language that bulimia is something separate from her. Bulimia is an "it." The other two individuals write about their bulimia as part of them. The therapist's assessment of the client's ownership and recognition of her symptoms allows for differentiating stages in therapy and determining the client's readiness for certain work. For example, the first woman quoted is not ready to begin giving up her symptom, but needs to focus on her lack of trust in relationships and feelings of powerlessness. In contrast, the third woman has some control over her symptoms and is ready to be more active in replacing her bulimia. In all cases, in order to begin controlling her symptoms, the individual needs to own her symptoms. Without ownership there is no control.

## SYMPTOM CONTROL

Symptom control or relief of bingeing and purging is the goal of most individuals and families seeking therapy. Some focus on the symptoms helps the therapy to make sense and is an important aspect of joining with the individual, family, or couple. If therapy does not make sense and the individual is not experiencing any change or relief, she will terminate shortly and look for some other type of help.

Most people cannot change their symptoms permanently without changing dysfunctional patterns in their relationships, lifestyle, or internal self-talk. While most people are ambivalent about giving up their bulimia, there must be a part of them that is motivated to give up their bulimia in order to begin working on symptom control with any chance for success. A simple and crude technique for assessing the client's ambivalence is as follows:

I know you are not sure about giving up your bulimia. To start controlling your bulimia you don't have to be 100% sure you want to give it up — but it doesn't make sense to proceed if we're both destined to battle with most

of your effort directed towards keeping your bulimia. Really think about it:
What percent of you *feels ready* to give up your bulimia?

We don't proceed with interventions to actively reduce bulimia unless the
person feels more than 50% ready. The therapist must also assess the degree
to which the family is ready to let go of the bulimic symptoms. If the
therapist determines that the family is set on keeping the individual bulimic,
this will help him or her set realistic expectations about symptom control
with individual therapy.

We follow four rules in helping people manage their symptoms. The
client's readiness to agree to some of these rules also helps us assess her
readiness to eliminate her symptoms. The rules are:

1) We never take responsibility for the bulimic's behavior. Even if we
   introduce symptom scheduling, the choice is always left to the client
   (see symptom scheduling below).
2) We never tell the bulimic she cannot binge or purge.
3) We do not ask the bulimic to monitor her food or calories.
4) We ask people not to "diet" while in therapy.

Below we outline several interventions we use to facilitate clients' control
over bingeing and purging symptoms.

Binge-purge behavior does not reflect a lack of willpower, as many individuals and families think it does. There are several things that set a person up to binge. Symptom control starts with education:

1) We educate people about the effects of dieting and how dieting actually facilitates weight gain. We provide bibliotherapy to help clients understand why dieting works against them and sets them up
   for bingeing (Schwartz, B., 1982).
2) We help people develop a vocabulary of feeling words (at least 75).
3) We ask people to write down what they are feeling before they binge
   (other than a conflict over whether or not to binge) in a journal
   specifically designed for increasing symptom control (Root & Fallon,
   1983c).
4) We ask people to be responsible for the part of their behavior they
   can control, such as cleaning up after themselves and replacing the
   food they have used for bingeing when they are living in a group
   situation.

Most people can accomplish the beginning steps of symptom control
within four weeks. By the time this control has been accomplished, two

things have usually happened. The therapist has joined with the client and the client feels more hopeful. As individuals demonstrate readiness, we introduce the intermediate steps:

1) We have people continue with monitoring their feelings associated with bingeing and/or purging.
2) Next, we introduce a cognitive component to treatment, which we will subsequently integrate into the family therapy at a distance. This involves introducing a set of beliefs common to bulimics. We help clients connect their frequent beliefs with the feelings they experience associated with bingeing and purging, such as depression, anxiety, hopelessness, responsibility, and frustration.
3) We encourage clients to develop alternatives to address the specific feelings they experience. For example, if they are tired, it would be reasonable to consider taking a nap, listening to music, or taking a bath. This intervention helps clients understand that there will not be a single alternative to replace bulimia.
4) We ask people to use the alternatives they have developed to delay a binge. Credit for successfully *delaying* a binge further supports movement away from all-or-nothing thinking commonly seen in bulimics.
5) We teach a brief relaxation method that can be used routinely, and as an alternative for different feelings. However, therapists should be aware that clients who have been victimized usually have difficulty with exercises or interventions which require them to close their eyes.

The time it takes for the individual to accomplish intermediate symptom control varies widely. If the individual has a difficult time controlling symptoms following the steps outlined above, we then have more leverage and incentive to explore other issues, such as the role of her bulimia in her family. We may intervene by asking the client to refrain from any further attempts towards symptom control. This may be the point at which we suggest another modality of treatment, such as family or group treatment.

Usually, by the time clients have demonstrated intermediate symptom control, they are also less depressed (because the cognitive component of symptom control simultaneously targets depression) and more confident that they will be able to get their behavior under control. Most frequently, their bulimia has decreased in intensity, as well as in frequency. They are encouraged to continue developing and using what they have learned from the previous two stages of symptom control, as the following steps are added:

1) They learn to predict and anticipate binge-purge situations by anticipating the feelings they are likely to experience in certain situations or with certain people.
2) They engage in planning alternatives to bulimia to deal with upcoming stressful situations.
3) When they have eliminated the symptoms, we may have them plan a relapse to confirm or disconfirm their symptom control.

The first two interventions require that the individual own her bulimia rather than dissociate herself from it. The planning and foresight reinforce the notion that the individual does have control over her bulimia.

An additional intervention for symptom control that we have found useful, though not appropriate for every client, is symptom scheduling. This intervention requires at least intermediate symptom control skills. There are many variations on this, including having clients plan bulimic days, e.g., Monday, Wednesday, Friday, and Saturday, or schedule binge-purge episodes within a day, e.g., they can choose to binge or purge from 2 to 3:30 in the afternoon. The effectiveness of symptom scheduling rests in clients' planning and awareness of their behavior, as well as the permission to have bulimic episodes.

After a client has achieved responsibility for her symptoms cognitively and behaviorally, i.e., she talks of "my bulimia" rather than "it" and cleans up after herself or replaces depleted food supplies in the group living situation, we consider the usefulness of a nutritional consultant. It is important that the nutritionist has experience working with clients with bulimia and anorexia nervosa. Working with clients with compulsive or overeating problems is not the same.

Many times the nutritional consultant is brought in for people who have had bulimia for over 10 years or have had their eating disorder since their early teens. The bulimic may need help to learn what constitutes a normal portion of food. In most cases, however, the bulimic is often cognizant of normal portions for others; her difficulty is in applying the same rules to herself.

When the individual has developed the skills associated with advanced symptom control, she has all the tools she needs to eliminate the simple habit part of bulimia. However, she will not necessarily have eliminated her binge-purge behavior. For example, a person may have her symptoms under control except for when she goes home to visit her parents or housesits for them. By looking at the types of situations and feelings that are most difficult for the individual to handle, the therapist is able to further explore relationships and patterns that contribute to the maintenance of bulimia.

## CONNECTING THE SYMPTOMS AND THE INDIVIDUAL

Most individuals entering therapy experience their bulimia as something that takes them over (powerlessness), over which they have little control (helpless), and which is alien to the way they see themselves in other aspects of their life (dissociation). Much of what the therapist can offer in individual therapy is to help a client connect her symptoms to herself so that she is not "victimized" by her bulimia. The simple interventions and guidelines offered below will help individuals to understand their bulimia as part of them.

### Facilitating Ownership of the Problem

Symptom control cannot be achieved by the individual until she has accepted responsibility for her behavior. By facilitating ownership of bulimia, the therapist empowers the individual. Additional attention to the internal dialogue and beliefs of the bulimic can provide her with increased control over her experience and greater understanding of her feelings, especially depression. A client wrote the following passage in response to the homework assignment to write about how she got herself depressed. This young woman had learned tools for cognitive restructuring and had tools for symptom control, but nevertheless would slump into very deep depression, which contributed to a vicious cycle involving her bulimia.

> It happens so frequently that I should actually realize exactly how I do it. I start with focusing intensely on the negative and bad aspects of my life. I then look at others and focus on their good qualities. I then proceed to compare myself (my bad qualities) to the others (their good qualities) and it ends up that I see myself as a nothing who really isn't going anywhere. I then start thinking so much about my own worthlessness that I can't really find any hope to go on.
> I say mean things to myself and I don't care about what happens to me. I feel like I have absolutely no control at all because I can't stop throwing up—I feel like an imbecile because I don't even know how to eat right. I ask myself why I'm doing this and I can't find an answer. I feel really sorry for myself and moreover, I feel sorry for the people that have to live with me—and then I really hate myself. I pretend that my life is great. I don't tell my family or friends how I feel when I'm depressed. I let them know by the messy room and all my time spent in my room and the bathroom. I cut myself off from friends and stay by myself for a while—sometimes days, sometimes weeks. I call myself names like "fat ugly pig." All I think of is food, food, food.

### The Cognitive Set of the Bulimic

Bulimics and their families share a dichotomous style of thinking which reflects the rigidity of their rules and all-or-nothing thinking. This style sets up a very narrow, unrealistic view of the world, others, and self. The bulimic's rigid beliefs are derived from the culture and from family messages that have been handed down in the socialization process. Family messages for each of the family types are outlined in Chapters 8, 9, and 10. The set of bulimic beliefs that we work with, discussed below, are derived from Ellis and Harper's (1974) irrational beliefs, Beck's (1976) cognitive therapy for depressed persons, and work with bulimic clients (see Table 6).

The bulimic beliefs are introduced as a set of beliefs commonly held by persons with bulimia and depression. The client is asked to pick out two or three of her most commonly used beliefs. Next she is asked to think and feel what feelings are likely to accompany her beliefs. For example, with the first belief, "I must be approved of by everyone for everything I do," clients may recognize accompanying hurt, rejection, anxiety, insecurity, and dependency. She is likely to be hypersensitive and exhausted and to feel failure in trying to please everyone all of the time. This may be the client's first experience understanding how her beliefs moderate her feelings.

Most clients are intrigued by the relationship of their thoughts to their feelings. This linkage can be a tool for empowerment. As she becomes clearer about the messages she gives herself, she can start to challenge them and replace them with healthier messages.

## CONNECTING THE FAMILY TO THE SYMPTOMS

Connecting the family patterns in relationships to the bulimia is necessary for the individual therapy to be systemic. This is an ongoing process that the therapist must teach the client. Questions such as, "Who would suffer most if you gave up your symptoms?" or, "Who in the family may need to have symptoms if you give up yours?" can intrigue the client and open the door to talking about symptoms of the family. Furthermore, these types of questions teach clients a way of thinking systemically about recovery. Clients from the perfect or overprotective families can have a difficult time with such questions, as they need to protect the family or uphold the image of perfection. However, if the therapist has been laying the groundwork by making observations about how the family and the bulimia might be connected, it is more likely that these questions can open up discussion.

Several simple interventions are used to help clients connect the patterns in the family with their symptoms. These include: family drawings, letters to family members, bibliotherapy, education on anger, and group therapy. With the exception of the family drawings (see Chapter 15), these are discussed below. With all these interventions it is important for the therapist to make observations and even predict changes in the client's bulimia (and depression) related to the work that the client is doing in therapy. For example, the therapist might repeatedly observe, "It seems that when your

TABLE 6
Bulimic Beliefs

1. I must be approved of by everyone for everything I do.
2. I should be in control and competent at all times.
3. If things do not go as I have planned, I am out-of-control.
4. I have no control over what happens to me.
5. The past is all-important and determines my life. There is nothing I can do to change my life.
6. Bulimia is just a phase and will pass.
7. If people really knew me, they would think that I was a terrible, weak, uninteresting person.
8. I should appreciate what I have and consider myself lucky.
9. I should be able to satisfy my own needs.
10. I should be productive all of the time.
11. I am responsible for everyone's feelings.
12. I should be considerate at all times.
13. I am destined to be miserable.
14. If anything goes wrong it is my fault.

bulimia gets worse, your parents fight less," or "It sure seems difficult to get attention in your family unless you're feeling miserable." Eventually, the client should be able to anticipate her own reactions and do her own predicting.

It is unrealistic to expect some clients to talk with family members about their feelings, particularly when there have been strict rules in the family about talking or when a parent has expressed anger explosively. The therapist can help clients prepare to break the code of silence by writing letters to particular family members that will not be sent or given to them. The letter can be a catalyst for jogging painful memories of abuse, neglect, and victimization experiences.

Anger is a difficult emotion for most bulimics to recognize in themselves, much less express. At the same time, most bulimics are very angry (or alternatively, very depressed). Work towards recognizing anger can be facilitated through education about how anger can simmer and boil, as well as how it is experienced and expressed. However, this is not beginning work. It is helpful for the individual to have some symptom control and understanding of her bulimia beyond a weight control tool before commencing intense work around anger, since there may be a temporary intensification of her bulimia. It is also important for the therapist to realize that the client from a chaotic family may have additional restraints on acting angry within the home. The therapist needs to provide additional information to this client to support her safety while helping her deal with her anger. Group therapy may be a more appropriate modality of treatment at this point.

A combination of experiential exercises and education can facilitate a client's awareness of her anger. For example, helping clients to identify how they physically experience anger increases their awareness of anger, while simultaneously helping them to connect more with their body. For example, one client, when asked to close her eyes and visualize the last interaction when she felt angry, was unable to do so, but reported a tightening in her chest and being close to tears when she was trying to visualize an incident. She was asked again to close her eyes and visualize her chest tightening and tearfulness. She eventually realized that she experienced these feelings when she was around her father. With repeated visualizations and descriptions of interactions with her father, she came to realize how angry she was at him, how demeaned she felt in his presence, and how the same feelings, in a slightly muted form, existed with her boss and boyfriend. Role-playing around expressing anger or difficulties doing so is helpful and can increase the client's sense of power. Group work can be particularly useful in giving clients permission to be angry.

Providing permission for the client to be angry is important because anger is part of the rebellion necessary for the client to psychologically and emotionally leave home. Part of leaving home involves separation, individuation, and rebellion (at least in this culture). However, for most bulimic clients rebellion and/or efforts to separate are not reinforced by the family. The therapist can reinforce and even encourage overt rebellious behavior, pointing out its positive aspects and relating it to the symptoms. Some clients need to learn how to be rebellious. Assigning acts of rebellion that are direct instead of covert, as their bulimia is, can be helpful. For example, one client, Jill, was uncomfortable with being "rebellious," so it was subsequently decided that she was to say "No" at least twice on odd-numbered days. As an overworked receptionist, she had numerous opportunities to do so, and reported a marked decrease in bulimic episodes on the odd days. This intervention helped to graphically portray for her the link between her bulimia and her lack of assertiveness.

## ENDING THERAPY

The ending of therapy symbolizes leaving home, growing up, being competent, and accepting the therapist's confidence in her recovery. Some clients (and therapists) may anticipate difficulty with this step and avoid dealing with the therapy relationship by terminating before they feel too dependent or too attached to the therapist. The way in which therapy is terminated is extremely important, as it provides an opportunity for a new relationship experience for the bulimic.

Most bulimic clients have a difficult time ending relationships because of the intensity of feelings associated with endings, the personal vulnerability they experience, memories of abandonment and loss, and/or past experiences of intense, unresolved anger associated with separation. The bulimic may have had very little control over the ending of previous relationships (as in the case of abandonment or loss), and the ending of therapy can challenge this feeling.

The decision to end therapy must be made by the therapist and client together. It is important that the therapist inform the client of her right to end therapy at any time. During the course of therapy, a delicate balance must be maintained between challenging the client who wants to end in a way that sabotages her work and supporting her right to end at any time. The following is from a client who ended therapy after 10 months. Both client and therapist agreed that it was time to end therapy, even though the client was not symptom-free. While the ending was also framed as an end to a phase of recovery, termination was conducted as though the client were not coming back, so that she was indeed free to leave therapy.

> I just have a lot of strong feelings about ending therapy. I know when I first started this all I felt real strange and I didn't want to become dependent on you; you know how I even brought up terminating a couple of times? It's like I was testing you to see what you'd do. The first time, I really couldn't believe that you weren't going to make me stay. I knew you wouldn't intellectually, but it was hard to believe emotionally. The second time was real hard for me because I wanted you to convince me to stay, almost as though this would prove to me that you cared. I was angry at first that you didn't try. I had to decide.
>
> But I am really sad to leave now even though I know it is time. Therapy has been a relationship like I've never had. I never thought I'd be able to have a relationship that I could trust. This has been the first relationship in which I felt that I really got listened to and respected. That's been important for me.
>
> You know how we talked that I might be holding on to my bulimia now so as to postpone ending therapy? I think you might be right. As a kid, I think some of my misbehavior was to hold my parents' attention. Part of me really doesn't want to end. Knowing that I can come back if I want helps, though. I am going to miss you.

This client's ability to express her feelings about termination was remarkable, given her chronic history of faded endings in relationships. Clearly, the therapeutic relationship had been beneficial.

Individual therapy is the most common form of therapy available to bulimics. It can be most helpful if approached systemically. The therapist needs to consider that recovery may entail taking breaks from therapy and changing modalities of treatment. Avoiding treatment failures requires attention to the therapist-client relationship and an anticipation and awareness of the issues that are likely to arise in the therapy.

# CHAPTER 14

# *Couples Therapy*

COUPLES THERAPY IS a possibility for any bulimic patient who is in a long-term relationship. We have found couples therapy to be very useful as either an adjunctive or even primary therapeutic modality. To treat the married bulimic client individually for her entire course of therapy denies the system of which she is a member. While within our framework even individual therapy is systemic, the availability of a partner and the additional opportunities that affords should not be overlooked. In this chapter we present the systems framework that informs the therapist and keeps the focus on the interaction of the couple. However, the actual techniques are borrowed from behavioral, strategic, structural, and family-of-origin approaches.

Here we address three issues: First, we discuss themes common to bulimic marriages and offer some suggestions for how to intervene in each of these areas. This is followed by a section on decision-making as to when couples therapy is useful. Finally, we present some considerations on how best to combine individual and marital/family therapy and the potential problem areas.

## THEMES COMMON TO BULIMIC MARRIAGES

The themes common to bulimic marriages parallel those issues that are discussed in the chapters on family types (see Chapters 8, 9, & 10). In fact, marriages will reflect or be a reaction to the family typology. For example, the individual from the perfect family marries the perfect partner, and they appear to have little or no conflict. Thus, they continue the family-of-origin rules. On the other hand, an individual from a chaotic family may duplicate the chaos and unpredictability in her relationship or strive for the opposite, which can result in a brittle perfection or overprotectiveness of children. The individual from the overprotective family often marries a partner who continues taking care of her and treating her as younger than her years.

Broadly speaking, two of the most common issues in bulimic relationships are power and intimacy.

*Power*

When we speak of power issues, we are speaking about a systems characteristic that is synonymous with the concept of hierarchy as it is used in structural family therapy (Minuchin, 1974). The parental/marital subsystem is assumed to be farther up the hierarchy than the child(ren) subsystem, and within each subsystem hierarchical differences exist. It is rare in clinical settings to see an egalitarian marital relationship. What is more common is for the bulimic partner to be lower in the hierarchy, at least overtly. The bulimic partner is viewed as less competent in one or more areas significant to the relationship. For example, one couple presented because the wife had been told it was fine to get pregnant by both her husband and an M.D. Although she was objecting, she was unsure that was her prerogative. The maintenance of the bulimic symptom perpetrates this inferior status. However, as communication theory so clearly illustrates, communication occurs on more than one level simultaneously (Watzlawick, Beavin, & Jackson, 1967). Consequently, it is not unusual for the bulimic partner to be competent in ways that both members choose to ignore, e.g., the wife is making significantly more income than the husband or the husband is seriously depressed and frequently suicidal. To recognize this competence could challenge the balance of power in the relationship.

In part, the power differential is a caricature of traditional marital relationships, with the male partner viewed as more powerful. The sociocultural influences inherent in the etiology of bulimia, which support women's being in a less powerful position, do not stop with the individual and do affect marital relationships. In systemic terms, the one-down position of the bulimic spouse serves a system-stabilizing function. What would otherwise be a tenuous relationship can maintain homeostasis and continue indefinitely — as long as both parties agree that all problems in the relationship are a direct extension of the wife's bulimia. Meanwhile, the husband's frequent job losses, gambling losses, and excessive drinking are ignored. It is not uncommon to hear statements such as, "He married me despite knowing I had bulimia — I can never thank him enough for that." Another woman failed totally to recognize how controlling her husband was and obsessed about suicide as being the only way to "release him from my bondage."

A particularly disturbing, and surprisingly common, power imbalance is manifested in the battering relationship. Bulimic women are frequently

groomed as "victims." Prior experiences have reinforced feeling powerless
and helpless, a victim stance. In a research sample (Root & Fallon, 1985),
more than 20% of the women had been physically battered in relationships.
While that might be expected in the chaotic families, the disabled, enmeshed
style seen in overprotective families seems also to facilitate its expression.
Anger and violence serve almost a differentiating function. Yet the result
is reached at too high a cost.

For example, Zach and Marcy would begin a cycle of intense closeness
and shared activities that would persist until, from their perspective, "We
were living inside each other's heads." Both would begin to underfunction
at work, and Marcy's bulimic symptoms would increase. Zach would drink
too much, strike Marcy, feel remorseful, and for a brief period, Marcy would
be symptom-free and both would get caught up in their jobs again.

Another common arena where power imbalances are seen is with the
eating disorder. For example, during an initial consultation with a recently married couple, it came to light that the husband would follow his wife
into the kitchen, restrain her from entering the bathroom to purge, and dictate what she would eat when the two went to a restaurant. Both reported
this as positive and desired behavior, neither could understand why the rate
of bingeing/purging was increasing, and both were convinced that, if the
husband stopped being controlling, the rate would increase. The two of them
had struck a delicate balance between her competence on the job and his
current underemployment by colluding to allow him to appear competent
and her incompetent at home.

What this particular case so clearly suggests is that power imbalances are
not necessarily what they overtly appear to be. The more likely scenario is
for the two parties to have worked out a carefully choreographed dance that
on an overt level allows the husband to appear elevated in the hierarchy,
but on another level is extremely discordant from the first and involves the
wife's parenting the husband. The discordance parallels the discrepancy between job competence and eating imcompetence that we see in our clients.

*Intimacy*

Power imbalances directly relate to the expression of intimacy in bulimic
marriages. What do we mean by intimacy? One way to conceptualize this
is to consider a continuum that is anchored on one end by total separation
and on the other by total fusion and loss of identity. Optimal levels of intimacy occur in those relationships where individual identity needs and interpersonal connection needs are both being met. Kegan (1982) explains it
as an evolutionary process where the individual, over the course of the life
span, alternates between the poles of inclusion and autonomy until even-

tually achieving a developmental level that is labeled "inter-individual." "Individuals and couples evolve not only to that place where each can guarantee to the other his or her distinct identity but which allows persons to share their identities as well" (p. 253). In general, bulimic couples appear to occupy one or the other of these extremes of closeness or distance. As Ackerman (1980) states eloquently, they establish "an early pattern of alternating extremes of intensity" (p. 159).

Traditional psychology equates maturity with a state of independence and autonomy and represents the male emphasis on differentiation. Feminist psychology (Gilligan, 1978) argues that integration gets demeaned by calling it dependency and immaturity. We have been impressed with the creative resolutions these couples have achieved that help to "regulate" how intimate or distant they are. The resolution achieved by bulimic couples tends to be one of three types: 1) rigidly overinvolved or a pseudo-intimacy; 2) rigidly distant or a pseudo-distance; and 3) a more variable fluctuating between closeness and distance. The first two types do seem to be somewhat similar to Wynne's (Wynne, Ryckoff, Day, & Hirsch, 1958) description of pseudo-mutual and pseudo-hostile couples. In each of these cases, some homeostatic balance has been achieved and the systems tend to be stable.

Various patterns or rituals serve as "emotional distance regulators" in bulimic couples. The rigidly overinvolved couple usually has a partner with a history of being in an enmeshed relationship in his or her own family of origin, and both are frequently able to create a closeness by banding together against a common enemy, e.g., mother-in-law who rejects their marriage. When the fusion becomes uncomfortably distant, the mother-in-law can be counted on to behave in a way that restores homeostasis.

Partners who are more rigidly distant often have clearly separate lives and use work or family most commonly as their primary source of emotional support, thus allowing for their "closeness" to be more superficial and transient. With these partners, the families of origin tend to be described as either perfect or chaotic — both family types where emotional distance is often the norm.

The more variable couples alternate between these extremes of closeness and distance. Enmeshment is the rule, but both the bulimia and frequently substance abuse and/or battering serve as the "regulators" to this overinvolvement.

The particular issue that one couple chose to use as a distance regulator was the issue of whether or not to have a child. (Other issues had served in this role before, and we want to remind therapists that the content of the issue varies widely but the process of distance regulation is very similar.) The husband, Harry, pretended he did not want a child when the wife, Charlene, expressed her noninterest. However, he covertly undercut his verbal statement with his comments about his nieces and nephews, although, when challenged, he replied that these were simply the comments of a loving uncle. Charlene saw that she would have to "give up" her bulimia if she decided to get pregnant and, in addition, "give in" to her husband's indirect requests and also her mother's request for grandchildren. At this stage in therapy, Charlene still felt that if she went along with someone's request, she lost her identity with that person and so her only recourse was to be noncompliant in almost everything. When Charlene finally resolved her bulimia and announced she wanted to get pregnant, Harry brought up the issue of finances and their inability to afford a child. This infuriated Charlene, who announced she wanted a divorce; then, when Harry backed off from his stance in a conciliatory move, Charlene accused him of being too untrustworthy to be a father but made no moves to divorce or separate. This unhappy balance remained for several months, with each party responding in a complementary way to the other's moves.

This couple did vacillate to a considerable degree between closeness and distance. In fact, a breakthrough was achieved when both finally were able to express that they enjoyed some alone time and to accept that as an acceptable component of their relationship, rather than to deny it and strive for an ideal that seemed equivalent to fusion.

Related to intimacy is the issue of expression of feelings. This is commonly seen as a problem area in families with a member who has an eating disorder. Even where feelings might be expressed, e.g., chaotic families, they often are not resolved or used as an avenue towards change. Enmeshed couples equate intimacy with a narrow, measured expression of feelings, with negative, hurtful comments edited out; if there are negative comments, both collude to frame them as "loving." We have all heard the following, "If I didn't love you, I wouldn't say this . . . ," or, "This is hard to say, and maybe I shouldn't say this, but . . . ." This is a common preface in the enmeshed bulimic couple's complaints.

## INTERVENTIONS

We are not wedded to any particular couples therapy style or approach. We are quite different as therapists and have very distinct styles. To be successful with a variety of clients demands the use of a variety of techniques. There are, however, some approaches that seem to be very useful when doing dyadic therapy where one partner is bulimic. Below we discuss some general guidelines from which we derive more specific techniques. Each of these seems to address some of the issues identified in the previous section.

*Rebalancing*

One general approach can be called rebalancing the relationship. This is directly reflective of the power imbalance mentioned earlier in this chapter. One member of the dyad (almost always the bulimic partner) is frequently reviewed as sick or dependent and hence the relationship is "unbalanced." The earlier the non-bulimic partner is included in the therapy, the easier it becomes to tip the hierarchy and allow a more egalitarian relationship to emerge.

A technique that is very effective is the use of a reframing or relabeling process. This technique, developed by strategic therapists, requires the therapist to place a different "frame" around a behavior so that the system understands it differently. Because our perceptions of another's behavior dictate our actions and reactions, a reframing of those perceptions can bring about a marked alteration in a couple's interaction.

We have found reframing to be incredibly powerful and useful from the very beginning of the therapy. It might be useful to begin with some simple examples. In a case presented in *Psychosomatic Families* (Minuchin et al. (1978), an anorectic adolescent is viewed as "bad" by the family, but Minuchin reframes her behavior as "stubborn." The difference between "bad" and "stubborn" is really quite enormous. The former implies hopelessness, and the latter implies that the daughter is willful and requires the parents to be more willful.

Let's bring the example closer to the topic. Consider a young couple, described earlier, who has been married for less than one year. The wife is bulimic and a successfully employed professional. The husband is underemployed and depressed and attempts to control his wife's symptoms. After listening to the couple for the first 45 minutes and hearing the wife berate herself for harming this wonderful marriage because of her uncontrollable illness, the therapist stated, "You know, it's interesting to me that you describe yourself in that manner. I have given some thought now to your situation, and while I realize that this may sound farfetched, I'm wondering if you (the wife) aren't having some problems with being too successful — like it's impossible to think of yourself as successful personally and also professionally. I almost worry more about what would happen if you didn't have bulimia. Not only does keeping track of your bingeing give Jim something to do, but I don't know too many couples, even modern ones, that know what to do with a wife who's more successful than her husband. I'm not necessarily saying that's true of you, but it is certainly a thought."

The rather complicated and lengthy nature of the reframing and the therapist's disclaimers embedded within it made it difficult for the couple to undo it, particularly since it was given toward the end of the session. The result was that for these spouses, it brought into the open their style, where overtly the husband appeared in control but covertly the opposite was the case. Another reframing the following session challenged the wife to "quit acting as if her husband couldn't handle her success — he doesn't look as if he needs protecting." This more than anything exposed the underlying conflict, and the couple had the first of many dialogues about her anger at his not working at her level and thus preventing her from taking time off to have children, and his anger at her putdowns of him and her sexual inhibitions. The desired goal of redistributing the symptom was achieved when the therapist ended the second session by stating that "it took a lot of bravery and trust in the relationship to get into these important issues and not get stuck just with the bulimia."

A strategic intervention, e.g., reframing, is not always necessary or appropriate. The more rigid the system, the more likely it is that we will use strategic techniques, e.g., symptom prescription. We choose carefully, and with some couples, we feel very comfortable about being quite directive in the session. We frequently will tell one partner to listen while the other talks, although even then a reframing is possible. Or, we thank a defensive husband for being defensive because it underscored that his wife was really serious about what she said and it gave her a chance to be assertive. Other directive interventions include having the couple contract for behaviors that are more respectful of each other's autonomy or power, e.g., the wife is directed to choose her own television channels.

Sometimes, a family-of-origin approach to rebalancing the relationship is very useful. This is particularly so when the partners appear very stuck and the therapist wonders where they learned this behavior. The couple is directed to examine how their relationship is the same and how it is different from that of their parents. This is not said in a pejorative way but matter-of-factly, with the expectation that it is natural for there to be both similarities and differences. Once they identify the similarities, we talk about it being very natural for them to exercise some options around which features they would like to preserve and which they would not. Inevitably, the partners do see parallels and then the therapist helps them redress those, again with a mixture of direct and/or strategic approaches.

Therapist: It seems like you are saying that Lee's questioning you about that sounds just like your dad.
Teri: Yes, it does, and then he wonders why I don't want to get close to him.
Therapist: Sorta like it's hard to be married to your dad.
Lee: But I want to help her out.
Therapist: Teri, have you ever tried to educate Lee how to be helpful in

a way that is different from your dad? It seems like he's motivated to do that—we can't deny that. And that's over half the battle. He just needs some lessons on the actual words and actions.

Physical abuse is frequently an issue in these couples and definitely demands rebalancing. A significant number of our clients report having been in a physically or sexually abusive relationship as an adult. The secretiveness pervasive in bulimia extends to physical abuse, and we have learned that this is something we must inquire about directly. This may be the most dramatic statement of an unbalanced relationship. It must stop if therapy is to continue. None of us has found that we could continue without such a guarantee from the abuser. What this necessitates in the therapy is a delineating the cycle of events that leads up to the abuse, making changes in this process, and also sometimes incorporating anger management techniques into the therapy at that point.

### Boundary Delineation

The issue of boundary delineation may be construed as very similar to rebalancing the relationship. For example, individuals with poor boundaries are going to act dependent and be one-down in a dyadic relationship. In all likelihood, they have been raised in families where individual identity was undervalued (most commonly overprotective and chaotic). Rebalancing the relationship includes delineating individual boundaries, redistributing power, supporting resolution of anger, and also reinforcing boundaries between the couple and their families of origin.

Sometimes the interventions used seem very concrete. For example, with partners who prided themselves on "no secrets," an intervention that proved to be quite successful was to schedule separate sessions and to have them arrive in separate cars. The husband in this case was quick to volunteer to "just sit outside the door," while his wife had her appointment. This offer was denied. Another quite direct intervention involves physical proximity. The seating arrangement in the room gives a sense of implied boundary and distance, as does helping them contract around personal space at home. When problems arise at home, we encourage them to tape their problem-solving efforts and bring them into therapy. This has a number of effects. In some sense, the anticipation of problems arising during the week is a symptom prescription and frequently has the effect of reducing problem frequency. Another effect is that the tape becomes the couple's "observing ego" and requires each one to do more thinking about the process as it is going on, since both know that they will be playing it back in the session.

Family-of-origin therapy has its place here also. A couple, both professionals, came in due to their ambivalence about commitment to each other. They were engaged but did not live together. The woman treated her bulimia as completely secondary and mentioned a six-year history only in passing. Recently, the man had had an affair that was discovered accidentally by the woman, who had a penchant for dropping in unannounced at his apartment. She would do this frequently and reported that the visits were in response to uncontrollable urges to see him and be close. The discovery of the affair created a resolve in the woman to prove she was better than the "other woman." Within a week, she promptly "discovered" the man again with the "other woman" and both expressed a lost of amazement that this still did not end the relationship. The man was unable to state directly that he wanted to end the relationship, so the session (our third) turned towards a discussion of "women in your family who chase after seemingly doomed relationships." The woman saw a parallel with her own mother's relationship to her father, whom she had married and divorced several times because of infidelity and alcoholism. She was told by the therapist that "Maybe there's still something you need to understand about your mother— this is one way for you to share a common experience. As your therapist, I certainly don't feel like I can say yes or no about ending the relationship." She responded to this reframing by spending the next several weeks ending the relationship and talking to her mother about her father, a previously forbidden topic of conversation. Her bulimia became a clearer focus at this time, when she commented how the frequency had reduced to less than one time per week now that the relationship was over.

A question that frequently arises when we consult with therapists has to do with the involvement of the spouse in the bulimia per se. For example, it is not uncommon for the husband to be a surrogate parent, superego, etc., to the bulimic, and this results in a highly controlling relationship. We actively discourage this type of involvement, seeing that more often than not the bulimia becomes a necessary boundary in these relationships and that it will not subside as a symptom when it is a primary focus.

Finally, boundary establishment frequently involves boundaries shared with family members. We have seen bulimic symptoms wax and wane in response to boundary violations by the family of origin. For example, one patient, fairly well stabilized as symptom-free, resumed a significant and daily rate of bingeing and purging when her mother moved to the city after her father died. The patient was married and an issue in the marital therapy had been her husband's depression, which the patient would assume as her own. Her mother was significantly depressed, and our patient had to learn all over again how to "shield" herself from her mother's depression and create her own time separate from her mother.

*Decision-Making*

In this section, we share some of our thoughts related to when and how to involve significant others in couples therapy. The options available to the therapist are to either involve the spouse in the first several sessions or to delay the couples therapy. By immediate, we mean somewhere within the first several sessions. For example, you learn either on the telephone when setting up the first appointment or in the first interview that the client is married, engaged, or in a committed relationship. She is clearly part of a dyadic system that is intense and needs to be considered in the treatment planning. Referring to the themes of bulimic marriages discussed earlier in this chapter, one realizes how essential this involvement will be. How do you decide whether to have the partner in or not? Let's first examine those characteristics that argue for immediate intervention.

*Immediate Intervention*

We have learned that there are several considerations that must be weighed very early in your history with the client. These are:

1) The degree to which the bulimia is out of control and/or getting worse.
2) The presence of concurrent couple problems that demand attention.
3) The involvement of the partner in the symptom. This is an indication of the absence of boundaries.
4) The degree to which the bulimic client is viewed as the "sick one" in the relationship.
5) The "ego strength" of the client. This may also reflect an ongoing battering relationship that needs immediate attention.
6) The availability of the partner for couples sessions.

Clients are going to vary widely in the degree to which their bulimia is interfering with their daily life. A recent client, married for over one year, began therapy bingeing and vomiting an average of six times per day and purging an additional one or two times. The daily frequency had been steadily escalating for the previous 10 months, and when she began treatment she was experiencing chills, had lost over 15 pounds in the previous four months, and was having regular dizzy spells. She had been bulimic for the previous seven years but averaged less than one binge/purge cycle per day for most of that time. A decision needed to be made. The remarkable increase in symptom severity seemed to be related to her marriage, although the client attributed it to a job change and a longer commute. Should the two of them be seen together or separately? Either format could allow for a preliminary focus on symptom relief. Over the telephone and in the first session (individual), the patient's description of her husband was positive, and he seemed to be generally supportive of her and not interfering or overly controlling. The decision was made to focus our attention on making the bulimia more manageable using individual therapy, and the husband was told by the therapist that his input would be needed in later sessions.

She was seen individually for 10 sessions. During this time, the binge-ing/purging was reduced to one time per day with the use of monitoring and hypnosis that reduced her anxiety. It did emerge that the bingeing/purging was directly related to fears that her husband would abandon her now that he was finally aware of how "awful" she was. In addition, her job change had resulted in a salary increase that exceeded his, and she perceived that both felt uncomfortable with this and were unable to discuss it. Now that she was able to be candid about her bulimia and was able to identify precipitants related to her fears of his view of her, the husband was invited into the therapy.

When her husband did come into therapy at session 11, the transition to marital therapy was fairly rapid. Although initially defensive, he was able to identify some of the problems she had earlier reported and began to acknowledge his role in them. *A key to his successful integration into therapy was the groundwork laid early on that his involvement was expected.* There was some initial difficulty with joining him and having him realize that the therapist could also be interested in his welfare, but overt demonstrations of empathy for his position facilitated his involvement. The two of them were seen for an additional 18 sessions. At termination, the wife had been binge/purge-free for three months.

What would have happened if the first session had been conjoint? This client was embarrassed about her bulimia and felt very vulnerable in the relationship. The efforts at getting her symptoms under control would have been diffused not only by her self-protective efforts, e.g., continuing to be secretive about her bulimia, but also by her protectiveness of her husband, e.g., trying to reassure him that he was not at fault and, in so doing, minimizing the severity of the problem. The fact that she came to see how the symptoms were related to the marriage during the first phase of therapy enabled her to get them under control and reinforced her resolve to involve her husband as soon as possible. Yet, given her protection of her husband, the way the bulimia kept her clearly one-down (balancing her salary in-crease), and her husband's personal strengths, a decision to initiate couples therapy from the very beginning could also be supported.

With another couple, immediate marital therapy began because the husband and then the wife called in the same day to express their panic at the seemingly irrevocable dissolution of their marriage. The bilateral concern from both husband and wife cemented the therapist's decision to begin marital therapy. The wife's binging and vomiting were escalating but problems with in-laws, finances, and a potential relocation of the husband were demanding immediate attention. With this couple, bulimia symptom management was secondary to helping them with decision-making around the relocation. The husband decided not to relocate after several sessions, and each was able to talk more candidly about the problems their respective mothers were presenting in their lives. For example, his mother was continually requesting sewing favors from the wife, a talented seamstress, and she was not only unable to say no to them but also unable to ask for fair remuneration. The husband had other complaints about his mother-in-law, and when each agreed that the other's position was equally valid, they were able to equilaterally set some limits with in-laws. During this time, self-monitoring of the bulimia was done irregularly, and the wife reported a significant reduction in the frequency. They terminated marital therapy after 11 sessions without any consistent focus on the bulimia symptoms, but yet there was clear progress in this area also. This was a case where the pressing marital issues were addressed initially with a marital focus. Not only did the couple request it but, referring back to our guidelines, concurrent couple problems demanded immediate attention.

In another case, the wife requested individual therapy for her bulimia and depression. However, at the initial telephone contact and particularly after the first session, the therapist expressed the desire to have the husband in the sessions as "a consultant." How was that decision reached? What unfolded during the first session was a scenario where the husband monitored the wife's food intake, followed her around the house to keep her from purging, and had taken to hiding certain favored binge foods in his car trunk. In addition, he would call her during the day to give her "pep talks."

The therapist made the decision that if the wife were seen individually, the therapist would be rendered useless by being caught in the middle of their controlling tactics. In addition, the husband was clearly involved in the symptom, and the wife's role as the sick one needed to be changed. During the initial conjoint session, after listening to the husband's concern about his wife and how his actions were prompted only by his love for his wife, the therapist complimented him on his love and also reminded him that sometimes the most loving thing a person could do was to let another person "find her own way." He agreed to a temporary moratorium on his activities, and the wife was told to test his love of her by really "making a mess of things during the next week." This symptom prescription created some increased differentiation between the two and a reduction in symptom frequency.

Gradually, it emerged that the husband's caretaking role with the wife was a mask for his own feelings of inadequacy as a graduate student on academic probation. This was in direct contrast to his wife's position as a highly successful CPA. The couple separated after seven sessions and both briefly stopped therapy. Two months later the wife returned to therapy. She had filed for a divorce and was determined to work out her feelings regarding the loss of the marriage and also to control her bulimia. In this case, then, clinical judgment regarding system interaction dictated conjoint sessions that prevented the therapist from being triangulated — a likely occurrence if individual treatment had begun. Individual treatment might have provided a temporary, unstable hiatus that marital therapy, with its greater intensity, did not allow to develop.

Discussing her binge/purge patterns is very difficult for the bulimic client. This seems to be more difficult in front of a spouse. Yet, when a husband calls to make an appointment for his "struggling wife, who is also so depressed," a decision must be made as to how to address the wife's obvious role as identified patient. A basic rule of systems therapy is to spread the symptom around to the other members of the system (Watzlawick et al., 1974). It is much easier to do that if a third person is present in the therapy sessions. However, this must be balanced by a careful consideration of how best to alter the identified patient's status in the relationship. The usual, most defensible position is to utilize couples therapy. Yet, on one occasion, I saw a client individually at an initial appointment that was supposed to be conjoint. Her fiancé was overbearing, dictatorial, and had forced her into therapy. He had agreed to come to the first appointment but was out of town on business for the first three appointments. The client used the sessions to discuss her ambivalence about the relationship and come to a decision to break the engagement. Seeing her alone had not reduced her identified patient role in her fiancé's eyes, but it had given her an opportunity for greater individuation and a chance to react to her situation in a more reasoned, mature way. However, her ability to reach that decision as rapidly as she did, on an individual basis, is unusual.

## Delayed Intervention

Each of the above rules/guidelines is useful to consider when deciding whether to delay conjoint treatment. Sometimes, marital treatment is delayed despite our wishes for it to be immediate. For example, a spouse may refuse, or a client may refuse to include a spouse at this point. You may feel that her problems warrant attention and since you have a relationship with her, you continue with treatment.

Whatever the reason, *your delaying marital treatment must be made with an appreciation of the systemic implications.* Clinical lore is clear that individual treatment of one spouse may distress a marriage or at least make the distress more overt. Individual treatment may also be the quickest route to maintaining the status quo in the system or preventing second-order change. Many of you know the feeling of seeing a client week after week with no change reported either in the symptom or in the barely tolerable marital relationship.

Delaying conjoint treatment may be a means towards clarifying a marital relationship or establishing a necessary boundary between the members of the marital dyad. The increased emotional distance that may result could be the precipitant to the couple's doing some changing in those areas that seem to perpetuate the symptoms, e.g., conflict.

While some therapists can facilitate rapid symptomatic relief and enhance marital relationships via immediate conjoint sessions, this may be more difficult for others. Finally, a reluctant husband may come to therapy only after concrete evidence that the therapist is competent; no amount of earlier cajoling or joining maneuvers will be successful at enlisting his involvement until his wife is noticeably improved symptomatically.

# CHAPTER 15

# *Group Therapy*

WE OFTEN UTILIZE GROUP therapy as an adjunct to family therapy, and in some cases as the principal modality of therapy in the treatment of bulimia While we do not intend to provide a comprehensive discussion of specific group treatment techniques, we will address a number of issues: therapeutic factors in group, indications and contraindications for group, facilitating family work in the group, sabotage, setting realistic goals towards recovery, and reducing dropouts from group therapy. This discussion will be illustrated with examples of family drawings and treatment interventions from a short-term group for bulimic women.

## THE THERAPEUTIC ASPECTS OF GROUP

Group therapy for the treatment of bulimia has been proposed by a number of researchers and clinicians (Boskind-Lodahl & White, 1978; Kirkley, Schneider, Agras, & Bachman, 1985; Lenihan & Sanders, 1984; Root, 1983). Group therapy has a number of unique therapeutic features, as outlined below.

Because the disorder has both psychological and physiological consequences, *education* can help the client to recognize aspects of her bulimia that are related to dieting behavior, as well as to assess the impact of her bulimia on her physical health. While we do not suggest that information alone will be enough to stop the behavior (unless the bulimia is solely related to dieting), education can allay client fears and anxiety. Yalom (1975) suggests that a lack of information can actually compound symptoms. We also offer information on the psychological aspects of the bulimia, including the experiences of "relapse" and "collapse" and of depression, as discussed later in this chapter.

194

In addition, group therapy can be a *cost-effective* way for clients to participate in therapy. While this should not be the primary reason for inclusion in group, it is sometimes an important consideration.

Yalom (1975) proposed unique curative factors associated with group therapy, including *hope, universality, and corrective emotional experience.* Without hope, clients rarely stay in treatment. In a group atmosphere, the members are able to hear the successes of others. Being hopeful reflects a significant change of cognitive state for many clients, who have been depressed and hopeless before the initiation of treatment. Universality, a concept that forms the foundation of many eating disorder support groups, allows the group members to share feelings, discover similarities, and reduce social isolation. A corrective emotional experience can occur in group when family roles are reenacted and worked through. Group offers a means of learning appropriate ways to resolve conflict, setting boundaries, giving and receiving feedback, and taking time for oneself. These are experiences that many bulimic clients have not had in their own families.

## INDICATIONS FOR GROUP TREATMENT

### Increasing Readiness for Family Therapy

Participation in a group can be an effective way to increase the readiness of the client for family therapy. The group can foster a climate in which the client is allowed, at her own pace, to look at the relationship between her family and her bulimia. Often clients, especially those from perfect and overprotective families, will initially strongly resist acknowledging the role of the family in the development and maintenance of the bulimia. The willingness of other group members to be less protective of family members can help such unwilling clients look at family issues and gradually make connections, as is illustrated in the treatment of the Long family in Chapter 19. We have seen many instances in which a client adamantly opposed to family therapy before group has become a strong supporter of family involvement by the end of the group experience. Group can also be a way to facilitate joining with a client or with the family. We often use the approach of combining group therapy with a series of family consultations.

### Working Through Victimization Experiences

The majority of bulimic clients have been molested, raped, or physically abused. The group provides a safe, supportive place to share and work through these experiences (although the work may occur metaphorically). Since others in the group have usually had similar experiences, they are able to understand and support the person who is talking. Common myths related to the victimization experiences are usually explored and challenged: "It is the fault of the victim," "She was asking for it," or, "The victimizer is not responsible for his actions." Challenging these assumptions and supporting the appropriateness of the client's anger in the group are essential.

## Providing Treatment When the Family Is Unavailable

The family may be unavailable for therapy due to several reasons: Parents have died, the family is geographically unavailable, or, particularly in the case of the chaotic family, parents are emotionally unavailable, e.g., because of alcoholism or depression. If the parents live some distance from the bulimic individual, it can be helpful to consider the possibility of group therapy along with family consultations. Often, therapists automatically assume that since the family lives out of town, this precludes family therapy. A consultation approach (see Chapter 12) combined with group therapy may be the treatment of choice.

Particularly with chaotic families, there is such disorganization and members are so needy that parents are emotionally unavailable for the children. To ask parents to participate in family therapy when they are unable to do so can lead to repetition of the patterns of emotional unavailability. The client may, in fact, find herself again taking care of her parents instead of getting what she needs. Group can be a place where she can get support, take time for herself, and begin to address the family issues in safe environment. Again, we suggest the use of concurrent family consultations, while warning the therapist to think this through carefully in terms of who is invited to the consultation.

## CONTRAINDICATIONS FOR GROUP

### Client Is Actively Abusing Alcohol

A number of clients with bulimia also have had or currently have alcohol or drug abuse problems. *If the client is actively abusing drugs or alcohol, this must be addressed first, before the bulimia can be treated.* If this is not done, the client is likely to increase her substance abuse when working on controlling the bulimia. In addition, the physical effects of alcohol dramatically decrease the efficacy of group treatment. If we have concerns or questions about substance abuse in a client, we will refer her for an alcohol/drug evaluation before acceptance into group.

## Group Would Sabotage the Family Therapy

In some instances, the involvement of a client in group might sabotage family therapy, especially if the family insists that the problem lies solely with the bulimic individual. If the family has been involved in family therapy, the therapist must be careful not to dilute the intensity of the family therapy by shifting too soon to group therapy. It takes careful assessment to determine whether group will increase the readiness of the client for family therapy, serve to facilitate the setting of appropriate boundaries, or, on the other hand, sabotage the ongoing family therapy.

## Client Is Too Different From Other Group Members

One of the therapeutic aspects of group is members' finding similarities among themselves. We have found that the risk of dropping out is increased when a client feels very different from others in the group. While this can be a common feeling among bulimics, we select the group members in a way that minimizes the obvious differences. Thus, we do not include males in our groups, or anyone who is a great deal older or younger than other members.

## The Client Is Not Ready for Group

Many clients, when first presented with the idea of group, express fear and hesitation. This is not a reason to exclude them from the group. However, if there are a number of signals which indicate that they have ambivalent feelings, the therapist should carefully consider the appropriateness of group. It may be that the client has been pushed into group therapy by the family and is an unwilling participant. In this case, it is unlikely that she will benefit from group treatment. Signals that the client is not ready for group include not returning telephone calls promptly to the therapist, canceling the screening session (especially if the client does not give a reason or does this more than once), taking a lot of time to return screening material, or verbally expressing hesitation about group a number of times.

Three minimal interventions we use to increase a client's readiness for group are 1) compliance with mail screening, 2) interview, and 3) wait-listing. If the client has invested time in filling out information, she is more likely to show up at group and less likely to drop out. In addition, an individual interview used as a prescreening for group increases commitment.

We have also found it helpful to put clients who are particularly ambivalent about group on a waiting list. Those who are still interested after the waiting period are less likely to drop out of the group.

In our groups, we include only clients who are currently bingeing and purging and who do not meet the criteria for anorexia. We exclude compulsive eaters, as well as those clients who are bingeing only and have not used purging techniques on a consistent basis. Our clinical experience has shown that the issues for compulsive eaters and anorectics differ, and other types of treatment or groups are indicated for these clients.

## REDUCING DROPOUTS FROM GROUP

Since this is a population that tends to terminate prematurely, the therapist must attend to ways to reduce dropouts from the group. We have been able to reduce our dropout rate to almost 0% by the following methods:

1) payment in advance for the entire eight-week group;
2) careful screening of potential group members;
3) setting realistic goals for group members;
4) discussion of sabotage;
5) providing tools for symptom control;
6) framing group as one phase of the work towards recovery.

While many of these ideas are discussed elsewhere in this chapter, two deserve further elaboration. We have found that requiring payment in advance for the entire group, as opposed to payment session by session, increases client commitment and decreases ambivalence. If clients pay by the session, they are more likely to miss a session or drop out of the group as the intensity builds. Framing group as one step in the recovery process can prevent clients from expecting too much or aiming for perfect recovery in eight weeks.

We encourage therapists who are planning to offer groups for their clients to carefully consider whether this is the appropriate treatment for the client. We have often seen members included simply because the therapist needed one more person to start the group. Including a member under these conditions is a set-up for premature termination.

## THE STRUCTURE OF THE GROUP

We spend a great deal of time screening potential group members, believing that the group can be set up to succeed or fail before the first member walks in the door for the first group session. The potential group member is asked to complete the BREDS (see Chapter 11) and the MMPI as the first step. Upon completion of these materials, the client schedules a screening interview. This session is used to assess the advisability of group therapy and to review relevant history. If it is mutually decided that the client will participate in the group, the client is given a journal in which she is to record thoughts, feelings, and situations related to her urges to binge and purge (Root & Fallon, 1983c).

Monitoring is a minimal intervention directed at decreasing dissociation of the client from her bulimia and increasing her awareness of patterns of thoughts and feelings associated with her bulimia. The client is asked to begin monitoring before the group starts, thus setting the tone for the cognitive work conducted in group. Oftentimes, this initial intervention has a positive effect, as noted by Kanfer (1975).

The client is also asked to set goals for group and to think of ways in which she might sabotage her work in group. Group members are asked to set three goals for the eight-week group, focusing on goals which are challenging but also realistic. We ask them to write down the goals and give a copy to the group leaders. We encourage realistic goals, stressing that what is realistic for one person may not be realistic for someone else. Some examples of realistic and unrealistic goals are provided in Table 7.

These initial goals are not set in concrete. Group members may decide to change their goals, to toss out ones that are not realistic, or to pursue additional ones. For the most part, the family work that is facilitated in group constitutes a substantial portion of therapy that is not set out in the client's goals. However, this is often the most important work of group, as one client relates:

> The most valuable part of the group experience for me was when we talked about families. I feel like, for the first time, I didn't present this perfect picture of my family. I was able to get mad and sad and the group was supportive. Hearing others talk about their families helped me to see how their bulimia was related and that made it easier for me to protect my family less than I have in the past. I know now that it will be important for my family to be involved in my recovery. Before group, I thought it was just me, just my problem.

An essential aspect of group is having members talk about ways in which they might sabotage their work in the group. We tell clients that all of them will sabotage their work in group in some way and ask them to talk about ways in which they will sabotage. Sabotage differs from client to client, and depends on family type. Sabotage and obstacles to treatment are discussed in length in Chapter 21.

The perfect group member may sabotage her work by not allowing herself

TABLE 7

Sample Goals

| *Realistic* |
| --- |

1) To eat a meal with friends.
2) To extend the period of time between binges.
3) To learn to determine when I am hungry.
4) To become aware of feelings related to my bulimia.
5) To give up my scale.
6) To say something positive to myself every day.
7) To reach out to others.
8) To go to the store for food without being anxious.
9) To better understand the purpose of my bulimia.
10) To take five minutes for myself every day.
11) To understand the relationship of my bulimia to my family.
12) To write in my journal *before* I binge and to make bulimia a choice.

| *Unrealistic* |
| --- |

1) To lose 10 pounds.
2) To stop eating sugar.
3) To stop bingeing and purging.
4) To stop wanting to binge and purge.
5) To run five miles every day.

to take time in the group and by refusing to admit that she has any "negative" feelings such as anger or loneliness. She may smile even though she is depressed or angry and miss a session if she has had a relapse in bulimic behavior. Often, she will report that everything is fine when it is not, since in the perfect family one is not allowed to feel anything but happy. She may feel guilty if she is not doing the homework assignments and miss the group rather than come "unprepared." She may not give herself permission to cry in front of others in the group.

The client from an overprotective family may pull for protection from the therapists and other group members as the intensity of the group builds. She may also try to rescue others from emotional intensity as she rescues her parents from conflict. As others talk about their families, she may try to point out the positive aspects of the relationship and smooth over the negative. It is likely that she will not take responsibility for either the changes in her behavior or the lack of movement. Wishful thinking that some event may happen to change her behavior is commonly seen.

The client from a chaotic family may feel very different from the others in the group. She may also "space out" when other group members express anger, since often her experience of anger has been violent and unresolved. Trust is extremely difficult; she may sabotage her work by being unwilling to trust either the group members or the leaders. Commitment is also difficult since consistency was lacking in her environment. This may be reflected in missing sessions or coming late to group.

Other ways in which clients may sabotage their work in group include: drinking before the group, not thinking about the group or doing homework assignments, focusing on weight as the only issue, focusing on being different from other members of the group, not allowing herself to feel or connect with others, or refusing to take time in the group. We encourage members to take the responsibility of confronting each other if they feel that someone is sabotaging. We also have members reflect on the ways in which they have sabotaged throughout the group, especially during the family work. Talking directly about sabotage from the beginning of the group can facilitate the work done in group and decrease the dropout rate.

The beginning treatment groups are eight weeks long and each member makes an advance commitment to attend all eight sessions. The group is closed to new members after the first session. Six to eight women are in the group and they are led by a female-female co-therapy team. Providing structure is very important, particularly in the beginning groups (Kirkley et al., 1985). Information is provided on the physiological aspects of the bulimia, tools for symptom control are offered, and the bulimia is linked to family dynamics. It is important for these areas to be addressed before moving into more advanced issues in recovery, such as body-image, sexuality, and relationships.

The work in the group is divided into three sections. In the first two sessions, members share goals, talk about ways in which they may sabotage their work, and receive information about the physical consequences of bingeing/purging and dieting. Building trust in each other and in the group leaders is an important aspect during this phase and continues throughout the eight weeks.

In the second phase of group, there is a focus on identifying thoughts, feelings and situations related to the bulimia, using a cognitive restructuring format and developing tools to manage bulimic behavior. A list of bulimic beliefs (see Table 6, p. 177) is used in this phase to help clients identify self-talk related to bingeing and purging. Later, when talking about families, clients are asked to relate the beliefs to messages that they received in their families. We have found that giving the clients some tools for managing their behavior is helpful before addressing the family work. The intensity and frequency of the bulimia often increases during the family work. We also begin to use prediction of the behavior and to relate these predictions to the family issues.

During the last half of the group, the focus shifts to directly addressing family issues. First, we describe the three family types and the relationship of birth order to vulnerability to developing bulimia. This introduction provides a fairly more structured, didactic approach to an intense subject. Clients are asked to share whether they can identify with any of the three family types and to briefly talk about the similarities. Then, to deepen the emotional intensity, we choose among several techniques, depending on the group. We may use family sculpting, letter writing to important family members, or family drawings. We have found family drawings to be a particularly powerful way for members to get in touch with issues in their families and will discuss this technique in more detail.

Members are asked, as a homework assignment, to draw a picture of their family. The picture can be set either in the present, or more frequently, in the past, when the client was growing up. We ask that family members be drawn "in motion," rather than simply as faces, or bodies in a row. Clients are encouraged to include all members of their immediate family, as well as any other important people (grandparents, aunts, uncles, etc.). Often when this homework is assigned, clients experience an increase in the intensity or frequency of the bulimia. When we assign the drawing, we also ask clients to predict how their bulimia may change and why. This supports the connection of the bulimia to the family issues. Clients are given time in the group to talk about their pictures and the way in which their bulimia is connected to their families. Figures 5, 6, and 7 are examples of client's drawings which illustrate the perfect family, the overprotective family, and the chaotic family. The next two drawings, Figures 8 and 9, were done by a client from a combined family type—both overprotective and chaotic. The chaos in this family is difficult to escape and leaving home comes at an incredible price. Recovery for this client has taken incredible effort.

Family drawings can be a powerful way to get in touch with family issues, both for the person who is drawing her family and for the other group members. The next step is for clients to talk about the ways in which the drawings will need to change in order for them to recover from the bulimia.

## TERMINATION

The time-limited aspect of our group allows clients to practice endings, something that many have not had a chance to do in their families. In addition, an eight-week group decreases the likelihood that clients will become dependent upon the group or the therapist and gives them the responsibility for progress towards recovery. We begin the process of termination in the seventh meeting by asking members, for homework, to assess how they have worked toward the goals that they set out in the first session. In the eighth

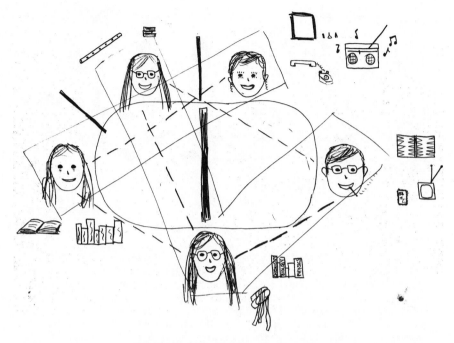

*Figure 5. A Perfect Family Drawing*

"Everyone in my family is always smiling, even when we are mad or upset. The way to tell us apart is by the things that we do. . . . I dance and study, my sister reads, my other sister plays the flute. . . . Mom and dad never talk to each other. Dad talks to me and my sister Fran because we are both planning to be doctors like him. Mom is always trying to get Ellen to talk more and be more outgoing. Sometimes, I feel like I am the conductor in the family because I talk to everyone but my mom. I think she gets jealous of my relationship with dad. He's always saying how proud he is of me."

session, each member is given time to talk about the work that she has done in the eight weeks. Members are also encouraged to give each other feedback in this session. It is important to stress that their work towards recovery does not end when the group ends. Rather, the ending of group reflects a change in the way in which they are working towards recovery. Thus, we also ask each member to think about her next step towards recovery. For many clients, this means family therapy or, if family therapy is not indicated, addressing family issues in individual therapy.

We offer two handouts at the end of the group to facilitate continuing symptom control. The first, "Relapse, Prolapse, and Collapse" (Fallon & Root, 1983), describes three experiences based on the way that the individual

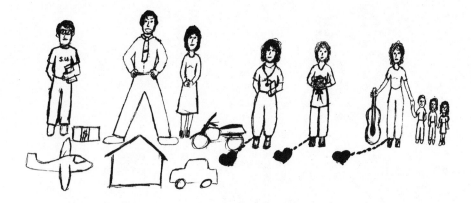

*Family Portrait*

*Figure 6. An Overprotective Family Drawing*

"I'm the youngest in the family, even though I am the only one that has kids (and is divorced). My dad is always upset about something, even though he is surrounded by his 'toys.' He and my brother are on one side of the family and we girls are on the other. Jack is the only one who went to college. We girls were supposed to find a good man and have kids. Even though I left home seven years ago, I'm still, like my sisters, bound to them by a chain and heart. They love us all so much. . . . We look independent on the outside, but I still feel attached. I've got to find a way to cut the chain and let go."

interprets urges to binge and purge. *Relapse* describes a temporary lapse into the old ways of behaving (i.e., bingeing and purging) but with the individual's having an understanding of the purpose of the behavior and being able to use the experience to gain new understanding of her bulimia. *Collapse* also refers to reverting back to bulimic behavior, but with little understanding for the reasons for the collapse. Thus, she may catastrophize and interpret one episode to mean that she will never recover. *Prolapse* is using alternative methods to cope with situations, thoughts and feelings related to the bulimia. Prolapse may involve identifying "warning signals" and predicting situations in which one is more vulnerable to bingeing and purging, using alternatives to feelings related to the behavior, or challenging bulimic beliefs.

The second handout, "Bingeing as a Learning Experience," encourages clients to ask themselves certain questions when they feel like bingeing and purging, such as "What are you thinking, feeling, and telling yourself?" Bulimia is framed as a choice; if they choose to binge, they are encouraged to learn from the experience, rather than to "collapse."

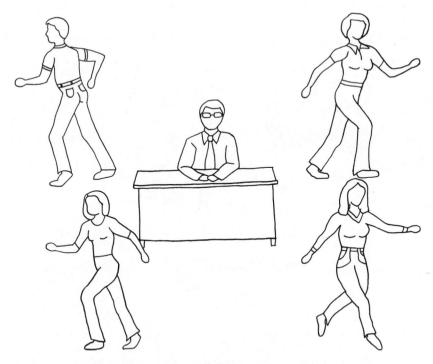

*Figure 7. A Chaotic Family Drawing*

"My dad has always been the central person in our family because everyone is so afraid of him. He used to beat up my mother — I can remember hiding under the covers, hearing her scream, and wondering if I would be next. He started molesting me when I was eight. He would come into the room that my sister and I shared and I'd pretend to be asleep. I was terrified that he would pick me. Looking back, I think that my mother knew that he was molesting us, but no one knew how to get away from him. The weird thing is that I still haven't really gotten away. He stopped molesting me when I left home, but now I work for him. We never talked about what happened; we both act like nothing happened. I know that part of my recovery will mean that I have to change jobs — and really get away."

These two handouts facilitate the continuation of the recovery process. In addition, we offer an individual follow-up session for the client to further reflect on her group experience, to obtain referrals for therapists, or to discuss her next step towards recovery.

Group can be a powerful vehicle to address family issues as well as to teach symptom control for the bulimic client. Mistakes are made in not screening carefully enough for the group or in becoming so invested in offering the group that members are accepted even if they are not appropriate.

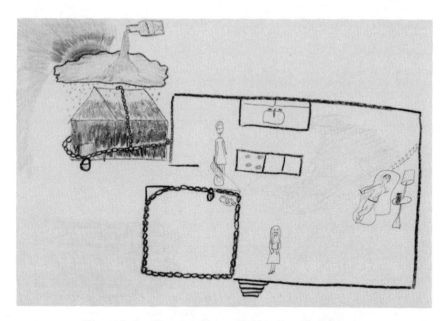

*Figure 8. An Overprotective-Chaotic Family Drawing*
"This is an outside and inside picture of my house. On the outside, the house is closed, locked up so that no one can get out or in. Alcohol pours all over the house, sealing us in as much as the lock that my mom puts on. Inside, my sister is getting ready to leave home. Even though I'm only two years younger, I'm trapped in my room, like a little baby. Dad is passed out from drinking and mom is outside my door, vacuuming. She would do that on Saturdays when she wanted me to get up. I couldn't leave the house so I felt trapped in my room. It felt like there was no way out. I don't know how my sister made it."

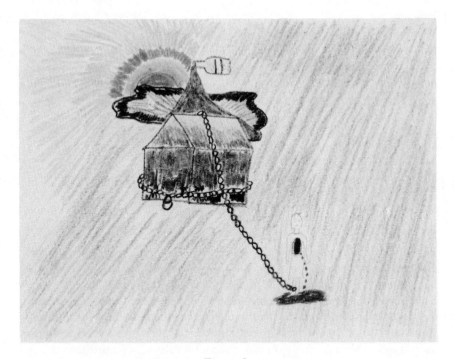

*Figure 9.*

"This is what it feels like now. I found a way out, but at a price. I had to break through the walls, but I'm still attached. I'm bleeding from the fight and now the alcohol is raining on me. I've been sober for two years now and at least I know that there is an inside to me, because I'm hurting. I still have to cut the chain and get out of the rain, over to the sun. I sometimes don't know if I can make it."

# CHAPTER 16

# Psychopharmacological Issues

BECAUSE OF THE POSSIBLE medical sequelae of bulimia, medical consultation is often advisable. The BREDS, described in Chapter 11, informs the therapist about the physiological symptoms the client is currently experiencing.

Psychiatric consultation, for the purpose of medication prescription, is a related issue. The medical model and the family systems model are presumed to be incompatible. Yet the current literature, both professional and popular (Pope & Hudson, 1984), makes a seemingly strong case for the use of antidepressant medication to treat bulimia.

This chapter has been written with two goals in mind. First, we want to increase therapists' awareness of currently popular drug regimens. We address this goal by examining the indications and contraindications for using medication with bulimic clients. Second, we want to emphasize that psychopharmaceuticals have systemic implications. Accordingly, we have included the summary of a very thoughtful and thorough letter written by a psychiatric colleague as part of a consultation with one of our clients. This letter illuminates the variety of issues that must be considered when making a medication decision.

However, before looking at these issues, let us briefly review the literature concerning the need for antidepressant medication with bulimia.

## BULIMIA AS AN AFFECTIVE DISORDER

The speculation that bulimia is related to major depression is based on several findings, including the frequency of concomitant depressive symptoms in eating-disordered clients, the response of some clients to antidepressant medication, client response to the dexamethasone suppression test (DST), and a higher family incidence of affective disorder in eating-disordered patients compared to control subjects (Altshuler & Weiner, 1985; Herzog, 1982; Hudson et al., 1982; Hudson et al., 1983). One hypothesis about the relationship is that eating disorders may simply be a variant of mood disorders; another is that eating disorders result in symptoms of mood disturbances.

Not surprisingly, as results from recent studies have been publicized, there has been increased interest in using antidepressant medication for treating bulimia. For example, in one uncontrolled trial (Glassman & Walsh, 1983), 10 of 12 patients demonstrated an impressive response to a monoamine oxidase inhibitor (MAOI), with reduction in both depressive and bulimic symptoms. In another study (Pope et al., 1983), imipramine was found to be superior to a placebo in the reduction of depression and bulimic behavior in a double-blind study of 22 bulimic women.

While the majority of bulimics, and especially those with a history of chronic bulimia, present with some depression, the exact nature of the relationship between depression and bulimia is not yet established. Some observations used to support the conclusion that bulimia is an affective disorder are not reliable indicators of depression. For example, the DST can be affected by low body weight (Gerner & Gwirtsman, 1981) and alcohol use (Swartz & Dunner, 1982). Stern et al. (1984) found no difference in the incidence of familial affective disorders between normal weight bulimics and a control group of women. Other studies have shown that antidepressant medications do not decrease the frequency of binge-eating or purging (Brotman et al., 1984; Kaplan et al., 1983). For example, in a study conducted by Sabine and colleagues (1983), a tricyclic (mianserine) was reported to be no more effective than placebo in the treatment of 40 bulimic women.

There is no research to date that has conclusively established that eating disorders are variants of mood disorders (Hatsukami, Mitchell, & Eckert, 1984). The depression and mood variations commonly observed in the bulimic are likely to be the result of cognitive patterns of thinking (Garner & Bemis, 1982), repressed anger (Root & Fallon, 1985), physiological starvation (Keyes et al., 1950), and powerlessness within the social system (Selvini Palazzoli, 1978).

Replicating the results of psychopharmacological research has not been easy. This difficulty may be due to the heterogeneous population to which the diagnosis bulimia is applied, as well as to flaws in research methodology. Follow-up with these clients has been minimal and frequently is compromised by the absence of objective or multiple measures.

Despite the equivocal findings, there is definitely an increase in the use of antidepressant medications with bulimic clients. We commonly hear from our patients that previous therapists have given them medications ranging from Lithium to MAO inhibitors to tricyclic antidepressants, with little or no effect on their bulimia. Given the equivocal nature of the research to date, and the fact that "everything that improves with an antidepressant is not depression" (Glassman & Walsh, 1983, p. 203), it is useful to consider how the nonpsychiatric therapist can best utilize psychiatric consultation when treating bulimic clients.

## INDICATION FOR MEDICATIONS

There are three situations in which psychiatric consultation for medication is indicated. However, let us emphasize that medication should not be the primary treatment of choice; also, before putting a client on medication the therapist should thoroughly read Chapter 21 in this book, where obstacles to treatment are discussed. Most often, the reasons therapy is stuck are related to problems in the therapeutic alliance and inexperience on the part of the therapist — not to the client's need for medication.

The first situation requiring psychiatric consultation is when the therapist becomes aware that the client has a history of recurring major depression occurring prior to the onset of bulimia. If therapy is not effective with either the bulimic symptoms or the depressive symptoms, and the therapeutic alliance with the client is well-established, a consultation with a psychiatrist experienced in working with clients with eating disorders may be useful.

A second situation in which psychiatric consultation is advised is uncommon: There has been a significant improvement in the binge-purge symptoms but no change in the depressive symptoms. This may be a signal that the depression is not related to the physiological aspects of the eating disorder and may indicate the need for medication. However, we caution against using medication without also addressing the person's depressive thought patterns.

The third indication for a psychiatric consultation is related to the first two: Therapy is stuck. Again, usually this is due to therapist inexperience or problems in the therapy relationship. Developing and enhancing the therapeutic relationship involve listening more closely, reflecting more accurately, being more active with the client and family, and preparing for the appointment by seeking consultation from another professional.

In general, a psychiatric consultation, if done correctly, can also enhance the relationship. The therapist needs to present a rationale for a second opinion that could have positive impact on the therapy, deal with the client's concerns about rejection, and discuss the necessity of professionals' working together in a team-like fashion. The therapist must also keep the avenues of communication open with the consulting psychiatrist; in fact, he or she may need to be present when the consultation occurs, so that the coordination of all parties is graphically illustrated. At the time of the consultation, the psychiatrist may address issues pertaining to medication, possible side effects, and the need for continued psychotherapy.

The question of whether or not to medicate in cases of depression is answered partially by studies comparing cognitive psychotherapy effectiveness with and without an antidepressant medication (Beck, 1976). Studies of this type commonly find that psychotherapy with medication has the best outcome, and psychotherapy alone surpasses the efficacy of medication alone. We certainly feel that this research supports our generally parsimonious approach to utilizing medication in the therapy of bulimia.

## CONTRAINDICATIONS FOR MEDICATION

There are a number of contraindications for the use of medications with bulimic clients, including the interaction between certain medications and eating behavior, the possibility of providing a convenient means for suicide, putting the client in a "sick role" in the family, and supporting a victim stance. Moreover, there is a lack of convincing evidence regarding the efficacy of medication.

One of our concerns pertains to the potentially negative interaction between medication and food behaviors. Certain medications aggravate already inappropriate food behaviors. For example, tricyclic antidepressants (e.g., imipramine, amitriptyline), the most widely prescribed compounds for bulimics at this time, have as potential side effects increased appetite, thirst, and constipation. They have also been shown to increase "carbohydrate cravings" (Paykel, Mueller, & de la Vergne, 1973). For individuals who are struggling with urges to binge, or who use laxatives to purge, tricyclics present potential problems. Other problems emerge with MAO inhibitors, which are not as widely used but appear to be more commonly used for individuals who have atypical depressions or do not respond to tricyclics. (Included among those who respond well to MAO inhibitors are individuals who are anxious and compulsive, characteristics shared by bulimics.) Certain foods are off-limits while using MAO inhibitors because dangerously high, even fatal, blood pressure elevations may ensue. MAO inhibitors should only be prescribed in those cases in which the psychiatrist and the therapist are confident that the client will be able to follow the dietary restrictions.

Lithium carbonate, a common salt used most widely in the treatment of bipolar affective disorder, is being more commonly used with eating-disordered clients (Hsu, 1984). The frantic behavior of some bulimics when bingeing or in acute distress may appear manic, though the etiology and function of the behavior are inconsistent with a manic or bipolar disorder. For bulimics who have electrolyte imbalances and who experience dehydration from purging, taking Lithium is potentially dangerous.

Our second concern is that tricyclic medications increase the risk of successful suicide in a high suicide-risk population. Some therapists have utilized suicide contracts or limited the number of pills that the client is given at any one time; nevertheless, the increased suicide potential adds to the complications of an already difficult therapy process.

Third, taking medication places the bulimic firmly in the "sick role" in the family, when the focus of therapy is to remove her from that position. Placing someone on medication has important systemic implications. It becomes much more difficult to make a case for familial basis for bulimia, to utilize such techniques such as "spreading the symptom around," or to reframe the daughter's behavior more positively. In addition, creating intensity in the system as an initial step in the change process is also more difficult. The effect this has on family dynamics is such that an already challenging therapy process becomes even more challenging. We have heard family members question the need for family therapy "now that Julie is seeing a psychiatrist." The sick role is perpetuated, and the therapist is apt to get caught between the client, family, and the consulting psychiatrist. Medication will not change the family system.

We have referred previously to the manner in which bulimic clients often present — as powerless, helpless, and out of control. Antidepressant medications can exacerbate these feelings, particularly supporting a feeling of being out of control of one's body and dependent upon an external force (the medication) to control behavior. Chronic depression is commonly observed in women who have been battered (NiCarthy et al., 1984; Walker, 1979), sexually abused (Briere, 1984; Herman, 1981), physically abused in childhood (Williams & Money, 1980), and/or raped (Burgess & Holmstrom, 1974). Since many bulimic women have been victimized, it is likely that their depression is a result of having been in actuality powerless and helpless. The victimization experiences need to be addressed in order for the client to let go of her depression and her bulimia.

The widespread use of antidepressant medications with bulimic clients is cause for concern, particularly given the equivocal results of the studies. Altshuler and Weiner (1985) take a dissenting view on depression and eating disorders, concluding that numerous uncertainties exist in the link between the two disorders and cautioning psychiatrists from leaping "on the depressive bandwagon." We certainly concur with that and are convinced that a nonmedical approach has at least as much possibility of being efficacious as a medical approach. Moreover, failure of medication to bring relief to a client's symptoms may further contribute to her sense of powerlessness and helplessness.

By way of illustrating the important considerations that the treating professionals must assess, we include a letter from a psychiatrist who conducted a thorough psychiatric evaluation on an adolescent bulimic client. This woman had persisted in depression and her bulimic symptoms despite several months of family and individual therapy, and her therapist was considering the advisability of antidepressants. After a consultation, the psychiatrist wrote the following summary and recommendations for treatment. The letter is very useful in that it reflects the degree of sensitivity to the individual and the system that is necessary when medication is considered. The summary begins:

Ms. B. is a young woman whose difficulties with an eating disorder occurred in the background of problems with separation from her family, heightened anxiety, and low self-regard. Her genetic heritage gives her a background of affective disorder, alcoholism, and psychosomatic symptoms in response to traumatic events. She developmentally seemed the most adventuresome of her siblings but is also the most prone to psychiatric symptoms when she was confronted with situations she did not like (for example, complaining of anxiety when she did not wish to go to her grandparents).

She has developmental traumas, including a fairly acrimonious divorce between her parents. She needed to leave her father and was clearly in conflict about this. On moving, her siblings were all adult enough to emancipate, but she had no clear route for this or for her feelings that a separate identity was possible with peers. She began in ninth grade to identify with peers with whom she began some mildly disobedient activities, and her mother was unable to cope with this and sent her to boarding school. B. is still very much in conflict and upset about this and it was perceived, I am sure, as punishment for emancipation, in that she was sent away, which was the most difficult thing that she could possibly be asked to handle. At school, I believe she developed a major depression and bulimic symptoms, which resulted in her being returned home and beginning psychotherapy.

Concomitant with her psychotherapy and reintegration with her family, she has maintained a weight allowing her to continue outpatient therapy. Her progress may have seemed slow but I feel this is not clearly abnormal, considering the age at the time she became symptomatic, the extent of her thought distortion with respect to her body-image and bowel functions, the function bulimia serves within her family and intrapsychically for her.

She has evidence at present of a sufficient number of symptoms to qualify her for a diagnosis of major depression, but I feel that she has an insignificant number of symptoms to start her on antidepressants for several reasons. First is her own reluctance to take medication. Second is the constipating nature of tricyclics and her preoccupation with her bowel habits, which may further her dysphoria and preoccupation with constipation and restrict her life even more because of the behaviors involved in dealing with her preoccupation. Third would be a further identification of Ms. B. as having a "sick" role in her family. Fourth, it would continue to perpetuate the idea in her family that there is a "magic bullet" for Ms. B.'s ailment, which is an unrealistic notion at best and also reflects her family's wish to deal with her symptoms in a hurry and their despair over the situation. Fifth, it would give her a route for impulsive suicidal behavior which would be extremely dangerous.

In the face of insufficient symptoms of both major depression and obsessive-compulsive disorder, I feel that it would be more prudent to wait until one of these diagnosis declared itself more fully prior to instituting potentially deleterious treatment. Clearly, under several circumstances, B. would benefit by tricyclic supplementation and that would be if she were to develop more severe or more prolonged symptoms of major depression, or her obsessive-compulsive rituals manifested themselves as a disorder, or if the behaviors themselves became dysphoric. I also feel it will be necessary to monitor her for possible panic-anxiety syndrome in the future, particularly in event of separation.

Ms. B. has done a large amount of work in psychotherapy. The extent of her symptoms of thought distortion concerning food and her body-image is such that I would have expected her to have needed inpatient therapy by this time. She has not, which is a testimony to her response to therapy and the therapeutic alliance she has. She is clearly also a therapeutic challenge because of the degree her thought patterns have been altered by her disorder. Her separation from her mother is also a trial at present, in that her mother responds to this with some dysphoria. It is clear that when Ms. B. has angry or frustrated periods because of separation, her mother will often bring up Ms. B.'s depression, rather than thinking of this as a part of normal adolescence.

I feel working with this family pattern, increasing normal peer activities, and working on her self-esteem are the paramount tasks in therapy at this time. I would suggest a continuation of family and individual therapy, working on these themes, continuing to work on Ms. B.'s distortions in terms of her body image, perhaps dealing with her behaviors around her bowels with some behavioral techniques, decreasing the time she spends at home, having her tolerate progressively longer periods away from the bathroom without her rituals. She could be re-referred for antidepressants if any of the situations described above occur.


In summary, a multidisciplinary approach to the treatment of bulimia can certainly be efficacious, as long as the meaning the system makes of the approach contributes to change rather than to a maintenance of the status quo. We find that a minority of bulimic clients, particularly those who present with a history of chronic major depression before the onset of the bulimia and those who do not experience a change in the depression when the bulimia improves significantly, may benefit from a psychiatric consultation. We encourage therapists to refer to psychiatrists who have an understanding of systemic issues and the way in which medication may interact with the family system. We have rarely found medication to be helpful with our clients but are convinced that psychiatric consultation can be helpful, particularly when the therapist is knowledgeable about the indications and contraindications regarding medication with bulimic clients.

# PART V

# *TREATING BULIMIC FAMILIES*

# CHAPTER 17

# *Principles in Working With Bulimic Families*

FAMILIES SEEKING TREATMENT pose a paradox. They enter therapy because a symptom has developed that is mysterious to the family and is more than transitory. Family members are distressed and genuinely want help to get rid of the bulimia, but they have a stake in keeping it because the bulimic person allows them to continue to function in a familiar manner. By the time families enter treatment, they have exhausted personal resources in efforts to get rid of the symptoms. They have tried to determine what event triggered the start of the bulimia, such as a diet or the breakup of a relationship — events which are external to the family functioning. Alternatively, they have blamed themselves (or have been blamed by other professionals) or someone else for causing the bulimia.

Therapists working with bulimic families can also get involved in looking for a cause-effect relationship in the development of the disorder. Our experience is that a linear approach to thinking can explain why an individual or sometimes a family is in treatment for a year or two with little progress. Each of us has made the mistake of taking a linear approach to treatment when we should have considered how the symptoms served the larger system.

Chapters 18, 19, and 20 illustrate our treatment approach with three families, each one representative of a different type of bulimic family — the perfect Gems, the overprotective Longs, and the chaotic Weisfields. While treatment proceeds differently with each of the three families, the process we go through as therapists in making our assessment and formulating the hypotheses that serve as the basis for our interventions has a common foundation. We refer you to the chapter on assessment (Chapter 11) for guidelines on determining the family type. Here we provide an overview of the thought processes that go into treating the families we present in the next three chapters. We offer techniques for joining with the family and common interventions for use by the treating professional. In all three case examples, adjunctive therapies, including group and individual, were helpful and necessary, although timing of these different treatment modalities varied with the three cases. The reader is referred to Chapters 13, 14, and 15 for discussion of these adjunctive modalities.

## JOINING WITH THE FAMILY

Joining is an essential part of negotiating the family's rules and boundaries. It starts with the first contact and continues throughout therapy. Several techniques for joining are discussed below, some of which are more effective with particular family types.

Joining starts in the therapist's head. If the therapist expects to dislike a family, it will be difficult to establish any therapeutic alliance. In addition, if the therapist has the attitude that the family is to blame for the bulimia, joining becomes impossible. In order for the family members to respond to interventions, they must feel that the therapist is working with them, not against them. They must feel that she or he accepts them and finds it possible to like them. Especially with chaotic families, the therapist needs to be able to accept that in most cases the parents have done the best that they could under the circumstances.

### Acknowledge the Family Rules

To join with the family the therapist must be able to assess the unspoken family rules, boundaries, and hierarchy. In families that are closed to outsiders by their implicit rules ("Don't tell anyone" or "You don't take your problems outside the family"), as perfect and overprotective families often are, the therapist needs to recognize the family's boundaries and respect the hierarchical system. For example, in collecting information about the family, the therapist may ask a mother who has established a pattern of speaking for her daughter, "Do you mind if I ask Jenny some questions about what she thinks about all this?" While many persons may object to this seeming collusion with family rules, one must demonstrate respect for the family structure in order for the family to continue to be involved in therapy. The therapist must join before being able to effect change in the system.

## Accept the Family's View of the Problem

Another effective way of joining with family members is to accept their view of the problem. Trying to convince family members that the bulimia is a family issue if they are resistant to this idea will end up in a wrestling match. Even if the therapist "wins," the family may not return to treatment. If they do come back, the therapist may have created major obstacles to treatment by setting up a power struggle. The therapist is advised to find out how the family members view the problem, accept this view, and then reframe it with systemic implications or positive connotations.

## Positive Relabeling

Positive relabeling, as described by Selvini Palazzoli and her colleagues (1978) is a technique that enables the therapist to recognize and support the family's view of the bulimia, while reframing the family's "offering." For example, a husband may observe that since his wife has been bulimic, she has become increasingly indecisive. The therapist may support the husband's observation by saying that she has noticed this with other people who have bulimia; the therapist can also relabel the wife's indecisiveness as a way of showing her trust in his decision-making. Positive relabeling of the bulimic behavior may be, in the chaotic family, "sacrificing to keep the family together," or in the overprotective family, "providing parents a way to feel needed." One must be careful in using positive relabeling because casting one member's behavior in a positive light necessarily has implications about another member's behavior.

It can be difficult to join with chaotic families because of their angry or out-of-control presentation. Recognition of the numerous crises the family has attempted to negotiate in its history or of how difficult it must be for them to face one more problem when they have so many can significantly relax the family and facilitate the joining process. You need to accept them instead of judge them. One can relabel the family's anger and gruffness as a sign of their recognition of the importance of the family, of their care and concern. In any case, sincerity is essential. Trying to positively relabel behavior or reinterpret the function of behavior in ways that the therapist does not believe will be detected by the family and ultimately serve as an obstacle to treatment.

## Acknowledge the Family's Efforts
## to Make the Appointment

Experience allows the therapist to join by offering guesses as to what the individual and family members have been through to get to the appointment. It is important to acknowledge their flexibility in organizing multiple schedules, the guilt and self-blame parents have had to deal with, and the humiliation or embarrassment the bulimic person may have encountered in telling her family, much less coming in to talk to a stranger. Even recognizing that the bulimic person does not feel that she needs help and therefore is angry and puzzled as to why she is here may facilitate a therapeutic alliance. Frequently, we ask families about solutions they have tried, recognizing that therapy was not their first attempt to solve the problem.

Bulimia usually serves several functions in the family, as discussed in Chapters 8–10. It should be a relief to therapists to know that they do not need to address all the functions of bulimia or all the dysfunctional patterns of the family in order for recovery to occur. The therapist has a difficult enough task in presenting a view of reality that connects the symptom to the family system in a way that makes sense to the family and motivates the family to change. We suggest that each of the chapters on family types and on the systemic issues of bulimia can be a useful reference for generating possible hypotheses about the function of bulimia in a particular case.

## DESIGNING INTERVENTIONS

Designing appropriate interventions requires that the therapist keep in mind the overall goal of therapy, which is to restructure the family system so that it no longer needs the bulimia to function. A common goal across bulimic families is to help them negotiate the life-cycle stage of "launching" or "leaving home." For example, the perfect family may need help in facilitating overt forms of rebellion typical of adolescence. In the overprotective family, the parents may need to focus on their own lives. The chaotic family may need help negotiating abandonment of the family by the oldest daughter, who has played the caretaking role.

The goals of therapy are guided by the family type and the systemic function of the bulimia. The goals of therapy may include (but are not limited to): establishing appropriate boundaries, increasing or decreasing the emotional availability of a parent to the symptomatic member, helping the symptomatic member disengage from her addictiveness to the family, facilitating a change in the family rules, helping the family grieve a loss, enabling family members to address anger towards each other in appropriate ways, negotiating a resolution to conflict, and facilitating direct communication.

Interventions are directed towards these goals. The interventions that we mention below are just a few available to the creative therapist. Some are clearly direct and others indirect or paradoxical. Most of the interventions that we describe are direct, because with these techniques the results are the most predictable and reliable. We offer some common interventions in the hope that they may spur therapists on to further creativity and to invent adaptations of these interventions geared to the specific needs of different families.

One of our direct interventions is to set realistic guidelines about the bulimic's behavior and the family's responses. Often we will ask the bulimic person to be responsible for replacing the family food that she binge-eats within 24 hours of a binge. This relieves the family members of their role of playing watchdog over the cupboards and refrigerator and gives the bulimic control over an aspect of her behavior that she can control. This intervention is not feasible if the bulimic does not have a job. Then we might engage the bulimic in devising a payback plan that is realistic but does not repeat the family's dysfunction. Along these same lines, we direct the bulimic member to be responsible for cleaning the bathroom in which she purges.

Often, in dysfunctional families, dyads triangulate a third person in order to carry on a relationship or conversation. Directing members to talk to — rather than about — each other can break the triangle. The therapist may simply say, "David, I would like you to tell that to Joan directly." This is not enough for families that have a difficult time talking about conflict. The therapist may need to physically restructure the setting by asking two family members involved in a conversation to pull their chairs apart from the rest of the family and face each other. Directing one member to talk and the others not to comment builds listening skills, breaks patterns of arguing, and initiates power shifts. The therapist may use nonverbal reminders such as pointing to one person to talk to another to reinforce direct communication.

Physically restructuring the seating arrangement can be a direct, nonverbal means of creating new lines of communication, setting limits, and establishing boundaries. It may be useful to seat the bulimic member between her parents if this is the source of tension that she attempts to regulate or if her parents generally talk through her. At other times, it can be useful to seat parents together to indicate they are a unit.

We have found bibliotherapy to be useful with families who tend to be intellectual but have a difficult time obtaining insight into family dynamics. Parents may be asked to read about the family life-cycle and to expect to be quizzed on what they read. Or a peripheral member may be asked to do the reading and to teach the others what she or he has read. Ironically, this intervention can establish the groundwork for intervention with difficult but intelligent families. If they understand what they have read and are invested in being "good students," it will be difficult for them not to apply what they have read to their own family.

When family members say they want to change but the therapist sees little evidence of this, it can be useful for the therapist to be direct about her or his observation. The therapist can even predict the occurrence of behaviors reflecting the family's ambivalence. However, in these cases it may be necessary to use indirect interventions to involve family members. Interventions may even be made to support the symptoms.

We stress that such interventions must be carefully planned. Some of the most "spectacular" interventions described in the family treatment literature are strategic or paradoxical. When examined carefully these are really not contradictory at all; they usually highlight an aspect of the systems's dysfunction. While we prefer direct interventions, paradoxical approaches are sometimes useful, especially with families that enter therapy defiantly.

Symptom prescription or paradoxical intention (Haley, 1973; Watzlawick et. al., 1974) is used to decrease the secondary gain accrued by the symptom, to help the individual take control of her symptoms, and to shift the punctuation in an escalating symptom cycle. Additionally, symptom prescription can actually help the family realize the function of the bulimia. For example, it was suggested to a 21-year-old woman living with her parents, "Your bulimia is a very good barometer of family tension. The family does not have another way to measure this. You are very helpful to them. It is important that you continue to engage in bulimia when you are feeling the tension in the family."

Another indirect intervention is to prescribe an interaction which recaptures some of the family life-cycle or exaggerates an aspect of the family's dysfunctional pattern. For example, one might ask a husband who treats his wife as a child to read her a bedtime story every night.

Family members might be asked to imitate other family members. Besides throwing a humorous light on a too serious situation, this can be very illuminating to the persons being imitated. For instance, two adolescent siblings might be asked to recreate a typical parental discussion about their symptomatic sibling. This technique provides a way of allowing family members to see themselves as others see them. Therapist feedback, as well as reviewing videotape segments of therapy, can also be used to tactfully point out interactional styles in the family.

Directing the bulimic individual to openly binge-eat in the kitchen whenever her parents are fighting can highlight the function of the bulimia. The bulimic may be asked in session to report on how successful she was in getting her parents to stop fighting and turn their concern or anger towards her. She may be congratulated by the therapist for being a "peacemaker" and holding the family together.

Whatever interventions the therapist designs, it is important to stay one step ahead of the family. One must keep in mind that, although the family members want help, they also have a vested interest in maintaining the system as it is in order to avoid upheaval.

In the next three chapters, we integrate the ideas and the thoughts that we have developed as we follow three families through treatment — the perfect Gems, the overprotective Longs, and the chaotic Weisfields. Several issues are considered: how we determined the typology of each family, how we decided whom to involve in treatment, how we formulated our hypotheses about the functions of the bulimia in the system, what risks the family faced by attempting change, the obstacles to treatment, and the development of and rationale for the interventions used.

We provide a brief guide for the reader for the next three chapters. Notice first how the families initally presented for treatment and the degree to which the bulimic individual was the family's vehicle to address considerable, ongoing distress that was most overtly seen in the chaotic family. In a variety of ways, family members other than the bulimic were in considerable distress. This distress in all cases appeared to have roots in multigenerational stress and estrangement from the family of origin. We direct your attention as you read to the function of bulimia and how it differed in each case, the enmeshed dyads in each family, the emergence of marital conflict as therapy progressed, and the continued reemergence of issues and the recycling of symptoms. The recycling of symptoms underscores that therapy with these families is hard and protracted. Very few of our families complete treatment in less than six months.

Adjunctive therapies, including group and individual, were also utilized. When employed as a systemic intervention, individual treatment has great utility. It marks the emergence of the individual from the family and is seen as a healthy steppingstone, rather than a sign of weakness. Group therapy can prepare the individual for family therapy, reinforce appropriate boundaries, provide support, and further the individuation process. Liberal use of seeing "part families" was done with the Weisfields in particular. This structural intervention was intended both to draw clear lines between parent and child subsystems and also to allow the siblings to derive support from each other in a family where support was not freely given.

If you keep in mind these foci, i.e., initial presentation, focus of therapy, systemic function of the symptom, and the uses of adjunctive therapies, the material in the next chapters should be more easily accessible and useful to you. It will then become easier to see how different in style bulimic families can be, despite similiar underlying structural features.

We chose families typical of those that present for treatment. None of these cases were "easy families" or "quick cures." Treatment of these families from our initial contact ranged from 9 months to two-and-one half years. Therapy sometimes included breaks and, as the reader will see, a variety of direct and indirect interventions was used.

# CHAPTER 18

# *The Gems: Treating the Perfect Family*

THE PERFECT FAMILY illustrates very well the existence of multiple levels and contradictory communications discussed in Chapter 4 on "Bulimic Family Systems." This makes the perfect family's dysfunction subtle and difficult to challenge. Oftentimes the sender of the communication is unaware of his or her own behavior; consequently, the therapist needs to address nonverbal communication frequently. Typically, the family has had years to practice and perfect interactional patterns involving rigid rules, restricted communication, and avoidance of conflict. Hand in hand with its overemphasis on achievement and appearance, the perfect family superficially appears happy and healthy in the tradition of the mythical All-American family.

Ironically, the development of bulimia in the perfect family contradicts the functional exterior, though it is usually kept a secret. The bulimic member is able to channel her anger through her bulimia while continuing her membership in the family, because she has adhered to rules of communication and expectations of achievement, appearance, and success. The bulimic from this family type often describes herself as living a "double life" or "living a lie" when she tries to meet both her own and her family's needs.

The Gem family is a typical perfect family. The family members are reserved and controlled, so that the impact is less intense, immediate, and urgent than with overprotective or chaotic families. Contradictory communications frequently occur. Anger is difficult to express; tones of voice communicate the anger while facial expressions contradict this communication. The result is that it becomes difficult for an individual to trust what is perceived to be true. For example, a parent may express words of concern while frowning or looking angry. Frequently, angry words or irritation may be verbally expressed while the sender of the message smiles. The receiver tends to respond to these confusing and incongruent messages in two ways. First, she becomes extremely sensitive to the incongruent communication and engages in approval-seeking behavior to avoid conflict. Second, she resolves the confusion and incongruence by ignoring one level of contradiction. In this case it is likely that the receiver will attend primarily to the nonverbal messages (Watzlawick et al., 1967).

## THE INITIAL CONTACT

Kristen, a 22-year-old woman, sought therapy for her eating disorder. She felt that she was "living a double life" in trying to uphold her successful image and hide her bulimia from her friends and family. When asked why she was seeking help now, when she had had an eating disorder for two years, Kristen stated that it had gotten worse in the past three months. She was worried that if she did not get her bulimia under control, she would have to drop a class, which would keep her from graduating in June.

Kristen came to the initial consultation straight from work. Dressed in a business suit and high heels, she was physically striking. Nevertheless, she appeared younger than her age, giving the impression of playing at being grownup. She admitted to feeling very nervous and scared about coming to the consultation. She was tearful throughout the interview, though she managed to maintain an almost constant smile.

In the course of the consultation Kristen mentioned her parents several times, reflecting on how disappointed they would be if they found out about her bulimia. When it was suggested that her parents might need to be included in the therapy, Kristen initially protested. It was proposed that she use four individual sessions to learn some tools for symptom control, explore the possible purposes of her bulimia, and gain a clearer understanding of what she would need to do to recover from her bulimia. Additionally, the relationship between her bulimia and work, school, graduation, and relationships would be explored. At the end of the brief individual therapy we would consider 1) continuing in individual therapy, 2) terminating, or 3) proceeding with an alternative modality of therapy—group or family.

The following information was gleaned from the consultation and four individual therapy sessions.

Kristen, named after her father, Chris, was the youngest of four children, three girls and one boy. She was the only one still living in the same city as her parents. She had lived away for two years when she attended college in California, but returned home after breaking up with her boyfriend. She continued school at the university, majoring in economics. She currently lived with a roommate and was able to support herself except for tuition and car insurance, which her parents paid.

She described her family as a close, All-American family. Her father's family had been established in the Northwest for several generations. Chris, the older of two children, was thought to be very much like his father. A successful businessman, he met his wife, Carol, while he was working for an accounting firm in New York. Carol, the oldest daughter of a well-to-do East Coast family, was graduated from an Ivy League school and worked as a journalist for a large newspaper. After a three-year courtship, Chris asked Carol to marry him and move back to Seattle, where he had been offered a promotion.

Carol quit her job and moved back to Seattle with Chris. Although she had planned to seek work, she soon became pregnant and assumed the responsibility of raising the family. The first child was Melissa, now 30, then Mark, 28, Penny, 25, and Kristen, 22 (see Figure 10). Kristen remembers Carol's talking about wanting to go back to work and her father's telling her that the children needed her at home. Finally, when Kristen was in college her mother started a restaurant business with the wives of other businessmen. The restaurant had taken much of Carol's time but was unquestionably successful.

Education was important in the Gem family; all the children had obtained at least a four-year degree. Mark was a successful businessman. Kristen's two sisters had followed a pattern similar to their mother's. Melissa had taken the bar exam and married in the same month. One year after starting her first job as an attorney, she became pregnant. She eventually quit her job and has since stayed home with her child, now two years old. Penny married her college boyfriend. When they were both accepted into medical school, they decided that she would work while he went to medical school first. Kristen said that she doubted that Penny would ever return to medical school. Kristen worried that she would repeat the pattern of her sisters and mother and not use her education.

Kristen had fond memories of growing up. The family was close and supportive. She remembered that childhood friends loved to be at their house and that there was almost always someone over for dinner from the time she was five or six years old. Even now, with the children grown, the family continues to plan a trip together every one to two years, visiting warm sunny spots such as Mexico or Hawaii during the winter months. Kristen notes that everyone has a good time but drinks a lot during these vacations to "keep up the good spirits." (See Kristen's family drawing in Figure 11.)

Kristen described herself as being much more like her father than her mother in temperament and looks. She felt very close to her father and special to him, describing their relationship as one in which she could do

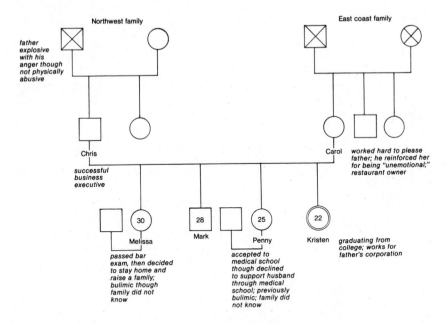

*Figure 10.* The Gem Family

no wrong. Her father had been very supportive in her career development and had helped her obtain a sales representative position with his corporation. Kristen described her position as a dream job that her peers "would kill for." She had worked for one-and-a-half years and had been offered a full-time position in management upon graduation.

Her relationship with her mother felt rocky, though the tension between the two of them was never acknowledged openly in the family. As a teenager, Kristen felt unduly criticized by Carol for things she thought were "none of her business," such as noting if Kristen had gained a few pounds, or had a blemish on her face, or had friends with "success potential." Kristen noted angrily that she did not remember her mother acting this way towards her sisters. It was during this time that she started to drink and use drugs, using speed to help her to keep from gaining and eventually to lose weight. During the last two years of high school she was high most of the time, but her parents either did not notice or did not say anything. When she was heavily into drugs, there was less tension in her relationship with her mother.

Kristen's parents encouraged her to go away for college, as her siblings had done. She was reluctant to leave her friends, but excited about going away to school. Together she and her parents visited schools in the summer after her junior year of high school. She decided to attend a private college

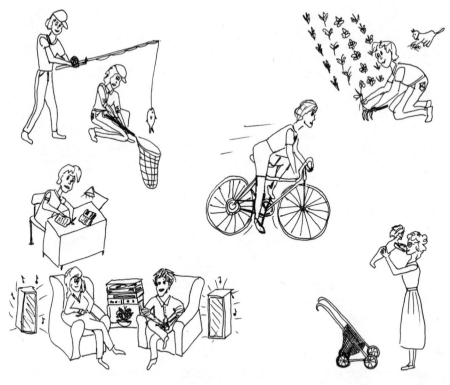

*Figure 11.*

in California. While Kristen said that she enjoyed her time away at school, she did have a difficult time adjusting. Her drug use increased and she struggled to keep her weight down through rigorous dieting and amphetamine use. Nevertheless, she managed to maintain good grades.

In her sophomore year of college, two events led to her decision to return home to finish school at a local university. A close friend overdosed on drugs and two months later her boyfriend ended their two-year relationship. During the next three months, before she moved back home, she tried to lose weight in an attempt to attract her boyfriend again. She significantly decreased her drug and alcohol use. Instead of using speed to suppress her appetite and lose weight, as she had in the past, she started using laxatives. She returned home after finishing her sophomore year. Within two weeks of moving back home she started binge-eating.

Chris, who struggled to maintain a trim weight, noticed and complemented Kristen on her weight loss. Carol did not mention anything until

Kristen had lost too much weight; then both parents expressed concern about her health. In retrospect, and looking at photographs, Kristen realized that she did not look healthy at her lowest weight. She was able to gain weight but started inducing vomiting for fear that she would become "chubby," as she had been as a child. She has maintained a "normal" weight for the year preceding therapy, though she still felt that she would look better if she weighed 10 pounds less.

During the course of the four individual therapy sessions, Kristen learned some behavioral tools to manage her eating and restructured her eating schedule to include three meals a day. She was using a structured journal to monitor the situations, as well as her thoughts and her feelings, related to bulimic episodes. Her bingeing decreased from an average of three times a day to once a day. She even experienced some bulimia-free days.

Over the course of the four weeks of individual therapy Kristen became aware that the toughest situations in controlling her bulimia were when she visited her parents, had dinner with them, or housesat for them. She admitted that it certainly looked like her parents had something to do with her bulimia, though she did not know what.

For the last individual therapy session Kristen was asked to write about her understanding of her bulimia and the role it played in her life and relationships.

> My bulimia makes me feel terrible and unattractive, while at the same time it helps me relieve tension. At times I think I unconsciously do it to escape everything I have to deal with or because I am angry at myself. Of course, being bulimic only makes me get angrier at myself; then I don't have to deal with anything else because I'm so into myself.
>
> Sometimes, I think I do it hoping someone will know. Although I tried to hide my bulimia, I think it's pretty obvious that I'm doing it especially around my parents. They ask me if something is wrong and I just say my contact lenses are bothering me. I get angry that they ask and I get angry that they believe my answer. I want them to know that I am just pretending that everything is fine. I am angry that they do not notice.

During the last individual session, Kristen concluded that she needed to stop pretending that everything was fine. She felt she needed to let go of her secret if she wanted to recover, though she was scared about upsetting her parents' image of her. Kristen was encouraged to explore the consequences of upsetting the family rules if she asked her parents to join her in therapy, as well as how she might abide by the family rules in the family sessions and subsequently sabotage the work she wanted to do with her parents. Kristen anticipated that the sessions would be uncomfortable for all of them because they did not discuss problems openly. She was worried that her parents would feel that they were to blame. Kristen also suggested that she might minimize the extent of her worry about her bulimia or the effect it was having on her life so that her parents would not think she was weak and disgusting. The therapist further suggested that it was possible she could feel angry in the sessions but avoid expressing her feelings because anger was an emotion that was not directly expressed in her family.

Kristen invited her parents into therapy. Therapy was conducted in eight sessions with Kristen and her parents. Subsequent to the eighth family session, Kristen requested four more individual therapy sessions. From the first consultation with Kristen to the last individual session, therapy extended over nine months.

Excerpts taken from six months of family therapy are offered to illustrate the family's patterns of interaction and the subtle rules governing their interactions. The family therapy was delineated by two stages: 1) letting go of the secret, and 2) exposing conflict. Both stages of therapy challenged the basic family rules governing conflict resolution. The first stage questioned Kristen's image as the perfect daughter; the second challenged the family's image as the perfect family.

Kristen's description of her family led to several hypotheses about the function of her bulimia in the family. First, a familial theme appeared to be that women were less important than men. Although the women had a repetitious pattern of sacrificing their needs for the men, there was a push for achievement through education. Kristen appeared to be trying to make up for the career interruptions the women in the family had experienced. Secondly, there was no evidence of overt expressions of anger in the family. Kristen's consistent smiling signaled the importance of supressing anger. Her bulimia appeared to be an outlet for her anger. (It was also possible that her bulimia was the conduit through which anger was expressed for other members of the family.) Third, as the youngest girl in this perfect family, it was difficult for Kristen to disappoint her parents. She revealed a pattern of behavior that was highly responsive to her parents' needs, thus effectively inhibiting the development of her autonomy and subsequent individuation.

## PHASE 1: LETTING GO OF THE SECRET

Kristen's parents, Chris and Carol, arrived at the first session separately and before Kristen. Kristen, normally punctual, was late. She apologized for her tardiness and from the beginning of the session appeared much younger than she had in any of the individual sessions. Despite smiles all around, it was obvious that Kristen was nervous and scared as she sat with her arms wrapped around herself between her parents. Neither Chris nor

Carol knew why they were invited to the session by Kristen. The following excerpt follows Kristen's initial disclosure to her parents that she has sought therapy because she is bulimic. Chris and Carol are attentive and look concerned.

Kristen: (Looking apologetic and anxious) I have been so nervous and afraid to tell you. I don't know why. I know you still love me and care. That's not true—I do know why. (She sits up and projects an adult image.) I just worry about what you think—that maybe I'm weak. I worry that you'll blame yourselves. (She sinks down in her chair.)

Carol: (With a frown on her face) Well, is there something we have done wrong?

Kristen: (Hesitantly and without a smile) No . . .(pause). But I felt I had to ask you in so that I could stop pretending that everything is so perfect. I've been having a hard time with school and studying because I start bingeing and throwing up and then I'm too tired to study.

Chris: (Turning to the therapist, sounding concerned) Is this related to anorexia nervosa? You know, Carol and I were concerned a few years back when Kristen had lost some weight and become thin. She's like me; she's got the kind of build where we can put on weight pretty quickly. Anyway, we thought it was a phase. She has been looking so healthy and beautiful, we had no idea anything was wrong.

Therapist: Kristen, you look like you're hanging on to every word your father says, but you also look confused or frustrated. I can't tell.

Kristen: (Imploringly and haltingly) Mom and dad, this isn't new for me. I've just been pretending for years that everything is okay. I didn't want to disappoint you. You've given me everything. But I've been having problems since I was 16. You know when I lost all that weight? I was obsessed with my weight. I've used speed; I've thrown up; I've starved so I could look just right. Dad, at first you said I looked better and then soon after that you both said I looked too thin. I thought better too thin than too chunky.

Chris: (In a comforting tone) Honey, you know we love you no matter what.

Kristen: I know it sounds silly—I sound silly to myself now. But I'm serious. This problem feels like I'm an alcoholic or drug addict. I can't stop. I'm scared.

Carol: (With little feeling) What can we do to help you, Kristen?

Kristen: (Looking at her father) Being here means a lot to me.

Chris: (Sounding puzzled) You know, I've thought something was going on because whenever you visit you eat so much but you never gain weight. I've wondered how you do it.

Therapist: What other clues have you had that Kristen had an eating disorder or that something was wrong? (There is a pause as Carol and Chris look at each other, then at the floor. They appear to be thinking.)

Carol: (Looking at Chris) You know, how I told you I thought something was wrong because she would go through my cupboards and eat things? (Sounding angry) Later, I would go to get something and it would be gone. But I didn't know what to say. (Turning towards Kristen) One time I tried to approach you, remember? But you became so defensive and angry. I'd rather see you when you're happy and pleasant so I haven't brought it up. (Kristen looks ashamed and angry.) (Continuing abruptly and quickly) I think you mentioned it to me once, but I didn't think it was anything serious. (Kristen tears up.)

Kristen: (Taking a deep breath) Well it's been going on for years and I'm tired of it, but I can't get rid of it by myself. I know I've got to stop.

Chris: Knowing when you need help can be a sign of strength. (Pause) Would you like some help paying for therapy?

Therapist: (Motioning Chris to stop) This is really serious for you, Kristen. Do you remember mentioning your bulimia to your mom?

Kristen: (Thoughtfully) Yeah, I do. I was so scared and then I regretted I said anything. It's never been brought up again until now.

Therapist: Was it a surprise that your mother didn't ask more questions? (Carol is looking at Kristen intently.)

Kristen: Yes and no. (Pause)

Carol: She got so defensive in those days if I'd ask her questions it just seemed better not to upset her. Then the visit would be so much more pleasant.

Therapist: Chris, do you ever remember Kristen approaching you about her bulimia or Carol approaching you?

Chris: (Thoughtfully, tilting back in his chair) No, I can't say I do. I hope she knows that she could approach me with something like this.

(At this point, the therapist turns to the parents and mentions some signals other parents have noticed with a bulimic daughter.)

Therapist: Knowing what you do now, are there any other signals you can recall that would indicate that Kristen has had bulimia? (After some thought, both parents shake their heads, no.) (Turning to Kristen) You are even better than I thought you were at pretending everything is fine. (Turning back to Chris and Carol) How do you think Kristen has learned so well to hide her problems?

Kristen and her parents were communicating in a contradictory fashion. While all families communicate on multiple levels using nonverbal cues, in this family type the nonverbal cues are both contradictory and difficult to point out. For example, Chris and Carol communicated concern and attentiveness, but maintained a reserve that contrasted with Kristen's intensity.

Chris' nonverbals, such as tilting his chair backwards, also communicated discomfort with the intimacy and intensity of the dicussion. Watzlawick et al. (1967) observe that the child listens to the discrepant nonverbal level of communication first. Thus, the nonverbal communication is often more powerful than the verbal communication. Direct interventions, such as asking family members to not smile when smiles were not appropriate and to sound angry, frustrated, irritated, etc. to match their words, were initiated at this stage of therapy.

The contradictory communication in the Gem family, coupled with Chris and Carol's reluctance to respond with intensity matching Kristen's desperateness, increased the distance between Kristen and her parents. It was their well-practiced approach to problem-solving that had become part of the problem. For example, Carol mentioned that she avoided asking Kristen questions when she thought Kristen would respond angrily or defensively. Carol's solution is an example of what Watzlawick et al. (1974) refer to as first-order change — an avoidance of behavior that resulted in the undesirable outcome (in this case overt conflict).

First-order change is not sufficient to eliminate the need for bulimia within the family system. Kristen's ability to decrease her bulimia after deciding to invite her family into therapy appeared to indicate that the disclosure of her secret was a step towards second-order or true systemic change. Her disclosure necessitated that she not avoid conflict and that she set the expectation that this is how the family members needed to communicate. The therapist's facilitating Carol and Chris' listening to her and dealing with how it came to be that she had learned to keep secrets so well also promoted second-order change.

In promoting further change in the family relational system, it was important for the therapist to respect the family's signals that intimacy was difficult. While Kristen continued to invite her parents to move closer to her, they had subtly avoided dealing with her desperateness and fear. A common sense approach to this family's difficulty would be to point out their difficulty and facilitate their increasing tolerance for intimacy by directing discussion in sessions and scheduling sessions more frequently. While perfect families often accept such therapeutic observations, they nevertheless ignore them and repeat their patterns. The therapist thought that the Gems, if forced to act intimately without a means of distancing themselves, would rigidly avoid conflict and insight and probably drop out of therapy. Consequently, the therapist regulated the intensity of therapy by lengthening or shortening the intervals between scheduled sessions. Towards this end, the sessions occurred at one-month intervals initially and then, as the family's tolerance for intensity increased, every two weeks. Another possible intervention to address the family members' need for distance regulation would be to discuss how they do it, so that they have a conscious awareness of what they are doing. Subsequently, the therapist may schedule sessions closer together, but direct the family members to employ their distancing techniques between sessions. This type of intervention is particularly useful with a family that is likely to do this anyway.

## PHASE 2: EXPOSING CONFLICT

Between the second and third family session the family took a vacation which included all the siblings and their spouses. Prior to the vacation, Kristen had determined that she was going to let each of her siblings know that she was bulimic and in therapy. In talking with her sisters she discoverd that both had been bulimic and had sought therapy but had kept their problems a secret from the rest of the family.

The following excerpt is from the third session. The tension between Carol and Kristen builds.

Carol: (Tentatively) Kristen, you seemed just fine during the vacation. More relaxed than I've seen you in a long time. It's really comforting to see you at peace with yourself.

Kristen: (Tearing) Yeah, I have felt a lot better and a lot closer to you. I've hardly binged at all since the first time you came in.

Carol: (Sounding irritated though looking supportive and earnest) I wish we could have done this sooner if it's been so helpful.

Chris: (Turning to the therapist) Is it possible for this thing, bulimia, to disappear just like that?

Therapist: That's a good question, Chris. What do you think?

Chris: Well, if as Kristen says this has been going on for years, I don't see how she could be sure she's done with it. I'm thinking about when I quit smoking. It took me quite a while to get to the point I considered myself a nonsmoker. There were situations that were hard — even now — luncheons where I was used to having a cigarette after the meal or smoking with a drink.

Kristen: Well, I'm glad you're wondering. I am, too. It hasn't been very easy these last two months. And I have had some relapses so I'm not done yet.

Carol: You just have to pick up and go on each time you relapse.

Kristen: (Angrily) Mom, how would you know? It's not that easy.

Therapist: Kristen, are you aware that you sound angry at your mother? Whatever you do, do not apologize. Instead, talk to her about the tension between the two of you.

Carol: (Unconvincingly) I don't know that it's that important. I can handle it.

Kristen: (Still sounding angry) Well, that's exactly what makes me angry. We don't talk about it. There's been tension between us since I've been a teenager, but we just sweep it under the rug and it just gets lumpier and lumpier until it starts to feel like I'm walking through a minefield when I come home to visit. Do you know that the only times I have binged and vomited in the last two months has been when I have come home to visit or have dinner or housesat for you?

Therapist: Carol, what do you hear Kristen saying?

Carol: That she's mad at me and that she binges and vomits in our home. (Turns towards Kristen) That makes me angry. (Sounding very angry, but looking concerned talking to therapist) Again, she took stuff from my pantry without asking me. Am I supposed to confront her about it?

Therapist: Carol, could you look angrier?

Kristen: (Raising her voice, looking surprised) Why didn't you say something? (Sounding frustrated) Why do you just pretend like everything's okay? We all play such a game at being the perfect family . . .

Chris: I'm not so sure that the two of you need to get so upset with each other. You can talk about this rationally.

Kristen: (Struggling not to smile) Dad, do you know what you're saying? This is part of why I've had this problem for so long. This is why I kept it a secret. I *was* trying to be "rational" and "in control," but I've been living a lie. I don't want to hurt either of you . . .

Kristen's direct confrontation of the family rules and movement away from satisfying her parent's needs are addressed by her father as he tries to get both women to follow the family rules about conflict. He reminds Carol and Kristen of the "family solution" by asking the two women to be "rational." It is likely, left to their own devices, that apologies would be made and the conflict would again be swept under the rug. Kristen has some insight that the solution has been part of the problem. She appears readier than either of her parents to try another solution, though she does not have the skills to continue or intensify the conflict between her mother and herself. Chris and Carol have used subtle ways of attempting to avoid becoming engaged in the intensity of the conflict. The next excerpt is from the following session, when again the tension has risen. Kristen and Carol were kept focused on their anger.

Carol: I don't know what it is that you have against me, Kristen.

Kristen: (Less tearful than previous sessions) Mom, I really don't know. (Pause) I just know I'm upset—I'm angry at you. (Pause)

Therapist: Because . . .

Kristen: Because you've been so critical of me since I was a teenager. You weren't critical of Melissa or Penny. I never heard you criticize what they wore or their weight or their friends. (Imploringly) Why are you so critical of me?

Carol: I haven't treated you differently from the others. I suppose you don't think your father has treated you differently?

Kristen: (Smiling at her father) He hasn't been critical like you have. I feel like he has respected me. (Pause) I couldn't have taken criticism like that from both of you. Dad has been real supportive.

Therapist: My guess is that it would be very hard for you to get angry at your father. Much more difficult than getting angry at your mother.

Kristen: (Thoughtfully) Yeah . . . I don't know why.

Therapist: Chris, has Carol ever criticized you the way she's criticized Kristen?

Chris: Not really. Oh, there's times when she's commented about my weight, but I'm glad she does that.

Kristen: (Sounding frustrated) But she has no right to do that! It's your weight not hers. That's why I sometimes get angry. (Turning to her mother) The things that you pick on are none of your business!

Carol: I just don't think I've treated you differently from the other kids.

Therapist: Carol, have you ever heard Kristen use the tone of voice she has been using with you with her father?

Carol: (Definitely) Rarely.

Therapist: Why do you think that is?

Carol: I don't know. (Pause) They seem to understand each other. They seem pretty close. I just don't have the same relationship with Kristen.

Therapist: Or with Chris?

Carol: (Tears, but does not cry) I'm not sure what you mean. (Pause)

Kristen: (Starts out incredulously, as though she has not thought of what exactly she is going to say) Mom, I think you have been jealous of me and dad.

Therapist: I think that's a pretty risky thing for you to have volunteered, Kristen, (Kristen lets out her breath and her shoulders visibly drop.) I think your mother can hear that. Carol, it looks like Kristen is waiting for you to explode.

Carol: (Seeming distant and choosing her words carefully. Her eyes are brimming with tears; she looks at no one) I think she's right; I have felt jealous of Chris and Kristen. They play together; they work together. Chris and I don't share that kind of time. Sometimes I feel that I'm just an acquaintance.

Therapist: It seems that the two of you act as parents but have forgotten how to be partners. Carol, it must be difficult to act as though things are just fine when at times you seem so lonely and depressed. You seem to have sacrificed a lot for everyone — at your own expense. (Carol barely nods to affirm this. Pause.) It also appears that it is hard to get Chris really involved with you. Both of you (Carol and Kristen) seem to avoid getting angry at him. Perhaps he really has quite a temper?

The family was approaching a clearer definition of the conflict as it involved the three of them. They were also demonstrating increased tolerance for intensity. The notion that Chris might have a bad temper later leads to direct discussion of anger and how it was learned in Chris' and Carol's respective families. Additionally, the idea that it was hard to get Chris' attention was introduced. This issue would come up again and be repeatedly observed to the family members.

At the end of this session, each person was asked to write down his or her explanation of the problem *as it involved all three of them* and to bring it to the next session. This was offered as an intellectual challenge (which often is the type of intervention that appeals to a high-achieving, perfect family) on a vulnerable and important issue. The next excerpt is from the fifth session.

Therapist: You've had a couple of weeks to think about the last session. I had asked you to write down your formulation of what the problem is, considering the conclusions from the last sessions. First, Carol feels that Chris does not treat her as a friend the way he does Kristen. Second, Kristen can't get mad at Chris but has felt angry at Carol for years. Third, Carol shows some of her anger to Kristen by being critical, but not to Chris. What do you think is going on?

Chris: That was a pretty tough problem you gave us.

Therapist: (Nodding affirmatively) I'm interested in how you put all this information together to define the problem facing you more clearly. I want to hear from each of you. Carol, how about you starting? (Carol acknowledges her willingness.) Before we start, Chris, would you change chairs with Kristen so that you are next to your wife? (A cooperative change of chairs with dad and daughter smiling at each other takes place; Carol looks out the window.)

Carol: (Sounding perturbed) Well, I don't know if I'm right.

Therapist: Carol, you sound perturbed. I don't know if that's because you want to be right or because of what you think is going on. If it's the latter, I encourage you to continue to sound perturbed. (Looking surprised, Kristen wraps her arms around herself protectively.)

Carol: Can I just read it? (Therapist nods yes. Pause) I have been competing with Kristen for Chris' attention. I should be angry about this, but it's difficult for me to express my anger at Chris for fear that he'll think I'm unreasonable. I don't feel much like a mother when this is going

on and I start bickering with Kristen when she hasn't really done much
to deserve my irritation with her. (Kristen is crying silently, trying to
hide her tears. Chris frowns.)

Therapist: What are your tears for, Kristen?

Kristen: (Trying to control herself from sobbing so she sound like she is hic-
cupping) It . . .it . . . feels right what you're saying, Mom. But it
hurts. I feel so responsible. And I don't know what to do.

Carol: (Leaning forward and looking across to Kristen) I don't think there
is anything that you are supposed to do, Kristen. I think that is between your father and me. (Therapist nods affirmatively.)

Therapist: (Chris is still frowning.) Chris, what have you written?

Chris: (Looking at Carol, then at his paper) Well, I had a very hard time
with this, like I said. (Pause) I started many times; I'm not sure I came
up with what you are looking for. (Looking up at the therapist) Should
I just read it?

Therapist: Whatever you prefer.

Chris: As far as I got was thinking that Carol takes out her anger towards
me on Kristen. In this way we don't fight and we keep up appearances
to everyone, including ourselves, and our kids. (Carol looks up at Chris,
looking angry and tearful. Therapist nods.) Though I don't know if
it's true that Carol has a hard time getting angry at me.

Therapist: What about Carol's feeling that she's not getting enough of your
time?

Chris: She's mentioned that before.

Therapist: Well, you've both indicated that Carol is angry at you. Carol,
could you try looking angrier? Good. that matches more how you have
been sounding. I'm much less confused when how you look matches
how you sound and what you say. (Turning to Kristen, who is smiling nervously) What does your smile mean Kristen?

Kristen: Oh. I wasn't aware I was smiling. I guess that mom has been sounding angry. It's less confusing to see her look angry, too.

Therapist: What did you write?

Kristen: (Taking a deep breath, looking up at both of her parents briefly)
What I've written is not that much different. I want to feel special.
Dad makes me feel special. It has been hard for me to feel mom's approval. I want to have both of you for friends, but it feels that if dad
and I are friends, mom and I can't be. Sometimes I just give up trying; I turn her off so she can't hurt me or I get angry so she won't talk
to me. Usually, I don't think we're even fighting about what's really
bugging us.

Dad really respects mom a lot and sees her as the perfect wife. I
think he makes her feel special. So she can't get mad at dad in case

he gets mad back. Mom wants what I have with dad but doesn't know how to get it so instead of being angry with dad she gets angry with me. (Kristen takes another deep breath, looking up at the therapist. Carol and Chris are listening intently without smiles.)

Therapist: The three of you have implied that it is your relationship, Chris and Carol, that needs attention, though I also hear you, Kristen, wanting to see their relationship as flawless. (Turning towards Carol) Kristen has been very loyal to you. She has actually supported you in your anger. (Looking back and forth between Chris and Carol) She has been loyal to both of you. Her bulimia has enabled her to continue every child's wish that her parents' relationship is perfect. It is important that you let her know that this is not reality. If you can help her to believe that you have difficulties like other couples, this may help her be more realistic about the difficulties she will encounter in her relationships.

   Kristen has already mentioned that the most difficult times she has with her bulimia, now, are when she visits you at home or housesits when you're gone. How do you think Kristen's bulimia is related to your relationship?

Several interventions are offered in a brief period of time. First, Kristen's behavior is reframed as loyalty to her mother, which aligns mother and daughter versus pitting them against one another. Citing her loyalty to both parents further removes her from the parent-child coalitions. Second, Chris and Carol's marital difficulties are reframed as desirable and normal — even helpful to Kristen — rather than as a flaw in the perfect marriage. They are then less likely to try to reassert a perfect image. Third, a very different perspective on the family's current reality is offered. Thus, the family members are likely to be confused. Confusion is often necessary for change. Subsequently, the therapist offers a way out of confusion, as the family is directed to reconnect Kristen's symptoms with the conflict between Carol and Chris. Towards the end of the session Carol starts to talk about family-of-origin issues, mentioning competition with her youngest sister for her father's attention.

Therapist: Carol, you have a younger sister. I wonder if the two of you used to compete.

Carol: (Pause, looking puzzled) I'm sure we did. We were only two years apart. Don't most sisters compete?

Therapist: You look confused. (Pause) Who or what were you competing about?

Carol: I'm not sure. It just seems like the usual stuff. (Pause) I remember feeling jealous of her. I was the intelligent one; she was the pretty, popular one.

Therapist: Were either of you more like one parent than the other?

Carol: Well, yes. I was much more like my mother. I look a lot like her. Elizabeth looked more like my father's side. My father doted on her; she was the baby of the family.

Therapist: (Kristen is tearing up.) How did you get attention from your father?

Carol: Well, he was proud of me for my grades, though he told me I was too smart for my own good — being a woman. I knew, though he seldom said anything about it, that he thought I was special because I was rational and didn't get very emotional.

Therapist: You have really been reinforced for holding back on your emotions, haven't you? (Carol nods. Pause) Carol, what do you think the connection is between what you competed for growing up and what's going on among the three of you now?

Carol was able to articulate the similarity between what she experienced growing up and what she was currently experiencing in her relationship with Chris. Chris subsequently took time to examine how he learned to be so rational. There were several indications at this time of important changes in Chris and Carol's relationship: 1) they arrived together; 2) they sat next to each other with no direction from the therapist; and 3) Carol appeared less depressed.

The evidence for second-order change in the family system noted above, as well as the family's increasing tolerance for conflict and intensity, suggested that what might otherwise seem like too quick or too perfect a recovery (a hazard with the perfect family) made sense. Nevertheless, a relapse was prescribed in order to assess the degree of change and to challenge the fragility of Kristen's elimination of her bulimic symptoms.

Usually, when a relapse is prescribed, the bulimic expresses fear and reluctance. It can be pointed out that a "planned relapse" is all the more important for her to determine whether bulimia provides the same satisfaction and outlet that it once did. In this way she can determine if her recovery is "real" (due to second-order change). If the changes in her bulimia are due to second-order versus first-order change, the bulimic episode will not have the reinforcing qualities of previous bulimic episodes.

In the next family session, Kristen reported that she had planned the relapse for a weekend when she was invited to dinner at her parents' house. She had started to go through the cupboards of her mother's pantry, but her mother confronted her. Kristen described her mother's confrontation as less confusing to her, since her mother not only sounded angry but also looked angry. At that time her mother asked if there was a tension between her father and herself to which Kristen was responding. Kristen said she almost forgot to follow through on the relapse. She tried to start a binge, which felt very alien to her. She managed to throw up, but felt no relief in the purging.

In the seventh session, the family was asked to talk about the family rules around anger and how Chris and Carol learned about dealing with anger from their parents. Chris described his family as one in which his father could be violently explosive, e.g., throwing things or putting his fists through walls. Although he never hit his mother, Chris, or Chris' sister, they were all afraid of him. Chris made a pact with himself to deal with anger differently and described channeling his anger into athletics and work. He noted that it now took an incredible amount of tension or conflict to make him angry.

Carol described her family as very proper and concerned with appearances. She was taught that it was not ladylike to get angry. She disclosed that she has felt that something is wrong with her because she does get angry. It was suggested that some of her depressed affect and appearance might actually be a result of her powerlessness to do anything with her anger. Carol admitted to feeling very depressed at times, but questioned her right to feel depressed when she had such a good life.

Kristen was able to relate to what her mother had learned, as illustrated by an excerpt from this session.

Therapist: Kristen, you seemed to be listening intently and nodding as your mom spoke. What are you nodding about?

Kristen: (Laughing) Mom, you just described what I feel like I've learned in our family. I feel like it's not ladylike to be angry and I've gotten real depressed at times. Instead of taking my anger out on people, I usually take it out on myself — I binged or purged.

Therapist: What have you learned from your father about anger?

Kristen: (Thoughtfully) I have to think of that a little more. (Pause). It's almost as though Dad knows what to say or do so people don't get angry at him.

Chris: I have a hard time with people being angry at me. (Pause)

Kristen: (Nodding at him) I'm afraid of people getting angry at me, too. I'll do all sorts of things to avoid getting people angry at me. I'll change my opinion, or usually I won't express my opinion. (Sounding disappointed with herself) I guess that's pretty sad.

Chris: (Shaking his head back and forth, looking down at the floor) I've done the same thing.

Carol: (Looking at Chris) Hmmm . . . I've felt somehow that I've had to protect you from my anger. (Chris looks at her questioningly.)

Therapist: What does Chris do, Carol, that makes it hard to be angry at
him?

Carol: I never really thought about it. Maybe it's just me—the difficulty
I've always had in expressing anger.

Therapist: Are you afraid of getting Chris angry now? (Chris looks attentive and concerned.)

Carol: (Shifting in her chair, cracking a smile) Maybe. (Pause) What does
he do so it's hard to be angry? . . . Well, . . . he looks so darned caring and concerned for one thing. It's hard to be angry when he means
well. (All three family members laugh uncomfortably.)

Therapist: Chris, how do you do it?

Chris: (Laughing) I wish I knew—it sounds like I'm pretty good at it whatever I do. (Therapist laughs and nods affirmatively.)

Therapist: (Jokingly) If you knew, you could teach it to Kristen and Carol
so they won't ever get angry at each other. (Kristen and her mother
exchange smiles at the joke.) Kristen, how does your father do it?

Kristen: Not get me angry?

Therapist: Keep you from *expressing* your anger at him?

Kristen: Some of what mom says. He looks like he cares so much. He just
doesn't say much controversial.

Therapist: It would be hard to have very in-depth conversation, I would
think.

It was obvious that the family was very uncomfortable around expressing anger. Old patterns of constant smiling were frequent and family members were more avoidant of risking anger and displeasure in the session. As
the family rule around recognizing anger was violated, the therapist experienced family members as less accessible and more uncomfortable. It was
tempting to wonder if they were making "something out of nothing" and
moved quickly away from this issue to avoid possible rejection by the family.

While the Gem family had been insightful up to this point in therapy,
they had much less insight into how they avoided anger. Unless the therapist
persisted and kept the family members focused on talking about anger, they
would have colluded to avoid talking about anger. Obviously, it would take
more than one or two sessions for the family to learn how to express anger.
The Gem's tolerance for conflict had been developed from the beginning
of the family therapy. Although it was still difficult for them to address conflict, they were able to demonstrate instances of overt and congruent expressions of conflict within and outside of sessions, which was another necessary
systemic change. Helping them to understand the origin of the rules they

had created for dealing with anger and how they currently applied those rules would allow them to make further changes.

Before the final session, Kristen requested an individual session to talk about her pervasive unhappiness with her job and her decision to quit. The therapist granted this session with some hesitation, but viewed it as an opportunity to determine by the way Kristen used the session if there was sufficient change to continue with the eighth family therapy session as the last in the series.

Kristen used this session to talk about dissatisfaction with her job. She felt that she was "window dressing" as the only woman in the sales department. Her coworkers always complimented her on how she looked, but seldom on her competence. She was always friendly but felt she had to be cautious so that her friendliness was not interpreted as sexual interest. She was dreading going to work. She was encouraged to look at whether she had requested the individual session for fear of her parents' reactions or disapproval.

The last excerpt is taken from this final family session.

Kristen: (Sitting up looking back and forth between her parents) I need to take time away from my job to do some thinking about whether or not this is the right track for me. I realize I haven't been happy in my job for a long time, but I didn't want to quit for fear of what you two would think, particularly you, Dad. I didn't want you to be angry or disappointed after all you've done for me (looking at her father). But, I've got to trust my feelings, which have been going on for a while. I wanted to bring this up in here so that if you are angry or disappointed in me, we can talk about it.

Therapist: You can handle it if they are disappointed? (Kristen nods yes.) If they're angry? (She nods yes.) (Pause) Do you need their permission to quit?

Kristen: No. I just hope they can accept my decision. It was not an easy decision.

Carol: Well, what if you take time off and when you want to go back the position is no longer there?

Kristen: Well, I've though about that. That would be hard, but then I guess, I'd have to get a job the way other people my age do. The experience has been valuable so I could probably start somewhere else. It might even be a good idea for me to work at a place that has nothing to do with the family so I can really feel like I'm on my own.

Therapist: What do you want from your parents?

Kristen: (Thoughtfully) I'm not sure. I just want to know what their— your— reactions are.

Chris: (Looking concerned, smiling) You know we're behind whatever is
    best for you.
Therapist: Chris and Carol, I'm confused because Kristen says she's not ask-
    ing your permission to quit, but her demeanor tells me otherwise.
Carol: Yes, it strikes me that way, too. (Adamantly) Kristen, you don't need
    my permission! You're a grown woman; you make your own decisions.
    (Looking at Chris) Maybe she wants your permission.
Kristen: (Waving her hand to get attention) Wait a minute. I don't want
    your permission. I've made up my mind. I already gave my notice.
    I just want to be clear on whether or not you're going to hold this
    against me or think less of me.
Therapist: Carol, I think you were right. Chris, I think this is really directed
    at you. Is that right, Kristen? (She nods.)
Chris: To tell the truth, I'm more surprised than disappointed. I'm wonder-
    ing if something has been going on that could be straightened out.
Kristen: (Assertively) No, dad, I don't want to straighten out anything. As
    I said, I've already given my notice. If either of you are interested I
    can talk to you about what has been bothering me about the job but
    you can't convince me to change my mind . . .

Ending therapy, with Kristen demonstrating a healthy separation from
her parents, marked the beginning of a new phase of the family life-cycle.
While the Gems had been successful in physically launching Kristen, she
had been tied to them through her need for their approval. The excerpt from
the eighth session demonstrated some of the individuation and separation
necessary for Kristen to be able to truly leave home. Although she still
wanted approval from her parents, she had made her decision to quit her
job before coming into the session and discussing it with her parents. Thus,
their permission was secondary. As planned, this remained the final family
session.

Although the family therapy was brought to a close, there remained work
to be done. For example, Chris and Carol had marital issues to address and
the family would benefit from continuing to increase their tolerance for conflict, intimacy, and intensity. Ending the therapy at this point demonstrates
a sensitivity to the family's tolerance for change. Several second-order changes
had started. To direct more changes might have been "too much too soon."

Kristen continued in individual therapy for four additional sessions over
a two-month period of time. She used these sessions to reflect on and stabilize
her personal changes, to adjust to her change of job, to continue her efforts
to relinquish a strong need for her parents approval, and to learn how to
be angry and less "nice" (with her family and in relationships with men and
her friends).

## SUMMARY

While the Gems had work left to look forward to, several important changes took place over the six months of family therapy that enabled Kristen to let go of her bulimia. It is doubtful that any one of these changes by itself would have been sufficient for longstanding symptom relief.

1) Kristen had challenged the family rules and exposed her vulnerability and current problems early in the therapy; she had broken the silence typically kept in a perfect family. Some of her ability to relinquish her bulimic symptoms early in the process of therapy was attributed to her breaking of these rules.
2) Family members had been given permission and support for their angry feelings; family-of-origin issues were exposed to help Chris and Carol understand why they avoided expressing anger. Kristen was able to realize that she had learned to cope with anger much in the way her parents did.
3) The therapy addressed how Kristen was triangulated in her parents' relationship and how this triangulation was related to her bulimia. Chris and Carol acknowledged that they had used Kristen as a buffer in their relationship with one another and subsequently started to act differently with each other.
4) Kristen's ability to quit the job her father had been instrumental in helping her to obtain was a sign of healthy separation from both of her parents. It was a movement away from the enmeshment with her father and a refusal to make up for the fact that the other women in the family had given up their careers.

Most bulimic families get stuck launching their last child. This transition leaves the couple to face being a couple again. Clearly, Chris and Carol had forgotten how to be a couple, but expressed interest in learning coupling activities.

In order to launch children and support their individuation, there must be room for anger. The Gem family was able to illuminate three generations of difficulty with expressing anger. In the women, difficulty expressing anger arose out of conforming with the definition of femininity they had been taught and subsequently resulted in depression. Females from perfect families, much more often then those from overprotective or chaotic families, have difficulty reconciling old and new definitions of femininity, which at times are mutually exclusive. This pattern is illustrated in the Gem family starting with the mother and extending to all three daughters. Carol, Melissa, and Penny have all been educated and then given up their educations and promising careers to take care of husbands and/or children. Kristen has a better chance at avoiding a repetition of this pattern.

It is apparent that there was more work that a therapist could have done with the Gem family. However, there are benefits to be derived from recognizing the earliest stopping point for therapy. With therapy being successful, the perfect family is more likely to seek brief help again in the future. In this case, Carol called six months later to ask for a couples therapist for her and Chris.

With perfect families, it is essential for the therapist to be active. Gradually, as the family's tolerance for ambiguity increases, the therapist can reduce his or her activity level and transfer responsibility for the direction of therapy to the family. It is not likely that the perfect family has had experience with therapy. The therapist's willingness to discuss the family's expectations of therapy and the role of the therapist provides a starting point for educating the family about therapy. Family members' expectations may also help the therapist understand their behavior.

In working with perfect families, it is helpful to remember that they would not be in therapy if everything really were so perfect. The perfect family is likely to appear calm and in control. A symptom such as bulimia signals difficulty. The calm exterior indicates a lack of practice in tolerating intensity, as well as rules about avoiding the expression of intense emotions. *The perfect family's induction can be very powerful; the therapist needs to be aware of his or her personal reactions to and needs from the family.*

The perfect family has subtle mechanisms for distance regulation. In this case distance regulation was choreographed by the therapist to increase the family's stamina for intensity. In this way, it was less likely that the family would resort to old, "nice" patterns of distance regulation. Flexibility with the length of time between sessions and psychoeducation are useful tools for regulating emotional distance and facilitating change.

# CHAPTER 19

# *The Longs: Treating the Overprotective Family*

THE OVERPROTECTIVE FAMILY bears a striking resemblance to other psychosomatic families. Minuchin's classic five signs of a psychosomatic family — rigidity, overprotection, enmeshment, lack of conflict resolution, and detouring conflict through the child — are definitely operative in the overprotective family. In fact, we believe that many therapists mistakenly view families of bulimics simply as a cross between the overprotective and perfect types.

The centripetal, or inwardly turned, focus of the overprotective family frequently keeps it and its children out of contact with a therapist until problems emerge in adolescence or the launching transition in the family life-cycle. This is the isolation that Schwartz et al. (1984) mention as an additional feature of bulimic families. One or both parents may be depressed, but this is rarely discussed or even very well-known to anybody but the family. This again echoes the common stance in the family of ignoring conflict and not discussing problems with anybody outside the family. A depression in the mother is, as mentioned earlier, frequently reflective of the chaos and loss in her family-of-origin, and the likelihood of her being an incest victim certainly exceeds the average. We have come to believe that the overprotection frequently represents a flight in the opposite direction of her family of origin; not only is a family created that is cohesive, but also the daughters are protected as the mother never was.

The Long family was chosen as illustrative of the overprotective family. The course of the treatment with one of the authors was 10 months, although there had been several other therapy contacts before that time. An enmeshed mother-daughter relationship, an extremely peripheral but controlling fa-

249

ther, and difficulty leaving home as the only child of the marriage capture the central dynamics in this family. Yet they differ from a perfect family in that connections with the outside world were not uniformly successful and members of the family varied widely in their accomplishments. The goals of therapy included rebalancing the power in the marital relationship, facilitating the launching of the symptomatic daughter, developing more appropriate boundaries, and addressing the multigenerational issues in both Mr. and Mrs. Long's family of origin.

While the daughter, Sara, participated in two bulimia groups and brief periods of individual therapy, the majority of the treatment course was family therapy.

## FAMILY HISTORY

Sara, 17, is the only daughter of James, 62, and Anne, 48 who had been married for 19 years. The genogram in Figure 12 illustrates the characters in this family drama. James was 14 years older than Anne and had been married before. He had two sons from that marriage, Frank, 31, and Sam, 29. Both had left home 10 years earlier. James' first wife, Cathy, had been abusive to the two boys and became overtly psychotic. James had taken custody of the boys after the divorce, but was uninvolved with either of them on an emotional basis. Both boys worked for their father in the family business, and each had serious psychological problems. Frank clearly had a major affective disorder, unipolar type, and Sam had a history of tumultuous relationships and was a "daredevil" — risking his life repeatedly in dangerous situations such as car racing, flying as a bush pilot, and hang gliding.

Anne and James had met while she was employed in James' business. Due to James' reluctance to get involved the courtship was prolonged before they eventually married. Sara was born one year later. Anne continued to work in the family business. The family employment arrangement both captured the overinvolvement present in the family and supported the authority hierarchy, with all members employed in some capacity by James.

James was an only child whose father ran a sporting goods business. His father was immersed in his work, and his mother focused all her attention on James. His mother had been very disturbed, and he left home abruptly in his early teens. A prevailing theme in his mind was that children make women crazy and needy and he was fearful of this happening again in his second marriage. As avoidance of conflict is typical in the overprotective family, this fear prompted him to "keep his hands off" his wife and Sara's relationship and facilitated their overinvolvement.

Anne came from a very large, rigid, fundamentally religious family. Her father was a minister, frequently gone — "ministering to everyone but his

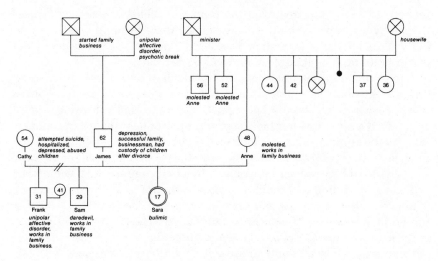

*Figure 12.* The Long Family

own family." She was the oldest girl in the family and was assigned major responsibility for the caretaking of the younger children. She was molested over an eight-year period by her two older brothers. Anne stated that she felt that her mother knew about it but refused to intervene. Too terrified to tell anyone, she felt guilty about the molestation and was determined to keep her daughter safe from men. James was aware of the molestation, but they had never talked about it in any depth. Later, as this issue was addressed in therapy, James stated that he felt that was the reason Anne protected Sara so much and that he thought she was afraid that he would molest Sara. This overprotection in this family reflected a "flight from chaos" in Anne's family.

## TREATMENT HISTORY

The Long family sought treatment for Sara's bulimia after a history of unsuccessful therapy. Her eating disorder began at age 16, shortly after her boyfriend broke up with her. She confided her binge-purge behavior to her mother, who urged her to use willpower to stop. When this was unsuccessful, Anne requested therapy from a psychiatrist, who prescribed antidepressants. She saw Sara individually for several sessions and then asked the parents to come in for a session. In the second family session, Sara ran out of the room and disappeared for several hours, effectively ending treatment. She was referred to our group treatment program and reluctantly agreed to participate in a group. She emphatically denied that her family had any role in the development of her eating disorder and reiterated her mother's view of her bulimia as a "lack of willpower" on her part.

Group proved to be a mechanism by which Sara was able to listen to others talk about the relationship of family to bulimia in an atmosphere where she was able to protect her parents less. Sara's family drawing (Figure 13) marked a move towards being less protective of her family and captured many of the family dynamics which surfaced during the family therapy. She drew her father involved in his work, with the telephone as part of his arm. There is a wall between her father and others in the family, with her mother providing protection to the children. Sara's attempt to join with her father is shown by the camera on her arm (an interest of her father's), which is similar to the telephone on the arm of her father. The picture was extremely difficult for Sara to draw — she made numerous attempts before bringing it to group. She was able to draw it only after an argument with her mother. This seemed to create enough separation for her to draw the picture.

After the group, she was referred to a male family therapist — again the request for therapy came from the mother. He saw the family for six sessions which the father attended only on a sporadic basis. The family "slid out of therapy," canceling numerous appointments and saying it wasn't helping the bulimia.

Sara attended a second bulimia treatment group, in which she was able to articulate both her anger at her mother for smothering her and her wish to get closer to her father. At the end of this group, Sara requested therapy with one of the authors (who co-led the group). This marked the first time that Sara requested treatment. While the group had facilitated Sara's understanding of the purpose of her bulimia, there had been no significant decrease in her symptoms. At the time at which she requested therapy, she was bingeing and purging three to six times a day.

## THE INITIAL CONSULTATION — WHETTING
## THE FAMILY'S APPETITE FOR THERAPY

The therapist agreed to see the family for a consultation session, rather than agreeing to see them for family therapy. This was due to several reasons. First, they appeared to be a family at risk for dropping out of treatment, based on their past therapy history. The consultation session was used to investigate: 1) whether the therapist would be able to join with the family; 2) the willingness of the family to be involved in therapy; 3) whether they would agree to conditions the therapist set for seeing the family; and 4) whether the therapist would be able to join with the family. James was 20

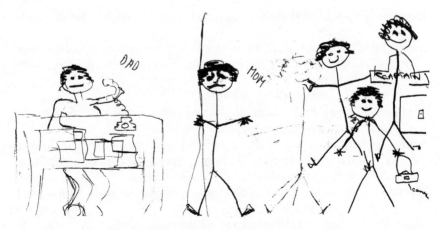

*Figure 13.*

minutes late for the consultation appointment. Anne suggested that we go ahead and start since she was unsure that he would be able to attend. The therapist decided not to start the session without him and informed her that the session would be cancelled and rescheduled if he did not come. After James arrived, Sara sat between her two parents, looking tense and angry, her head down. We pick up the dialogue early in the first session:

Therapist: This isn't the first time the family has been asked to come in for therapy. Can you fill me in on what has happened in previous treatment?

Anne: Well, Sara got really upset with the psychiatrist we saw and didn't want to go back. I think she was right, because the bulimia got worse when we went. Actually that happened with both therapists. We had a hard time scheduling appointments — James is out of town a lot and we just couldn't work out a time for us all to come. (Looking at her husband)

Therapist: It seems like everyone who has worked with Sara feels that it is important for the family to be involved in therapy.

James: (arms crossed) I might as well tell you from the beginning. I'm the bad guy in all this (smiling). (Pause)

Therapist: How's that?

James: I just don't understand the girls. It's probably my fault since I'm not home much — at least that's what they tell me (gesturing to Anne and Sara).

Therapist: So you think that Sara's bulimia is a way to tell you that she needs you?

James: I don't think she needs me except to feed her and put a roof over her head. Her mother is the one she's really close to. I've never known how to talk to Sara.

Sara: (angrily) You haven't ever tried!

Therapist: I always think of bulimia as a way to say something to the family. What do you think that Sara is trying to say?

Anne: That she is unhappy with herself and wants to lose weight. I don't think she really is angry at her father. She knows that he works hard to give us some advantages that he never had.

Therapist: If my hunch is correct and Sara is trying to say something to you, what do you think it might be?

Anne: Maybe that she's not ready for all the responsibility that goes with going away to school. I think she worries about her grades, boyfriends, and making friends at school. Isn't that right, Sara?

Sara: (Looks down and nods.)

Therapist: Does your mother have your voice, Sara?

Sara: No, but I don't know for sure what my bulimia has to do with the family. I just know they have to be here.

Therapist: I think you are right, Sara — having both your parents here will help us figure out what you are trying to say and to help you say it in a different voice or way.

The dialogue illustrates the roles of the family members — the father even admits to being the "bad guy" off in the distance. The enmeshment of Anne and Sara is evidenced by Anne's speaking for Sara. Anne works to protect both Sara and her husband. The consultation continued with the therapist offering her concerns about taking the case. She asked each person to talk about why she should see the family, expressing doubt about the family's commitment to therapy. This worked to put the family in the position of asking for family therapy, essentially helping to frame the bulimia as a family issue and whetting their appetite for therapy.

There were several indications in the consultation session that this was an overprotective family: the mother's speaking for the daughter, the mother's telling Sara that she wasn't really angry at her father, and the fact that the parents clearly had difficulty communicating. Almost paradoxically, James' admitting to being the "bad guy" protected the family from further, potentially dangerous, discussion. Sara's leaving for school would leave the parents to deal with their issues as a couple. Sara established control in the family by her protection of her parents, which was an important function of the bulimia.

The therapist decided to see the family for four sessions, under several conditions, at which point a decision would be made about whether or not to continue. The conditions were reinforced in the following letter, which was sent after the consultation:

Dear Anne, James, and Sara,

I have spent some time thinking about the issues that we discussed in our first consultation session. Your family has requested that I work with you to help Sara and the family to recover from the bulimia. I support your commitment to continue to work on the bulimia, even though at times it is difficult for you to understand the purpose of the behavior and how it fits into the family relationships. My concern is that we set up the conditions of therapy so that it has the greatest chance for success. I know that it has been difficult for the family to stick with therapy before, but I admire your willingness to continue to try.

There has been an important reason that each professional who has worked with Sara has asked the family to be present for sessions. This is not because the family is to blame for Sara's bulimia. James and Anne, you are an important part of Sara's recovery. Your support of her and of the therapy can speed her recovery from the bulimia and can help the family to adjust to Sara's leaving home.

As we discussed in the consultation session, I have several conditions for accepting the family for treatment. *First of all, all three of you must be present for the first four sessions.* As we talked about in the first consultation, I am aware that this will mean rearranging work schedules and making the therapy a priority. Each of you agreed that you would be willing to do so. If only two of you come to the session, it will be cancelled and there will be a charge. If this happens twice in a row, therapy will be ended. We will be meeting weekly for the next four weeks. I will try to be flexible in working out times to meet. However, it is important for the continuity of therapy that we meet on a regular basis. That is my second condition of therapy. *We will meet weekly, unless one of the family members is out of town for more than a week.* When we talked about this in the first session, you did not anticipate that this would happen in the next month. If there is more than one week during those four weeks that all three of you are unable to attend, therapy will be ended. My third condition for treatment is that *all family members must stay in the room during the session.* If the session begins to feel too intense and one of you wants to leave, you need to let me and the others know this. The last condition is that *if I ask you to do something outside the session in order to facilitate the therapy, I ask that you follow through on this request.*

I realize that it may be difficult for each of you in different ways to follow through with these conditions. I also feel that the family can meet these conditions and will help Sara to begin the recovery process. You may also need to be prepared for Sara's bulimia worsening as treatment begins. This can be a way for Sara to test whether you are tough enough and committed enough to stick with her. It can also be a way of expressing that the work is hard and stressful.

Each of you in your own way may try to protect the others when therapy gets intense. James, you may try to protect Anne and Sara by not being able to attend the sessions. Anne, you may protect the family by trying to keep things calm and smooth between James and Sara. Sara, you may try to protect your parents by accelerating your bulimia, or by running out of therapy or away from your family. It will be important for you to work to protect each other less.

You have many strengths as a family which will help to carry you through therapy. Your willingness to continue to seek help is an indication of the family strength. If each of you makes a commitment, you will be able to follow through with the conditions for therapy. We will reevaluate at the end of the four sessions.

Please make sure that all three of you have a chance to read this letter before our next meeting. I appreciate your willingness to be involved.

The letter formalized the conditions agreed upon in the consultation and set up therapy on the therapist's terms. The therapist let the family know that she was serious about ending therapy if the conditions were not met. She chose to capitalize upon the desperateness of the family and the strength of the relationship with Sara that had been built by the group sessions. The therapist did not set up any conditions that she did not feel the family could meet and attempted to set as few conditions as possible in order to keep the family invested in therapy. The initial consultation indicated the direction for the first phase of therapy: joining and setting therapy on the therapist's terms. It was clear that if these two goals were not accomplished, the family would probably end treatment, again unsuccessful in addressing Sara's bulimia and the family dynamics.

## SYSTEMIC FUNCTIONS OF BULIMIA

When we see families, we routinely assess the role the bulimia plays in the system. The purpose of the bulimia may vary in degree from family to family, but an understanding of it provides the therapist with a look into the process and patterns that are operating in the family system. Since a number of our intervention techniques are derived from structural family therapy, understanding the family system is essential.

An important function of Sara's bulimia in her relationship with her mother was that it established a boundary in an otherwise enmeshed relationship. Anne was a compulsive dieter and would involve Sara in the diets, as an active participant or as her "conscience" or an auxiliary source of willpower. Sara would encourage her mother to "keep trying"; this aspect of their relationship reflected the role reversal and overinvolvement of the mother and daughter. The daughter was involved in the mother's personal struggles with her body-image (which reflected her self-image) and coached her mother to success. Sara would binge, eating both for herself and for her mother. The purging was a way to reverse the enmeshment by creating distance and a difference between herself and her mother. She would leave visible signs of her vomiting in the bathroom, demanding that her parents take notice. Anne had no real friends other than her daughter. A common complaint by Sara was that her mom should "get some friends." This would have served to reduce the intensity of Anne and Sara's relationship, and performed a boundary-establishing, enmeshment-reducing function by itself.

Sara's bulimia played an important distance-regulating function for her father in the family system. James' being pulled into the system by the demands of the symptoms had problems and benefits. The problems were related to too much closeness. Anne could never totally trust her husband with her daughter, given her own history of incest. Sara's bulimia served to reinforce the idea that women in his life were crazy and that it was somehow his fault. Thus, he maintained a distant stance, allowing his wife to contend with Sara. The bulimia necessitated his involvement, paving the way for benefits, but exemplifying the potential problems. The symptom of bulimia reflected unresolved multigenerational issues in the parents' family of origin. It represented the craziness of the women in James' family and the overprotection generated by Anne's molestation experiences in her family.

Lastly, the bulimia served as an important conflict-detouring function, as it allowed Sara's parents to engage in detouring via their support of Sara. As they worried about Sara, they could avoid addressing their marital conflict, but yet would still be together as a couple. The bulimia served to draw the parents closer together, at least fleetingly. The parents would stop fighting because "Sara would get upset." During the therapy sessions, Sara seemed regularly on the verge of running out of the room, particularly when the focus was more and more on marital issues. Her role became redefined as the conflict barometer, and she was told to raise a finger when parental conflict was becoming too intense and she felt that she had to leave.

## PHASE 1: JOINING AND ESTABLISHING THERAPY ON THE THERAPIST'S TERMS

The first phase of therapy comprised eight sessions. The family decided (along with the therapist) after four sessions that they wanted to continue therapy. The therapy continued with the therapist setting a certain number of sessions after which they would reevaluate. This again helped the family feel that they had a voice in the process and some control over the therapy. The focus of this first phase was the joining process and some initial efforts to interrupt the mother-daughter coalition, decrease the distance of the father from the other family members, and reframe the bulimia as a family issue.

The first phase of therapy was shaped by two broad themes. The first of these was a continuation of the therapist's setting the therapy on her terms, which began with the first consultation. In a rather curious way, this battle also served to facilitate the therapist's joining with the Long family. As Sara put it, her father enjoyed "throwing his weight around" and control was clearly an issue. The fact that the therapist (who was female) did not back down and continually pushed him seemed to evoke a grudging respect. One of the battles was fought quite early. James used the therapist's telephone to make a business call immediately after the session. This behavior was a metaphor of his peripherality and disengagement, an illustration of the blurring between family and work, and an assertion of his importance to the therapist and to the family. After this occurred once, the therapist informed him that he could no longer make calls from her office. The assertiveness of the therapist with James challenged the family's sense of him as someone who would always do what he wanted. It also was a model of a female interacting with him in a powerful way and empowered Anne and Sara to begin viewing their relationship with him as more open for negotiation.

The second theme in this phase of therapy pertained to the enmeshment in the mother-daughter relationship, and its connection to the estrangement of the couple. This was reflected in the difficulty that the family had in launching Sara. Several interventions and directives from the therapist were made to address the enmeshment.

Therapist: You call them "the girls."
James: Yeah, I know it bugs them (Anne and Sara exchange glances) but that's what they are—two girls.
Anne: That makes me so mad. He treats me like a child.
Sara: Mom, sometimes it feels like you're my age. You borrow my clothes, wear my makeup, you even talk to my friends on the phone when they call like they're your friends.
Anne: Sara, I thought you were proud of the fact that I can wear your clothes.
James: (To therapist) See, I told you—two girls . . .
Therapist: How could your mother be more like a mother, Sara?
Sara: Well, she doesn't have any friends of her own. It's like she lives through me and my friends. Neither of them have anything but me and the business.
Therapist: It seems like the bulimia is the one thing that you have that's all yours—that your mother doesn't have. What will you have when Sara leaves home? (Turning to mother)
Anne: Oh, I'll be fine.
Therapist: How can you, Anne, and how can you, James, convince Sara

that she doesn't need to stick around any longer — that the two of you can take care of yourselves?
Sara: They can't.
Therapist: Anne? James? Sara isn't convinced yet.

The issue of leaving home was central during the entire course of therapy. The therapist needed to continually push the family to see the interrelatedness of the symptom to the family dynamics. This was done in several ways. First, the situation was reframed as one in which the parents had failed to give Sara the message that they could take care of themselves and each other when she left. Secondly, the parents were challenged to give Sara evidence that they would do so. As the therapist came back to this over and over again, Sara was pushed out of the middle of the marital conflict and a different view of her was established.

As there was more pressure on the marital relationship, this was reflected in the first major crisis. James had his wife call to cancel since he had a business trip. He was unsure how long he would be gone, and Anne mentioned that James had suggested maybe it would be helpful to see just the "two girls." The therapist refused and asked them to call when the three could come in together. Sara's bulimia worsened significantly and the family called for a session after a week's absence.

James: (Arms folded) I had to cancel an important meeting to be here today.
Therapist: It must be important for you to be here.
James: Well, if I didn't come, I never would have heard the end of it from those two.
Therapist: Does that mean that you've decided not to be the bad guy today? I think it is important for the family to have a bad guy.
James: (smiling) Well, maybe I just won't talk.
Therapist: Then you could still be the bad guy. Any other ideas of what you can do in the session to be the bad guy?

The session continued with James offering other ways he distanced himself from his wife and daughter (calling them "the girls," telling them that they are too emotional, making "joking" criticism, yawning). The therapist instructed him to try all these things in the session, saying it would be important for Anne and Sara to learn to challenge him. This facilitated two of the goals of therapy — to rebalance the power in the family and to decrease the emotional distance between James and other members.

By the end of this phase, Anne was no longer speaking for Sara in the session, the two were not exchanging clothes, and Sara was directed not to listen if her mother wanted to talk about anything personal or intimate.

Anne began to make some attempts to renew old friendships with other women her age, which were supported strongly by the therapist. The focus of this phase was maintained by the therapist's greeting the couple each session with "What have you done this week to convince Sara that she can leave home?"

## PHASE 2: FAMILY-OF-ORIGIN ISSUES AS A SOURCE OF MARITAL DYSFUNCTION

As Anne and Sara began to function more autonomously and independently from each other, it was anticipated that the marital dysfunction would become more overt, as Anne would need more from James. Therapy still included the daughter because of the anticipated buffering role she could play between her parents to sidetrack the conflict.

In this phase of therapy, the focus shifted to Anne and James as a couple, enabling the therapist to explore family-of-origin issues as a richer context for understanding the three-way matrimony among Anne, James, and Sara.

Anne: Well, he hasn't done any of that. I mean, the filling in you keep asking about.
Therapist: He hasn't, huh?
Anne: No.
Sara: No, he hasn't.
Therapist: It will be important for you not to fill in for your father, Sara. Anne, what do you need from your husband? Can you tell him?
James: I've been gone all week on business.
Anne: It doesn't matter if you're home or not. It's the same. I feel so alone in that house.
James: Well, I feel alone too.
Sara: Dad, you've . .
Therapist: You don't need to bail your parents out here. Why don't you move your chair out of the circle—over there. Anne, what do you need from him?
Anne: I want to spend some time with him. I only see him at work and that's not enough (starts to cry).
James: We've been over and over this. Besides, what does this have to do with her throwing up all the time?
Sara: Dad, can't you understand . . .
Therapist: Sara, why don't you move your chair back further. I know it's really hard not to jump in but your parents need to learn to solve this without you. I can tell you've had a lot of practice jumping in. Could the two of you tell Sara that she doesn't need to jump in, and that she should sit over there?

This particular segment illustrates very clearly the marital conflict. The daughter interrupted several times on behalf of her mother, and the therapist had to be alert and direct so as not to get caught up in either allowing that to happen or losing momentum by answering the father's questions about why this is all relevant. There were two additional challenges. The first was not to get overwhelmed by the rigidity and despair evident in the marriage — the rigidity from all parties' seeming unwillingness to change and the despair from the hopelessness that they projected, e.g., "It's been this way a long time." It is easy to see how Sara was pulled into the marriage.

The escalating of the marital conflict continued along the lines of:

- "What are you going to do to fill the gap?"
- "I don't know if you've convinced Sara yet. What else are you planning to do to show her that when she leaves she won't be leaving the two of you to rattle around in that big house, each alone?"
- "Do you think you can put the relationship back on the right track so she feels that she can leave home?"

Repeatedly the daughter will assume her previous role, and the therapist and the parents need to watch for this and resist it. It is important that the therapist continue to monitor her integrity within the system. The enmeshment of the overprotective family is much more pervasive and insidious than what we see in the other two family types. Therapists are not immune to this pull. A concrete indicator of losing perspective is if the therapist fails to create intensity around the marriage for more than one session in a row.

An important focus during this phase of the therapy was addressing the family-of-origin issues for both parents. This allowed for a more indirect avenue towards the conflict, still allowing for intensity, but making it a bit easier for the parents to confront. James maintained his distance from his wife in part because he was scared by her neediness. It was helpful for the therapist to direct her involvement with others outside the family (e.g., other women her age), so that, as Sara left home, the father would not be expected to fulfill all of her needs.

Anne: I'm afraid that Sara won't be able to go away to school if her bulimia doesn't get better.
Therapist: The bulimia would be a way for her to stay home?
Anne: I'm not sure, but I know I'd worry about her if she's throwing up all the time. She doesn't take very good care of herself.
Therapist: So you watch over her, and help to take care of her.
James: She watches over her like a hawk — I don't know why.
Therapist: When a parent protects a child in the way that Anne protects Sara, I find that usually something has gone on in the family or in the

family of the parents that has taught them that children need protection. Anne, how did you learn that children need so much protection?

Anne: (tearing up) I don't know, well, maybe it's because no one protected me when I was growing up.

Therapist: (gently) How were you left unprotected?

Sara starts to interrupt and the therapist gestures for her to be quiet.

Anne: (tears streaming down her face) My two older brothers, they, they bothered me and no one stopped them (starts to sob).

Therapist: Your brothers molested you.

Anne: (nods)

James shifts away.

Therapist: (gesturing to him) It's important that you stay near your wife right now.

James: I know that's why she protects Sara so much. Sometimes I think she worries that I'm going to get funny with Sara.

The therapist directed Anne to talk to her husband about the molestation. While he knew about it, they had never talked directly about it. The therapist supported and directed the talking, keeping the interaction between the couple. It was essential that the therapist had joined strongly with the family at this point because the discussion touched on major themes in both parents' families of origin. The molestation helped the family to make sense of the mother's protectiveness and allowed her to express her fears about having James get close to Sara. It challenged James' fears that talking about the molestation would make his wife crazy or plunge her into a depression. The session marked a shift in the family, with the parents functioning more as a couple. It allowed for a discussion of what protection was appropriate for a 17-year-old, framing to the mother that she could not have learned what children and teenagers needed in terms of protection because of the lack of appropriate protection in her family of origin. The therapist predicted that Anne would be sad after talking about the molestation and said that this was normal and appropriate and not a sign of craziness. It also allowed James to get closer to Sara, after Anne was able to voice her fears directly.

This session also marked a significant decrease in Sara's bulimia. The family was encouraged by this improvement. They could see that they had made changes which were reflected in a decrease in the symptoms. The therapist could use this improvement for more leverage and also as another way to support additional changes.

It was also around this time that the therapist directed the parents to come and leave the sessions in one car and for Sara to come and leave in a separate car. This request was designed to concretely reflect the "coupleness" of the parents and to support Sara's movement away from home.

## PHASE 3: LAUNCHING

For the Longs, the third phase of therapy built directly on the work of the first two phases, and enabled the therapist to get the family to focus exclusively on facilitating Sara's leaving home. With high school graduation a reality, an out-of-state university chosen, and Sara spending more time with friends her age, there was a reemergence of symptoms. Sara's bulimia became worse as the time to leave grew closer, Anne became more overtly depressed, and James began a pattern of coming late to the sessions.

This reemergence of symptoms is very common in working with rigid family systems and can make therapists question their judgment, become discouraged, and lose perspective. It can be hard to see anything positive about the family, particularly in the face of symptom regression. Yet it is essential that the therapist continue to restructure, anticipate the reemergence of family symptoms, interrupt old patterns, positively connote the reemergence of symptoms when possible, and compliment the family for the changes they have made. The reemergence of symptoms must be framed as something that is totally understandable, even an indication that change has been made. The family is faced with the option of choosing again whether they are serious about change.

For example, it would have been easy to ignore Sara's occasional attempts to speak for her parents or to attack her father. After all, the communication was much better. This phase took a great deal of energy and self-examination on the part of the therapist in order to continue to be direct, to address obstacles in treatment, and to encourage the family. A technique the therapist employed with the Long family in this phase was prediction of relapses. This laid the foundation for telling the family that the relapses made sense, that families change slowly, and that relapses often precede another period of growth. Thus, if there is a relapse in the bulimia, the family does not panic. If there is no relapse, the family can be praised for their increasing ability to handle difficult situations in a healthier manner.

With the overprotective family, the issues of personal autonomy and leaving home are recurrent themes. James and Anne were asked to talk about how each of them left home, and how they could help Sara leave home in a way that she wouldn't be cut off, but would be free to leave. The treatment modality changed during this phase of therapy, with Sara being seen individually and the parents coming in every three weeks. The father's lateness to the sessions was framed as his way of helping Sara detach; he was also asked to think of other, more direct ways he could help her leave. He and Sara visited the school she planned to attend, marking the first time that they had ever gone on a trip without Anne.

Individually, treatment was aimed at providing Sara with cognitive behavioral tools that she could use to help her control her bulimia on her own.

The individual sessions were also a way to mark Sara's separation from the family. The changing format reflected the family's launching of Sara. Prediction of relapses at school were made and techniques were described that Sara could use to manage the behavior.

It was explained to the family that leaving home for Sara had two parts—the physical and the emotional—and Sara was still not convinced she was no longer needed emotionally. It was anticipated that the stress of Sara's leaving would elicit a relapse to old longstanding relationship patterns among family members. The following dialogue reflects the movement of the family towards successful launching of Sara.

Therapist: James and Anne, I'd like you to talk about how much you're going to miss Sara when she's gone. I'd like you to also try to get her to jump into your conversations like she used to. Sara has become much better at staying out of your relationship so this is not going to be easy. One way you could do this, James, would be if you said things you think would make Anne cry.

Sara: No way—you can try as hard as you want but you can't get me to jump in (as she moves her chair back and crosses her arms).

Therapist: Sara, I think your parents can do a better job than you are giving them credit for.

Sara: I can still do it (defiantly).

Therapist: James and Anne, take three minutes to think of what you want to say to each other about Sara's leaving. Let's see if Sara can take the tension.

(Sara does very well; towards the end of the three minutes she avoids looking at either parent.)

Therapist: Who'd like to start?

James: Well, I know Anne is going to be most affected on a day-to-day basis because she and Sara *were* like best friends (Father is speaking in the past tense.)

Therapist: James, talk to Anne.

James: Anne, I know you are going to miss Sara and feel lonely. Sara will probably miss you too.

Anne: (Nods, lips trembling.)

(Therapist nods to James to continue.)

James: You won't have to tell her to pick up her wet towels in the bathroom or give her a backscratch. (Anne starts to cry.) (Sara is biting her lip.)

(Pause)

Anne: Yeah, it's really going to feel lonely, but I'll manage. It would make it easier, James, if you would spend more time with me. I know you are going to miss her too. It seems that just as the two of you are get-

ting closer, she has to leave. I've had her all these years.
(Pause) (Sara moves slightly towards her father, then leans back into her chair)
James: I feel closer to both of you, in different ways.
Anne: I'm afraid you're going to throw yourself into your work when Sara leaves and we don't come here anymore.
(Sara gets up and looks out the window — as though she doesn't hear.)
Therapist motions couple to continue.
James: Maybe I will. You'll just have to learn to take care of yourself.
(Sara walks over to her purse and starts to look through it.)

The dialogue continued as James and Anne attempted to pull Sara into their discussion. Sara worked hard to stay out of the marital interaction and the therapist praised her for not jumping into the conversation and reflected on the changes both she and her parents had made.

Sara's bulimia worsened significantly about six weeks before leaving, and then about two weeks before she left, the bulimia stopped. She was symptom-free for the first two months of college and had a minor relapse during finals which she was able to understand and control.

## SUMMARY

The Long family presented a challenge to the therapist — how to join with the family so that they would be able to stay in treatment in order to address the family issues connected to the systemic function of the bulimia. An overinvolved mother-daughter dyad and a markedly peripheral, although powerful, father kept the family from being able to successfully launch the daughter. The fact that two group treatments, using both cognitive techniques and a family focus, had not been effective in decreasing the bulimic behavior significantly indicated that the family needed to be involved in order for Sara to recover. However, the group had provided a necessary step in treatment, in that it helped Sara to join with the therapist and to see the need to involve her family in therapy. Also, as a result of group, she became less protective of her parents. It may be that in order to stay in family therapy, the Longs needed the previous treatment failures. This accentuated their desperateness and willingness to meet the conditions set by the therapist. It is also our assessment that the female therapist provided an important dimension in the therapy. She was able to provide a model to Anne and Sara as a woman who interacted with James in a powerful way.

The most critical phase of therapy with the Long family was setting the therapy on the therapist's terms, an issue that is discussed in Chapter 21 on obstacles to treatment. James would have preferred to stay as peripheral as possible, but effective treatment was predicated on getting him actively involved and committed to therapy. It took experience on the part of the therapist, a great deal of consultation with other professionals, and a belief that her assessment of the necessity of involving all family members was correct. The therapist had to be willing to risk that the family would not be able to meet the conditions and that they might drop out of therapy. Insisting on conducting therapy only with all three family members continually present forced the parents to confront their marital problems. It also required the therapist to respond to James in as powerful a manner as possible.

In some ways, the Longs did not even appear to be married — the father had two daughters who did their dieting and socializing together. The bulimia was a natural extension of the joint mother-daughter dieting and enmeshment. All of the family members were in distress, not just Sara. The multigenerational roots and subsequent emotional cut-offs as they related to Sara's bulimia surfaced as therapy progressed. It was essential that therapy address the molestation of the mother as it related to both the distance between Sara and her father and the distance in the marital relationship.

Individual treatment, framed as a systemic intervention, was employed as a marker of Sara's launching from her parents. In addition, it provided an environment in which Sara could discuss the bulimia and learn techniques for controlling it in an atmosphere separate from her mother, who was overly involved in the behavior. It was important that the individual therapy was used only in the third phase of treatment. If this had been initiated earlier, it would have been much more difficult for the parents not to see it as identifying Sara as the patient.

The rigidity, enmeshment, overprotection, and conflict-detouring in the Long family clearly illustrated the issues that can arise in treating the overprotective family. The emphasis on appearance as a measure of self-esteem and the isolation of each of the family members, the parents in particular, are frequently observed in this family type. Consistent escalation of the marital conflict, decreasing the enmeshment between mother and daughter, and engaging with the father in a powerful and genuine way that acknowledged his loneliness and distance from others provided the framework within which therapy was conducted.

# CHAPTER 20

# *The Weisfields: Treating the Chaotic Family*

TREATMENT OF THE CHAOTIC bulimic family has not been addressed in the literature on eating disorders. This absence is striking considering the number of persons with bulimia who come from multiproblem and/or alcoholic families — hallmarks of the chaotic family. Chaotic families' tendency to have multiple problems and to operate from crisis to crisis contributes to both their contacts with numerous professionals and to premature termination once the precipitating crisis that prompted help-seeking abates. They also demand an enormous amount of energy from a therapist; consequently, many therapists do not accept such families. Simply put, it is difficult for the therapist to keep the chaotic family in treatment and difficult for the chaotic family to maintain the motivation necessary to stay in therapy.

The Weisfield family is an atypical chaotic family in that they remained with treatment. As we have pointed out previously, the chaotic family may have a very low tolerance for therapy, so it is usual to approach treatment in a consultation format. The Weisfields were not particularly insightful, but they remained in therapy through many difficult periods of transition for the family and its individual members. This was a difficult family: Besides multiple problems and alcoholism, cultural differences had to be resolved. Cultural factors were subtle, but salient in conceptualizing the purpose of the symptoms, the need for symptoms, and the approach to treatment.

Therapy with the Weisfield family spanned a two-year period, after which therapy with the bulimic daughter continued for six months. Therapy modalities utilized were family, group, and individual therapy. Consultations and alcohol evaluations, in addition to bibliotherapy, Al-anon, and seminars, were part of treatment. Regardless of the modality of therapy, treatment was aimed toward establishing appropriate boundaries, helping the two youngest children assume more age-appropriate self-care, enabling the family negotiate the launching of the two youngest children, teaching individual members how to get some of their needs met within and outside of the family, reducing the pressure for the family to maintain the appearance of a happy family, and helping individuals to act more powerfully in controlling their lives. This last aim was central to enabling the two youngest offspring to relinquish their protection of their parents.

In this chapter, excerpts are taken from family and individual sessions during the active phase of family therapy. The sessions were selected for their illustration of the common themes and types of work that take place with these families. The work with the Weisfield family took place in three stages: 1) information-gathering; 2) restructuring the family; and 3) leaving home.

## THE INITIAL CONTACT

The therapist first had contact with the bulimic daughter, Nina, one year before the family sought therapy. She had graduated from high school and was getting ready to take a trip to Europe. Nina had called wanting information about group therapy for bulimia. Her therapist had suggested that this might be a useful approach to treatment. Her planned trip, however, made it impossible for her to be part of the group. Approximately one year later, Daniella, Nina's mother, contacted the therapist. Nina had recently returned from Europe, looking thin and having lost a considerable amount of weight. Relatives had called from Israel expressing concern about her eating habits. Nina also contacted the therapist at this time, asking for a consultation and freely admitting her distress—primarily over her family's uproar and panic over her health.

During the initial telephone contacts with Nina and her mother, there were indications that this was a chaotic family: 1) Daniella sounding very desperate and frustrated (mothers from perfect or overprotective families usually do not let out simultaneous desperateness and anger as overtly); 2) both Daniella and Nina disclosed a tremendous amount of personal information on the telephone with little prompting (which suggested both boundary problems and isolation or disengagement in the family); and 3) Nina had disclosed some descriptions of her father which indicated that he might have an alcohol problem.

Several consultation appointments were conducted with the entire family, except for the oldest daughter who lived in England. There were several goals in the first few interviews, including: 1) determining the extent and nature of the family's problems; 2) obtaining information about the current and past functioning in the Weisfield family and in the parents' respective families of origin; and 3) forming hypotheses about the function of bulimia in the family. Additionally, information was sought on substance abuse patterns in the family and signals of physical and sexual abuse.

## PHASE 1: INFORMATION-GATHERING

### The Consultations

The assessment and evaluation of the family started out in a consultation format which included family members: the father, 56-year-old Phil, the 55-year-old mother, Daniella, her 30-year-old daughter from her first marriage, Sarah, 19-year-old Nina, the older of Phil and Daniella's two biological children and the only son, 17-year-old Guy (see Figure 14). Daniella's other daughter from her first marriage, Elizabeth, 33, was absent from the therapy.

It was not difficult to join with members of this family, primarily because they were all so emotionally needy. Because of the tendency of family members to talk over each other and interrupt, it was difficult for them to be heard or acknowledged. Simply acknowledging and reflecting back what members had said was enough to establish some connection. Phil was the most difficult member to join with, though he, too, was overtly needy. Nevertheless, joining with him was accomplished in the same way by offering him acknowledgment and respect.

Family members tended to talk quickly and increasingly loudly in an attempt to be heard above other family members who were talking simultaneously and interrupting each other. The family members had a difficult time focusing on a particular issue and appeared scattered and unable to finish thoughts, give information, or express feelings because of their tendency to interrupt one another. Daniella and Nina, who bore a striking resemblance to each other, interrupted most often, especially in their attempts to expose other family members' problems. Daniella and Nina tended to finish each others' thoughts and sentences. Phil and Guy acted similarly with each other, but not to the same extreme degree.

Generally, Phil and Guy were very silent, volunteering little information or emotion, appearing to be present physically but not emotionally. When they did show emotion it tended to come out as irritation or anger. Sarah adopted the role of the referee, also tending to interrupt her mother and Nina. She often acted parentally towards her mother; she would tell her not to interrupt and to slow down, sometimes instructing her in their native language. On the surface, the family seemed to revolve around Daniella,

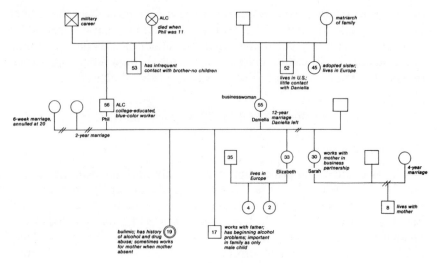

*Figure 14.* The Weisfield Family

though Phil seemed to exert a silent control by his capacity for anger.

Boundaries were clearly lacking and marked by both enmeshment and intrusion, particularly between Nina and her mother. Additionally, Phil seemed to confuse Nina with his wife, and Daniella tended to confuse Guy with her husband.

The organization of the family was inconsistent. Daniella and Phil did not function as a parental unit during the consultations, except when attention was focused on Nina as the symptomatic family member. Otherwise, there was an absence of effective executive functioning by parents. Rules seemed to change within the family from time to time with little reason. At times, Daniella was clearly head of the family during the consultations and therapy, as well as the source of financial stability for the family. At other times, Daniella appeared as an out-of-control adolescent, similar to her daughter Nina. (When she adopted a less powerful role, Phil would make an attempt to act as the head of the family, but he could not maintain this role.) Thus, it was difficult to sort out how much of Nina's style was modeled after her mother's and how much of it was the result of stress and her eating disorder. It was striking how Nina and Guy alternated between acting as brother and sister and reenacting their parents' relationship when they talked accusingly with each other.

The Weisfields' history as a family began when Daniella met Phil on a

vacation to the United States from her home in Israel. At that time she was
having difficulty in her marriage of 12 years. Phil and Daniella had a whirl-
wind romance for two months, one month of it being through an exchange
of letters. Phil asked Daniella to marry him and join him in the U.S. Daniella
agreed to marry him and left her husband—a move uncommon in her
culture. Daniella brought her two daughters, Elizabeth and Sarah, at that
time 10 and 8, respectively, with her to this country.

Daniella's leaving her first marriage greatly affected her relationship with
her parents. Her mother disapproved and both parents were saddened.
Though her father refrained from expressing his opinion, her mother interpreted his sentiments to Daniella. This was a close family; culturally, it was
unusual for family members to move far from one another, much less out
of the country. Daniella reported feeling a need to get away at this time,
as the family was too close and too involved in her life, but she felt guilty
for wanting to be farther away.

Phil had been married and divorced twice to foreign women (no children)
when he met Daniella. The first marriage lasted six weeks, the second two
years. His developmental years as the oldest of two boys were turbulent,
since his alcoholic mother died of tuberculosis when he was 11, at which
time he went to live with an uncle and aunt for approximately two years.
His father was unavailable due to military service. From age 13 to 16 he
lived with his father, and at 16 he joined the Navy. By age 20 he entered
his first marriage.

The first few years of Phil and Daniella's marriage were stressed by the
need to adjust to married life and to the cultural differences between them.
Phil taught both Daniella and her daughters to speak English, spending
hours with the girls each day after school. During these years, Phil continued
to work and completed a college degree in engineering. Three years into their
marriage, Nina was born and a year and a half later, Guy. While Daniella
was initially dependent on Phil to help her negotiate the new culture and
language, she learned quickly and began to show more independence and
interest in developing a career.

Five years into the marriage, the marital discord started to emerge as
Daniella became more independent. Phil and Daniella's fights became more
frequent; Phil began to drink heavily and to have extramarital affairs. He
was more and more verbally abusive and physically threatening. Shortly
after Nina and Guy entered grade school, Daniella started her own business.
Phil had made a career change, which Daniella viewed as a step down. His
change in job marked a decrease in his responsibility and level of functioning. Increasingly, the children and Daniella covered up for Phil when he
was drinking.

As Daniella worked on her business, Phil spent more time at home with the children. He appeared to dote particularly on Nina and lavished her with special presents that seemed to display a sensitivity and insight into what a child her age would like. During much of this time, Nina and Guy's older sisters acted as surrogate parents.

During the next three years, Nina and Guy experienced several changes. By the time Nina was eight and Guy was seven, Daniella had established her own business that required most of her attention. Phil was starting to assume the role of both mother and father (much as he had when the two older daughters were newly arrived to this country). In the next year and a half, both Elizabeth and Sarah left home, though they continued to live in the same city. Elizabeth began working and Sarah started college. Thus, within three years, Nina and Guy lost three mothers. Phil was more available to them during this period than at any previous or later time, though his drinking interfered with his ability to be consistent with his children.

Marital difficulties were more prominent in the marriage after the two older daughters left home. Daniella considered separating from Phil, since his drinking and abusiveness, including battering, were getting worse. However, as she seemed to move close to making this change, Phil experienced a severe depression, during which he made suicidal threats, and Daniella postponed her leaving. During the consultations, all the children were able to talk about the possibility that they and their parents might be better off if their parents divorced or separated. These disclosures came out as Nina and Guy remembered times when their father had either threatened their mother with a knife or hit her.

Despite the ongoing marital difficulties, the family was invested in presenting a successful image in the community. While the children expressed their confusion over their parents' unhappiness with each other and their inability to live with or without each other, outsiders and the extended family either chose to ignore or were unaware of the family's problems.

Both Nina and Guy were perfect children in many respects; they did well in school, got along with people, and were popular with peers. Teachers did not know they were having difficulties at home. Their use of drugs and alcohol in their mid-teens was invisible, as it did not interfere with their school performance. Nina started experimenting with drugs at 14 and Guy at 13. Guy started to use alcohol and marijuana regularly during the next year when Nina was away for school. At first Guy's drinking was not recognized by his parents. When he began drinking at home, Daniella's attempts to forbid this were not supported by Phil, who continued to drink. Also, during this period of time one family member always had some symptom requiring medical attention.

Shortly after her mother had visited her during her year of school abroad, Nina became very conscious of her weight. Her mother, especially attuned to physical appearance (she owned a modeling agency), had commented that Nina needed to lose weight. Nina started trying to lose weight before her return home to the United States for her junior year in high school.

The year that she returned home, her oldest sister, Elizabeth, moved to England with her husband. That same year she was gang raped while under the heavy influence of drugs. She had foggy memories of this trauma, and even had doubts about the reliability of her memory. By the end of her junior year in high school, Nina started experimenting with bulimia.

While there were elements of the dynamics of the perfect family (keeping symptoms invisible to outsiders) and the overprotective family (Daniella's extreme though inconsistent protection of her children), there was no question that the Weisfield family was primarily chaotic (unavailability of parents, physical abuse, marital discord, alcoholism, and the overt and abundant anger). The family had a history of increased difficulty when Phil and Daniella were compelled to engage with each other. This difficulty started when the two older daughters "left" home when Nina and Guy were nine and eight years old, respectively. Elizabeth and Sarah continued to have frequent contact with their parents and were financially dependent on their parents.

### The Systemic Function of Bulimia

Nina's development of bulimia provided many functions in the Weisfield family. Structurally, her bulimia alternately served a detouring-supportive function, as it enabled her parents to act as a parental unit as they worried about her, and a detouring-attacking function, as they blamed her for stressing the family. Both of these functions diverted Phil and Daniella from addressing their marital difficulties. Nina's bulimia allowed her to remain loyal to both parents (joining with her father's powerlessness and depression and joining with her mother's helplessness in the marital relationship) and to have both parents available to her at the same time.

On an affective level, Nina had developed symptoms which allowed her to comfort herself for her losses without having to tax the emotional resources of her parents or jeopardize their relationship. At the same time a very important function of Nina's bulimia was to express her anger while protecting herself from the family's abundant anger — particularly her parents' anger towards each other. By being bulimic, she was able to express her anger towards her father, but with the helplessness of a child, so that she did not threaten him as an adult woman.

*Spreading the Symptoms*

The following excerpt is taken from the first session after a series of three consultations with the family. This session served to further illuminate the function of bulimia in the family, as well as the need for continuous symptoms in the family over the previous five years.

Therapist: We've been talking about your symptoms, Nina, but from what the family has been telling me all of you have taken turns with symptoms.

Daniella: (Jumping right in and gesturing) Oh, I get these terrible headaches. I never used to get headaches. But they're so painful I have to take off work and go home to bed.

Therapist: You have always had these headaches?

Daniella: No, just for the last three years or so. But I manage.

Nina: (Turning to her mother) How about your ulcer? (Turning to the therapist) Mom has to take medication for her ulcer.

Daniella: Yes, I got it five years ago but I have medication. My back also gets pains. But what about Guy?

Guy: (Looking directly at his mother, sounding irritated) What about me?

Daniella: Your stomach.

Guy: (Squirming in his chair) Yeah, but I haven't had a problem for a while.

Therapist: Guy, what's the problem?

Guy: I first had it three years or four years ago (coincidentally when Nina was abroad). But nothing's happened now for four months. So I guess I'm all cured.

(Daniella has interrupted Guy, talking simultaneously, to say that it has been four years.)

Phil: (Interrupting, questioning gruffly, responding to Guy shrugging his shoulders looking annoyed) Did you go in for your appointment?

Guy: Naw, I've been feeling fine. Aren't we here because of Nina. (Nina looks intensely at Guy, with a look to kill.)

Therapist: She seems to be indicating that it might be helpful to her if other family members shared some of the burden of having symptoms. (Several family members asking, "What do you mean?") What are the other symptoms?

Sarah: I get constipated. That's it. (Pause)

Nina: How about all the drugs Guy does? Does that count as a symptom? (Guy looks back at Nina very irritated and annoyed.)

Daniella: (Jumping in, pointing at Guy before he has a chance to respond) His drinking! All those beer bottles I pick up downstairs. He drinks too much.

Therapist: Guy, Nina must be worried that you won't speak for yourself. Your family thinks you have more symptoms than just your stomach. It is OK with you, Phil and Daniella, that Guy drinks?

Daniella: No! It's not OK but I can't stop him. He tells me I nag him. Then he yells at me just like his father. I worry that he will get an alcohol problem.

Therapist: You've been very quiet, Phil.

Phil: (Bluntly) I have nothing to say. (Rescuing Guy) I don't see how any of this has to do with helping Nina get better. I thought that's why we're here.

Therapist: What is your symptom?

(Phil looks as though he has taken a stance not to say anything. Daniella smiles, slyly, and then seriously says . . . )

Daniella: He drinks, too. That's why he won't say anything about Guy.

Phil: Here we go again. (Phil has shifted his position, his face has reddened. He has raised his voice and is inappropriately loud.) So now you're going to call me a fucking alcoholic!

Daniella: You're the one who said it. (Turning to the therapist, gesturing emphatically) This upsets me so much. Can't you smell it? He has been drinking today. He gets loud when he has been drinking and he uses foul language. I am very sensitive. I can smell it across the room.

(Nina is shrinking in her chair, sliding down, with her arms folded across her chest.)

Phil: (Interrupts Daniella, gesturing, and talking very loudly) So now I'm a drunk, just a fucking drunk!

Nina: (Covering her ears and whimpering while sliding down in her chair) I can't stand it. Make them stop.

Phil: She's the one with the problem. I can control my drinking. (Addressing this to Nina) What's wrong with you? Sit up in your chair.

Nina: NOoooo. (Gets up and crawls behind her chair, hiding)

(Guy looks as though he has left the room, even though he has not changed position. Sarah is tearing up, crying.)

Daniella: Get up, Nina. You're acting like you are six. Act your age. (Turning to the therapist) See, a girl her age shouldn't be acting this way. Nina, why are you acting this way? She should be working and responsible and . . .

Therapist: (Daniella is gestured to stop.) Nina, perhaps you are six?

Nina: (Still huddled) This always happens. I don't want to be here! They can just fucking leave! I don't care if they all leave.

Therapist: Phil and Daniella, you were getting very angry at each other. I almost forgot that when Nina distracted me. Nina, do you always protect your parents this way? You are very effective. You must get

very tired from working so hard to protect them from each other's
   anger. My guess is that you are employed full-time protecting them.
Nina: (Looks up, a slight smile crosses her face; then she sits in her chair
   facing away from the family.)
Daniella: (Flustered, voice raised) What . . . what . . . do you mean she
   is protecting us? Look at her, do you call that protecting? She is helpless; she can't even take care of herself. How can she take care of us?
   I can take care of myself. (Muttering in a lower voice) I always have.
Therapist: Daniella and Phil, your children, espeically Nina, are showing
   me that you need protection so I won't look at your problems too closely. They keep protecting you with their symptoms, especially Nina and
   Guy. It sounds like right now Nina is working very hard to protect you
   two while she's trying to find someone else in the family to share some
   of the responsibility. Nina, you were trying very hard to get Guy to
   help you. It is very hard to get someone to help. You must feel stuck
   and angry that you are stuck. Guy has taken a turn with his stomach
   symptoms and drinking, but doesn't want to admit that he's still trying to help your parents, too.

The therapist's last statement summarizes the information gained from
the session. Nina is diverting attention away from the marital discord, while
sacrificing herself to keep the family pretending it is a family. Nina's bulimia
kept her young, giving Phil and Daniella a child to worry about, which in
turn would postpone the necessity of their dealing with the difficulties in
their relationship.

All the kids in the family had a history of protecting their parents both
physically and emotionally. As Daniella and Phil's conflict escalated, Nina's
symptoms got worse. *It became clear in this session that it was going to be
very difficult for Nina to let go of her symptoms.* Despite the family members' willingness to be involved in treatment to help Nina, they tenaciously
supported her symptoms — for example, by requiring her to cook, asking her
to model, or continuing to give her feedback that she had gained or lost
weight despite specific directions for these activities to cease. Her symptoms
satisfied the needs of the family too well while simultaneously enabling her
to be a child. At this point in the family's functioning, one of the children
needed to remain at home for the parents to stay together.

The next excerpt demonstrates the subtle and powerful way in which
Nina's symptoms divert the family from attending to long-standing problems, such as lack of privacy. It becomes clear that another function of Nina's
bulimia is that it affords her privacy in a family that has a difficult time
respecting personal boundaries. At the same time it keeps the family engaged
with her intensely, when there is a family tendency to disengage from
members who are not in crisis.

Guy: (Addressing Nina) I can't stand the mess you leave in the bathroom. It stinks from all your throwing up.

Nina: (Starting to shrink in her chair and tear up) Why are you always yelling at me? Someone tell him to stop.

Daniella: (Turning to the therapist) She is always using the upstairs bathroom when we have given her her own bathroom by her room downstairs. She even uses my bathroom when I tell her not to.

Therapist: I see a couple of things going on here. (Turning to Nina) One, Guy is insisting that the family focus on your symptoms because he does not want them to look at his symptoms. And, the family wants you to have your symptoms more invisibly. You're still letting them know things aren't right in the family?

Nina: (Talking in a whimpering high voice) Why do I have to stay downstairs? Perhaps you don't want me to live there at all. The upstairs bathroom is nicer and has a bathtub. I like to take baths.

Phil: Damn, she uses all the hot water. She can stay in there for a couple of hours in the middle of the night. She gets cold so damn easily that she's turning up the heat in the house all the time. She has no sense of what it costs for her comfort.

Therapist: It sounds like the bathroom is a comforting place for you.

Nina: (Pouting and sounding angry) It's the one place where I have privacy most of the time and can drown out everyone's noise (glaring at her father).

Phil: (Chuckling at her) What's that supposed to mean, kid? (Nina turns away, looking angrier and older.)

Therapist: (Turning to everyone) The noise gets this loud that it invades your privacy no matter where you are in the house?

Guy: Yeah.

Therapist: What do you do?

Guy: I try to go downstairs to my room, but it doesn't matter because they're loud. Dad throws things. So I just leave.

Therapist: How else do people invade each others' privacy?

Daniella: Nina takes my clothes.

Guy: (Simultaneously) Yeah, like my shirt. Nina, you took it, didn't you?

Sarah: (Before the other two are finished) She interrupts, she takes things from the agency, she borrows my things without asking.

Therapist: Everybody is pointing the finger at you, Nina. (Nina is sliding down in her chair.)

Nina: Yeah. (Raising her voice and lifting her head up) But they don't say how mom goes through my room and my drawers, or how Sarah borrows my things without asking, or dad barges in my room!

Therapist: Clearly, people do not know how to treat each other with respect for privacy and personal space. Whenever you interrupt someone in

here, you are not respecting this space. Nina is not the only one in the
family who has this problem

Several different types of communication were taking place in this excerpt. Anger from Nina was discouraged by her father's laughing at her and
calling her "kid." Family members were colluding to keep Nina the scapegoat. In working with the chaotic family, preparation before a session can
be important. In this excerpt the therapist decided to focus on the lack of
boundaries. It would have been easy to follow numerous other issues, but
if there is not a plan with this type of family, a session can become overwhelming and out of control.

Lack of boundaries was an extreme problem in this family. It was as
though there were no doors; a closed door meant very little. The loudness
of family members' yelling penetrated the doors. Intrusiveness was extreme.
Merely making suggestions or instructing the family to do things such as shut-
ting doors was not enough. It was recommended that Nina participate in
a time-limited group therapy program. This was a way to continue the family work while helping her to have some separate space.

## PHASE 2: RESTRUCTURING THE FAMILY

Restructuring boundaries and realigning more appropriate subsystems
were the next steps of therapy. Meanwhile the therapist continued to interpret and reframe the systemic function of the symptom. While the children's
role in protecting their parents had already been pointed out, very little had
changed in this regard. Clearly, a different intervention was necessary.

In the session excerpted here, all five members are present once again.
The session highlights the role of the offspring in their parents' relationship
in a concrete way.

### The Third Chair

Therapist: Phil, Daniella, and Nina, you have sat down in the right chairs
    because Nina is sitting between you. You seem to need her there very
    much.
Daniella: (As Phil harrumphs, and chuckles) What do you mean?
Therapist: Phil, you look like you recognize why I make this observation.
Phil: (Challenging) Yeah, I guess you're going to say it's because Daniella
    and I have problems.
Therapist: How long will you need Nina to sit there between you?
Daniella: (Sounding irritated, looking down at the floor) I don't need her
    to sit there. She can leave! It doesn't matter where she sits. You know

she is still throwing up and using those pills. She hasn't gotten any better. And look at her color. She is turning yellow. (Therapist holds a hand up to motion Daniella to stop.)

Therapist: What would the family do if you did not have symptoms, Nina? Whom would they point to when things were not going well or if your parents were angry with each other? Nina, how long do you think you will need to sit there between them?

Nina: (Smiling, talking slowly in a hesitant voice) I don't know. (Seriously, without smiling) I guess until they can deal with their own problems.

Sarah: (Laughing and confidently offering) Nina, you could be sitting there forever. I'm glad I'm not in your chair.

Nina: (Her smile fading, and tears welling up) I want to leave, but I can't.

Phil: (Gruffly) So, what's stopping you? (Nina turns away with her arms folded across her chest.)

Therapist: Guy, you have been in that chair many times. Why is it hard for Nina to give up that chair?

Guy: (Looks down at floor, and states matter-of-factly) Because she doesn't want them to kill each other. She probably can't trust them to be rational. Mom says she's going to leave; Dad says he's fed up, but they never do anything. So she thinks she can keep them from killing each other.

Therapist: You're not protecting your parents right now. I wonder if you feel guilty. (Guy tilts his head to the side with a "uh huh" but avoids looking at either parent.) Do you really have to worry about their killing each other?

(Daniella is tearing up. Phil is looking challengingly at Nina. Sarah is tearing up.)

Guy: (Pauses) Maybe. (Staring back at his father) (Nina is looking back and forth between her parents.)

Nina: Guy had to protect mom.

Therapist: Guy, change chairs with Nina. (He does so.) You are now in the middle protecting your parents from each other. How have you kept you father from hurting your mother.

Guy: (Looks like it is difficult to say this, maybe fighting back tears) It's a while ago . . .

Nina: (Interrupts) Guy stopped dad when he had a knife on mom. He told dad that if he ever did it again he'd call the cops.

Guy: Yeah.

Therapist: (Turning to Nina) One isn't enough? You seem to think that your parents need not just one but two chairs between them?

Phil: (Voice raised, shifting in his chair) Oh, come on. It wasn't that bad.

(Nina is adamantly shaking her head that it was that bad. Sarah looks as though she has exited even though she remains in her chair.)

Daniella: You see, this is terrible that they see this. (Pointing her finger at Phil and then turning to the therapist) It's because of his drinking.

Sarah: (Sitting up in her chair, angrily addressing her mother) Then why don't you do something about it instead of just talking? It's just as much your responsibility. (Sounding parental) Stop buying him beer! (Sounding frustrated) You're just as bad as he is.

Therapist: Be careful, Sarah; you want Guy's chair? Change chairs, Guy and Sarah. Sarah, this way you can be reminded of where you don't want to sit.

Nina: (Pointing her finger at Sarah, laughing with some glee) See, see! You got caught, too!

Sarah: (As Nina speaks, Sarah moans and tries to ignore her.) I have tried so hard to stay out of their relationships, but they do such a terrible job of it. They're like kids. They need a referee.

Therapist: Sarah, this is your role in the family, huh? Referee between your parents? Referee between your brother and sister? You must get tired, too, like Nina. (Nina is looking very tired; her eyes are half closed.) (Pause. Turns to Daniella and Phil) The two of you can't have a relationship without a third chair between you. What do you think, Daniella and Phil?

Daniella: Like I said, they can go wherever they want. I don't need them to protect me.

Therapist: Phil, you are not so sure that you can let go of their protection?

Phil: Naw, we don't need them. We've got to deal with our problems sooner or later.

Therapist: (Incredulously) You are ready to deal with your problems now, after all these years? I'm not so sure you know what you're saying. I'm not convinced that you can really do this. You still have a third chair. Do you know what it is?

(Pause, family looks puzzled. Phil looks like he is tensing up. Nina slides down in her chair, crossing her arms across her chest.)

Sarah: (Directly to the therapist) It's Phil's drinking.

Therapist: Yeah, it's the alcohol. The whole family seems to hide your drinking, Phil. (Looking back and forth between Phil and Daniella) If you don't — (Daniella starts to interrupt. The therapist motions her to wait.) — if you do not deal with the alcohol differently, I think you will need Nina and Guy to live with you forever. (Phil shifts in his chair, looking disbelieving; Daniella is smiling. The therapist turns to Nina and Guy.) Which of you is willing to sacrifice your life to stay at home with your parents so they continue to stay together?

Daniella: (Shaking her head) I love them very much; they can stay as long as they like. Phil's drinking is something else and separate from them.

Phil: They've got to have a life of their own. There's nothing more I'd like to see than for them to leave home and make it on their own. (Briefly looks up at Nina, but he starts to tear up) They've got to let go. Nina, you've got to figure this out and get past it without me. We can't solve your problems for you.

Therapist: (To Phil) They've got to let go or you and Daniella have to let go?

The exercise with the third chair enabled Guy, Nina, and Sarah to see how they were protecting their parents both physically and psychological-ly. The third chair was symbolic of the difficulty the children were having leaving home. It was a metaphor that was used repeatedly throughout therapy.

We returned to Phil's drinking, which was linked to the marital dysfunc-tion; Phil and Daniella were directed to seek a consultation with an alcohol specialist. Phil asserted that he did not have a problem while Daniella in-sisted he did. It was suggested to them that if Phil did not have a problem, a specialist would be able to see this and explain this to Daniella.

While it may have been a mistake not to force the alcohol issue earlier in the therapy, as there were certainly openings, it took several months for Phil to be engaged in the therapy. Phil and Daniella went to the evalua-tion, which was upsetting for both of them. The specialist gave them feed-back that they certainly acted like a couple that had an alcoholic member and that Daniella was acting as a co-alcoholic. Phil temporarily refused to return to the therapy. Daniella was told that she could not be helpful to her kids until she got help for herself to address her co-alcoholism. She was directed to attend Al-anon. This step took her three weeks, and she tried to get one of her children to go with her. The children supported her attend-ance, but refused to go with her.

Therapy shifted to supporting the recognition of the sibling subsystem in an attempt to help Sarah redefine her relationship to Nina and Guy as a sister instead of a parent. The three were also seen in therapy to establish bound-aries between the marital system and the sibling system. The therapy focused on helping them to understand how the alcohol had affected the way they experienced emotions, their tolerance for abuse, and their attempts to have control in their lives and to shut out the chaos: Nina through bulimia and Guy through drugs. Sarah had accomplished more separation. She was in-cluded in the therapy in hopes that she could teach Guy and Nina how to stay out of the middle of their parents' relationship.

After six sessions together, Sarah was encouraged to step out, so that she could stay a sister to Guy and Nina rather than falling into a parental role due to the ten-year age difference. Five sessions attended by Nina and Guy were spent helping them realize the similar struggles they were having in recognizing their feelings, coping, trusting themselves and other people. The following session illustrates some of this sharing, as well as their tendency to cope, like their parents by bringing in a "third chair."

Nina: Dad's been really moody since they went to see that alcohol person.

Therapist: Your parents' problems are very difficult for you to stay out of even when they are not here, huh?

(Smiling as though in realization, Nina nods vigorously, an affirmative.)

Guy: Yeah, dad was pretty mad. But he hasn't had a drink since. So maybe it was good. Maybe he doesn't have a problem.

Nina: (Sounding and looking angry, as though she is responding to Guy as her father) Huh! You don't think he has a problem? Just because he hasn't had a drink for a month. Just wait. Within two weeks he'll start drinking again. Mom and dad are just pretending. This is just like a honeymoon. They'll be fighting before long.

Guy: Don't get all mad at me — and maybe you shouldn't be so pessimistic. Mom's been better since she's attended that meeting. She's not bugging him as much.

Nina: It just seems so hopeless. They do this over and over again. Pretending, then going back to fighting and hating each other. (Matter-of-factly) They're going to kill each other one day. (Pause) They sure have discouraged me from wanting to get married. No wonder I'm afraid of relationships.

Guy: (Addressing therapist) Do you think this is maybe why I have such a hard time being with girls? I want a girlfriend, but just as I really start liking someone . . . (Choking up) I just worry that I'm never gonna be able to have a one. I don't know how other relationships are supposed to be except what I see in the movies. I just get so damned mad (punching his fist into his other hand) that I don't know how to have a relationship. I don't even think I know what love is. Sure I love my family, but so much other stuff is mixed up with it I'd rather not feel it. (Nina appears to be listening intensely, and nodding her head assertively in agreement.) I don't think that's how love is supposed to feel.

Nina: (Shudders, while nodding her head) I don't even know if I wanna get close. I can be friendly and nice. But as soon as someone starts to like me — oh no — I back off. I can't let them do that because then I might get hurt. I just know that is the way it is. If I let my guard down, I'm gonna get hurt. It always happens that way.

Guy: Yeah. Sometimes I feel so embarrassed or retarded because I don't know how to react. So I don't say anything. Then maybe no one will know that I don't know what to do.

Nina: (Nodding, and gesturing with her hands to get Guy's attention) Yeah! Do you ever find yourself watching your friends and trying to figure out what would be the normal way to act? Like what feelings would be normal or what you would say? I wonder how they know how to act or if they're watching everyone else to see how to act, but I don't think so.

Therapist: You both seem to know exactly what each other is talking about. Have you talked about this before?

Guy: Nope. I don't like to think about it. So I've never talked about it. One thing I know is I'm scared that I'm going to end up like my parents. Isn't that what they say? (Therapist responds with questioning look.) That people end up a lot like their parents?

Therapist: Like your parents' relationship? (Both Guy and Nina nod.) Maybe that's why it has been hard for the two of you to have a relationship as brother and sister these last two years. You have been busy acting as your parents. (Both Guy and Nina look at the therapist, directly.)

Nina: (Thoughtfully, as though gaining some insight) Yeahhh. (Guy utters 'hmmm.")

Therapist: What is the third chair for you two?

Guy: (Looking puzzled and confused) I'm still trying to see if I see things the same way you do. (Pause) I don't want to see myself doing that. That's the last thing I want to do is be like either of them (sounding disgusted).

Nina: I know what the third chair is (sounding angry and very deliberate). It's my bulimia. Guy, you treat me like both mom and dad, bossing me around and telling me what to do. (She turns to the therapist and says in an accusatory voice) Guy is like both of them, treating me like a little kid.

Guy: (No longer sounding intimate but defensive) Then you're like dad. You don't want to face up to things and take responsibility for your problems. You get all angry and loud whenever I bring up your bulimia. Just like Dad.

Nina: (Sitting up and becoming animated, gesturing) Hah! Look who's talking. You're just like dad. You drink too much but you don't think you have a problem (pointing her finger at him intensely). You're probably going to be just like him. (Guy flinches, his face colors, and eyes water.)

Therapist: Nina, maybe you fight with Guy when you start to feel too vulnerable to him? Guy, what is your reaction to what Nina just said?

Guy: It hurts. I don't want to be like Dad. I love him but I don't want his problems. That's what I'm scared of. That just feels like a low blow. (Turns to Nina and pauses) You know you just attacked me like mom attacks dad.

Therapist: It seems that you have also just done what the two of you were
  describing earlier in the session. That just as you start to let yourself
  get vulnerable and open up you get hurt or attacked. The two of you
  need to practice how to be Nina and Guy instead of Daniella and Phil.

Nina and Guy completed five sessions together. This appeared to be their
tolerance for intimacy with each other. The focus of the five sessions alternated between exploring their relationship with each other and their mir-
roring of their parents' relationship. Nina seemed able to tolerate more work
around relationships and her expression of anger. After concluding the five
sessions with Guy, she participated in a ten-week time-limited group for
women with bulimia; the group focused on relationships, anger, body-
image, and sexuality — all areas that Nina was able to work on more directly than at the beginning of family therapy. The group gave her some objectivity and distance from the family and allowed her to examine family
relationships with support from other group members.

Within a month of Nina's completing the group, the three siblings were
invited into a consultation as their mother prepared to leave on a two week
vacation. Daniella's vacations, though they were often justified as business
trips, also coincided with times of heightened and intense conflict with Phil
over his drinking. Predictably, Nina was becoming more involved in her
parents' problems again.

The siblings met for two sessions, after which both Guy and Sarah took
a turn being absent. Nina again talked about feeling abandoned. She made
a decision to exclude her siblings from another consultation. She asserted
that she did not need Sarah as a babysitter nor Guy as a parent. The following excerpt is taken from the session at which both siblings failed to show.
The therapist failed to predict this attendance pattern by Sarah and Guy.
In retrospect, because Nina was no longer in crisis *and* trying to spread the
symptoms in the family herself, the intensity was too great for either Sarah
or Guy, especially with their parents' concurrent marital difficulties.

Nina: (Sounding angry but trying to contain herself, also sounding hurt) Did
  either of them call you? (Therapist shakes her head, no.) Oh, that's
  just fine! They can't even be responsible for getting here. They just
  leave me not knowing.
Therapist: You sound angry. You have reason to be angry.
Nina: (Appropriately angry and assertively) I sure have a right to be angry.
  They are doing this just like mom and dad. First Sarah can't come for
  a lame excuse and then Guy forgets. And now they both can't come.
  Well, fine! I don't want them to come. They're the ones who will lose
  out because they have their own problems. I'm not going to take care
  of them and try to get them to come in.

Therapist: When you are angry like this you make so much sense and are easier to understand. I think you need to stick to your decisions here and let them know that you do not want to be stuck between them. This will be good practice for when you will want to leave home.

Nina: You're damned right I'm going to let them know! I'm sick and tired of everyone pretending to help me. Fine, I don't need them.

This session marks the first time that Nina is asserting more independence and control over her interpretation of events. She is not blaming herself for the failure of her sister and brother to attend the session. This session is important because it indicates that Nina is closer to being able to leave home. She will need some of her anger to leave home. Thus, at this point in time, the therapist could support a move toward individual therapy with Nina, although the focus continued to be on Nina's relationships and coping in the family.

Therapy shifted to an individual format in which family members were invited in for periodic consultations. The therapy progressed over a one-year period. Nina showed a noticeable increase in power, appropriate expression of anger, and confrontation with family members towards resolving conflict. During this time she quit a job that her mother had obtained for her without consulting her parents, and she decided to go back to school. Before she quit her job she had started volunteer work with disturbed adolescents despite her family's discouragement and the therapist's concerns. The volunteer job eventually worked into a paid position; it was the first work she had obtained without her family's help. Her ability to take this job and continue in it for over two years was a significant step towards establishing confidence in herself, individuating from the family, decreasing her enmeshment with the family, and establishing a credibility that had little to do with her appearance.

Two weeks before she started school, her family planned a trip to Europe from which she was excluded. Daniella provided a reason for every member to go except Nina. Phil would be returning in two weeks while Daniella stayed for an additional six weeks. Nina was angry. She interpreted the family members' trip without her as their need to pretend that everything was okay. Although she was angry, she was also able to reframe the situation as a vacation *from* her family. The therapist was also aware that if Nina had not been in therapy, the family would not have left her alone. Thus, the situation seemed reminiscent of leaving Nina with a babysitter.

The following excerpt is from a session before the trip. Daniella was invited in to remind her of Nina's symptom's connection to the family. During this session Nina anticipated how the family needed her symptoms. Although Daniella was reluctant to see the connection between a possible relapse for Nina and the family situation, she was unable to remain as blind as before.

Nina: I'm mad. It doesn't feel fair that everyone is going without me. I'm
the one who would really enjoy it. I don't want to be left behind all
by myself. And then have to deal with dad coming home in two weeks.
It's going to be awful (pouting and overwhelmed). (Angrily glaring
at her mother) I'm not going to babysit him!

Daniella: You don't have to.

Nina: Then why are you staying longer and making him go home six weeks
before you?

Daniella: Because I have business and he has to work. (Nina shakes her head
no.)

Therapist: Nina, how will your family know you are having a difficult time
while they're gone?

Nina: (Slowly) I guess if I lose weight, or get real sick.

Daniella: (Interrupting Nina, loudly, firmly) Don't lose weight! You are doing better. You don't need to lose weight!

Therapist: Well, I don't know. I worry that Nina could lose a lot of weight
while you are gone; she did the last time. (Daniella sighs . . . )What
could it mean if Nina loses weight?

Nina: (Sinking in her chair, starting to tear up, her voice getting higher)
I don't want my bulimia to get worse.

Daniella: I don't know. (Gruffly) That she has too much to handle.

Therapist: What is it that you are leaving her to handle?

Daniella: Herself. Nothing else. She's starting school. She just needs to do
that.

Nina: (Interrupting) Nothing!? But if there's any problem with the business,
they'll call me. And then when Dad comes back, I don't want to take
care of him, but he's going to drink and I dread it.

Therapist: It sounds like you don't want to play musical chairs while your
mother is gone.

Nina: (Assertively) You're damn right I don't! Just as I feel like I'm getting
out of the hot seat, she sticks me back in it.

Therapist: Nina, explain to your mother some more how she is asking you
to play musical chairs.

Nina's ability to express her anger to her mother and state her anticipation of the pressure she would feel to take her mother's place while she was
gone indicated that Nina had reached an understanding that her mother did
not want to see. By leaving Nina alone with her father for six weeks while
the rest of the family was gone, Daniella was supporting the confusion that
already existed in which Phil would mix Nina up with his wife.

Her mother's and family's absence came at a difficult time in her life, but
may have been fortunate, as it gave Nina some practice acting for herself

without having to mediate between her parents. During this time there were additional indications that Nina was maturing emotionally. She was menstruating for the first time in two years while her family was gone, although she had not gained or lost any weight. She had been able to stay away from home, spending the night with a friend, a few times after her father and the rest of the family returned; she had received an award of recognition for her outstanding work with disturbed adolescents. Additionally, she was struggling with school.

To complicate matters, Phil was diagnosed with cancer while the rest of the family was still in Europe. Nina expressed in therapy feeling angry that, although she was trying to get out of the role of playing "wife and mother" to her father, she had been set up by the family's departure to really be put to the test. She had called her mother in Europe several times to let her know how distressed and overwhelmed she was by all that was happening and that she did not feel that she could play musical chairs any longer.

The time alone without her family and her mother ended up being a catalyst for Nina to act more independently. Soon after the family returned she reflected on her need for her bulimia during an individual session.

Nina: (Thoughtfully and questioningly) This sounds weird, but I feel that I didn't lose enough weight while mom was gone.

Therapist: Maybe that is not so weird.

Nina: (Softly, but adultlike) They don't seem worried about me. Maybe I should have lost weight so they would feel sorry for what they left me with.

Therapist: You are telling me that your bulimia has a purpose in this family, to let them know how you are doing. Now you worry that they will expect you to handle as many things all the time as you handled while they were away?

Nina: Yeah. (looking up), that's it.

Therapist: You have been so much more responsible for yourself, working to grow up and be more independent, and so hardworking that I would think that you would be very tired from these last four months. (While Nina had bounced into the session, her eyelids started to droop as the therapist talked about her being tired.) It is important for you to let yourself feel tired because that is how a person feels when the work she does is exhausting. I think you need to let everyone know that you are so tired; whenever you are having more difficulty sleeping it means that you are starting to slide into the third chair. Who has been in that chair the most lately?

Nina: (Sleepily) Guy. Though I still do it, too, but not nearly as much.

Therapist: You have been doing much better at protecting yourself rather than your parents. That has been hard work for you. I am concerned that if you continue to fool your parents with all your energy, when Guy goes away to school you will take the third chair. After all, you'll be the only one left at home. It will be very hard to stay out of their relationship.

Nina: Oh yeah? Why?

Therapist: Why do you think?

Nina: Hmmm. Because I'll get in between my parents, again? (Pause) You know, I could see that happening. Hmmm. Maybe I should go away with Guy to school (laughing). (Seriously) I just feel panicked thinking things could get worse again.

Therapist: Nina, how do you think you could let them know that you are tired?

Nina: I guess I could tell them (quickly quickening the pace of her speech), but they don't listen.

Therapist: Well, I wonder if they get confused if you tell them you are so tired but continue to take care of them and keep getting stronger and stronger.

Nina: My bulimia could get worse. (Smiling and gesturing) I could leave them all and take my own vacation — after all they left me. I could use a vacation. Yeah, I could go see my friend or I could go someplace warm. I kind of like that idea. (Slowing down) Though I don't know if I could with my job.

At this point in the therapy, it was clear that Nina had a much better understanding of some of the systemic functions of her bulimia. However, because she was emotionally stronger, the family was more disengaged from her and her parents were starting to use her again as a conduit for their anger at each other. Nina also had a difficult time leaving her parents alone. As long as she lived at home it was doubtful that she would be able to get rid of her symptoms because her parents' neediness was so great.

## PHASE 3: LEAVING HOME

Since the thirteenth month of therapy, Nina had demonstrated more appropriate responsibility for herself and increasing independence from the family — and importantly, less destructive, but more appropriate rebellious behavior towards testing her and her parents' readiness for her to leave home. It was necessary for the therapy to reflect and support her demonstrated movement and preparation for leaving home.

The following excerpt is taken from the first session that Nina and Daniella had together after Daniella returned from Europe. Prior to this session,

Daniella had requested and been granted an individual session with the therapist to help her to develop some ways to confront her daughter. While granting such a session is unusual, the way in which the request was made indicated that Daniella's request was in line with skill-building. In that session, Daniella referred to Nina's forging of her signature on checks and credit cards which had been ongoing for several months, though Daniella has not known how to confront her daughter. Phil was not included in the session excerpted here. His continued drinking made him unable to act as a parent. The session is striking for how mother and daughter stay in role as a mother and daughter.

Therapist: I'd like the two of you to spend this session as mother and daughter. Daniella, Nina needs your help in guiding her towards being a young adult. Daniella, you told me that you are getting confused because Nina is showing responsibility in being able to choose her job, go to work, and go to school, but there are other things she is doing that aren't responsible. Talk with her about these things. Nina, I would like you not to respond to what your mother is saying, but just listen.

Daniella: (Leaning forward toward Nina, looking at her directly) First of all I want to say that you should forget about your daddy; he is not going to stop smoking, bitching, drinking, or yelling. I have given up on trying to change him. We are just living like roommates. I cannot handle making a major change — not financially, not morally, and not family. We do not have a husband-wife relationship. When he gets angry at you, he is getting angry at me. I can handle this. You need to worry about yourself. You are not responsible for my life or your father's life. You should be responsible for your life. Another thing . . .

Therapist: Daniella, what you are saying is important. You do not need Nina to be responsible for you. She needs to continue to stay out of the middle. You have made a decision not to make any changes at this time.

Daniella: Right, I am not ready. I cannot make any right now.

Therapist: You have decided not to pretend anymore?

Daniella: That's right. I am just waiting for Nina and Guy to grow up before I think about the changes I want for myself. They come first right now. One of the things that I want to talk to you about that I did not come to you before now, Nina, is that I am doing the same things with you that I did with Phil and that this is not helpful to you. But I did not know how to approach you. I love you very much; I care for you; I worry about you. So I had a session myself. The things I am talking about are how you are writing checks and signing my name and using my credit cards. I have been covering by trying to hide these things from other family members, stores, friends. I do not know for sure what to do. You are very responsible in some ways but not in this way. In this way you are acting like a juvenile.

Next, I would like you to take responsibility for your car's gasoline. I am not asking you to pay rent or food like other parents might do. I want you to take care of your own things. So if you want to go to a restaurant or do something for your own self you need to take care of this. If you need to borrow money from me, I want you to ask; I will try to help you.

Therapist: Daniella, you are wanting to help Nina practice taking on some of the responsibility she will have when she leaves home.

Daniella: Another thing I talked about was the cost of your therapy. I will be willing to share with you, but it is important for you to start taking some responsibility by paying for part of it. I don't want to feel that everyone is sucking from me and taking from me and taking me for granted.

Therapist: You want her to assume responsibility for treatment. If Nina was willing to pay for some of the therapy this would be a sign to you that it was important to her and that she is not taking you for granted.

Daniella: That is right. I do not want her to be upset about this because I am doing this to help her, not to punish her (responding to Nina tearing up but otherwise not indicating a reaction to her mother's statements). Because what if something happens to me? I want to know that she will know how to take care of herself.

Therapist: Nina, what is it that your mom wants to change?

Nina: She doesn't want to cover for me anymore. But she's probably just doing this because she can't do it with dad.

Daniella: (Assertively, and loudly) No! I am not covering for him anymore, either. I have to start taking better care of myself. How can I expect you to take better care of you if I am not doing this for myself?

Nina: I can't listen to this because Sarah is probably making you do this.

Daniella: This has nothing to do with Sarah. I just don't want to cover for you anymore. This is how I can help you. This is so our relationship doesn't go bad like your father's and mine. I worry that today you take from me, but what if tomorrow you take from someone else?

Therapist: Nina, do you worry that your stealing could get worse?

Nina: Yes, I've thought about that and worried, too.

Therapist: Daniella, it is important then that you are talking with Nina like this today.

Nina: I am doing a lot better than I was (in tears).

Daniella: Yes, you are doing much better. That is why I can approach you now. You are better now. But I had to put this out because this was bothering me. I don't want you to cry or get upset.

Therapist: You would not have talked with Nina like this six months ago.

Daniella: No, I couldn't have. Because I was afraid that she would run away. (Turning to Nina) You are doing much better. You are stronger. You are working and going to school, but why don't you have a boy-friend? . . . (Daniella catches herself and looks embarrassed back and forth between Nina and the therapist, smiles and starts to laugh.) I guess I'm wanting too much too fast. And I must not push you.

Nina: (Laughing) That would be too much too fast.

Therapist: Nina, your mother is clearly trying to support you towards gain-ing practice in being a young adult. One of the ways she can support you is not to cover for you. She would also like you to assume consis-tent responsibility for your personal expenses. She is also being clear that she has made a decision to stay with your father.

Daniella, your decision to stay with Phil will be helpful to you and to Nina because you are finally giving a clear message about your inten-tions with her father. She knows what she can expect. I would also suggest you buy an inexpensive safe in which you can put the checks and credit cards you are not using. I think this will help both of you because Nina is indicating that she is not sure that she can control her stealing behavior from you.

This session was followed by a letter to both Daniella and Nina con-gratulating Daniella on acting as a mother and supporting Nina's readiness to grow up. Nina was congratulated for her ability to listen without inter-rupting her mother and her readiness to take on more age-appropriate responsibility.

Transferring some financial responsibility to the bulimic individual who is a young adult by age is a good diagnostic intervention. If she can assume this responsibility, it indicates readiness to leave home and let go of the fami-ly. In Nina's case, it would not have been therapeutic either to have her take on all the financial responsibility or to go on much longer without confront-ing her stealing and offering her the opportunity for this responsibility.

Nina continued to be more direct about her anger and less destructive toward herself after this session. This session also marked a turning point in Nina's ability to reduce her bulimic symptoms.

Additional interventions during the session included reframing and re-peating Daniella's messages to Nina. This is an intervention used with chaotic families to help reduce the distortion that can result from the history be-tween two people. Another intervention involved instructing Nina not to respond at first, but just to listen. This decreased her need to respond defen-sively, and increased the amount of her mother's messages that she could hear.

The next step towards leaving home took place six months later. Nina had continued working and going to school part-time. Her brother had left for school three months earlier. She adjusted to being the only child at home. In fact, this experience seemed to provide her with some of the attention and special acknowledgment that she had been wanting all along from her parents. The increased distance between Nina and Guy allowed them to move closer to each other from a distance as they exchanged letters. This closeness played an important part in Nina's ability to further individuate from her parents.

In the following session both parents are included, for the first time in a year, at Nina's request. She expressed confidence that she would not feel overpowered by them and that she would be able to stay out of the third chair—most of the time. At this point she was considering buying a small house with a friend and was ready to initiate her goodbyes to her parents.

Nina: I've been wanting to move out for a year now. It started when I started to stay away from home—sometimes without letting you know. You know how the two of you would get so worried. I got a certain satisfaction out of that; I don't know . . . (Pause) (Thoughtfully) I really wanted to leave when Guy left for school, though I kind of liked being the only child. But I was so afraid that I was going to get stuck between the two of you. I knew my bulimia would get worse if I did that. So I stayed away even more. But it was hard to stay away because I always worried about you.

Daniella: What are you worried about? It is good that you want to leave (gesturing for her to leave). You do not have to worry about me—or your father.

Phil: (Gruffly) Damn, you start worrying like that and it means that nothing has changed. (Nina starts to tear.)

Therapist: I don't think your parents know what you worry about so much that you stayed home longer than you wanted to.

Nina: I think they know. At least they should know.

Daniella: What, that we will divorce?

Nina: (Matter-of-factly) No. I can handle that.

Daniella: What then, tell us.

Nina: (To her mother) I worry because dad is sick. I worry that I won't be around if he needs me. Sometimes I can cheer him up. And he can feel really lonely. I'm not ready for him to die.

Therapist: What else, Nina?

Nina: (Here voice starts to quaver) I worry about two things mostly. Mom, I worry that dad will hurt you. (Therapist: Physically?) Yeah, and that I won't be there to do anything. He doesn't know his own strength and when he's out of control I really think there are times that . . . (turns to father) that you want to kill her. I get really scared.

Therapist: What else do you worry about?

Nina: (Looking at the floor) Nothing, but — well it's not nothing or anything — it's the thing I have worried about for years. I'm afraid he'll kill himself when I leave, to get back at mom.

Therapist: Nina, turn to your father and tell him directly again what is worrying you.

Nina: (Directly and loudly) I'm worried that you'll kill yourself. (Father and mother start to tear.) I know you think about it, especially since this last summer when you've been sick. (Gently and softly) And I know what it is like to think about it. I know you could do it, too. I would be so mad at you if you killed yourself and so sad.

(Louder and sitting up more) You know how guilty I would feel if you didn't take care of yourself, mom, and you got hurt, or if dad tried to kill himself. I know you tell me not to worry about you but it is really hard not to when I think I could lose one of you like I worry about. I know I need to move out, but I still don't trust that the two of you can handle each other without someone getting hurt if no one is at home at all.

Therapist: You are really struggling to let go of your parents. You say it is difficult to trust them or to trust yourself. You will all remain connected by some of your fear Nina. In order to leave home you will need to give up your seat in the house and your belief that you can control your parents' relationship. You must be responsible to yourself. You cannot make your parents' choices.

If your mother does not know when things are heating up so that she gets hurt or if your father hurts her or himself, that will stick with you. You will wonder "What if?" But they could do these same things with you at home. When do you think you will be ready to fold your chair and move out?

Nina: I'm ready now. It's just hard. There is really nothing they can say that would make it any easier for me. (Sounding angrier) I am actually getting angry that this is why I have stayed for so long.

Daniella: You have already given up too much. You need to go now.

Phil: I'm really proud of you. I've been telling you you could do it without me.

Therapist: You have risked your life for them. It is time for you to leave. How would you like to start saying goodbye to them, Nina?

This session marked the end of family therapy. Nina moved out within two months. She allowed herself to gain some weight and broadened the scope of foods she would allow herself to keep down. At her request the frequency of therapy decreased to every other week six weeks after her move.

Therapy focused on helping her to deal with the rape she had experienced as a teenager. During this period of therapy, she was able and willing to predict relapses in her bulimia. Six months after she moved out she was able to terminate therapy, having been binge-purge-free for three months.

## SUMMARY

The function of Nina's bulimia in the family over the course of treatment changed, though certain elements were central throughout treatment: Her bulimia kept her parents together, allowed her to express her anger at them, and helped her establish some boundaries in a family where privacy was devalued.

Treating the Weisfield family required an active and frequent reassessment of the family's functioning and need for symptoms. A significant shift took place in the family's need for Nina's symptoms when Daniella decided to stay with Phil until she had launched her two youngest children. Because of the function of bulimia in the family (kids stayed home to allow parents to stay together), it was important for the therapist to assess if Daniella's decision would continue the need for Nina's symptoms. Her decision was a turning point because it was followed by a marked decrease in her ambivalence and powerlessness in her relationship with her husband. She needed less protection from her children.

Therapy with the Weisfields aimed to create more appropriate personal and generational boundaries. The alcohol evaluation was a big step for Phil and Daniella. It pushed the limits of their tolerance and need to address the alcohol in their relationship. Although Phil was unwilling to take further steps to address his alcoholism, other family members did. If everyone's behavior had remained the same, Nina would not have been able to let go of her symptoms.

The types of interventions that were used with the Weisfield family were not particularly creative or strategic. The interventions were kept simple: repeating interpretations (e.g., a third chair being needed), giving the family responsibility for interpreting the symptoms, instructing one family member to talk and another not to talk, teaching people to paraphrase, talking about a family member (with the member present) to other family members, circular questioning (e.g., asking Nina what she thinks her mother's reaction will be, then asking Daniella what Nina's reaction may be), and taping sessions. This last intervention works with many of the chaotic families that stay in treatment because they tend to be more concerned than other such families about appearances and making a good impression. Watching a videotaped session helps them exercise more control in their tendency to interrupt, be irrational, or explode. It is important to exercise the right to terminate a session if family members cannot control their verbal abuse or if they threaten physical abuse. This intervention communicates that this behavior is unacceptable.

The therapist needs to be consistent, and yet flexible, in setting conditions for therapy. Following up important, intense sessions with letters can be helpful in clarifying what happened in the session. People will hear only what they want to at times like these. Written contracts can be useful, particularly in families where accountability is low.

One should not expect members of the chaotic family to be particularly insightful. Furthermore, as in the perfect and overprotective families, persons without the symptoms initially have little to gain by being insightful. In fact, Nina's insight in the Weisfield family was a source of frustration and doubt for her, since her reality was not supported by other family members. Therapy helped her learn to trust her insight and her feelings. This support was a major purpose of group therapy.

Taking breaks during the course of therapy can be therapeutic, though initially difficult. There is seldom a "good time" to take a break; the therapist almost always worries about initiating a crisis. With proper preparation therapeutic breaks give the family or individuals practice in separation and pave the way for termination. Furthermore, a break challenges the reality of abandonment, which individuals from chaotic families have come to expect at every turn. Lastly, a break may be timely when the therapist assesses that the family is reaching its limit of tolerance. A break may avoid premature termination or treatment failure.

The therapeutic relationship with the chaotic family is more tenuous than with perfect or overprotective families. The chaotic family has more difficulty establishing commitment and trust. It is important to accept that working with the chaotic family will take much energy and will tend to take longer than working with perfect or overprotective families.

# PART VI

# PLANNING FOR THE INEVITABLE

CHAPTER 21

# Obstacles and Sabotage in Treatment: Challenges to the Therapist

THIS CHAPTER HAS been a challenge to conceptualize. As systemic therapists, we do not believe in the concept that has traditionally been labeled "resistance." Originally, resistance was viewed as an intrapsychic process and was one further manifestation of the pathology of the individual. Yet we repeatedly observe systems acting in ways that interrupt or slow the progress of therapy. Helping us to understand this process is the work of Watzlawick and colleagues (1974), who have very clearly indicated that the change process carries with it two seemingly opposing "forces"—one advocating for change and the other for sameness. This is a universal characteristic of systems and is related to the concept of homeostasis.

When working with rigid systems, the family therapist needs to be continually aware of those events and interactions posed by the family members, the therapist, and the larger social system which interrupt, slow, or even sabotage the progress of therapy. In Chapter 2 we outlined the obstacles that our culture sets up which hinder the recovery of individuals from bulimia. The therapist, as a part of the therapeutic system, contributes to the presence or absence of these obstacles. Sabotage is a part of the therapy process and by anticipating and predicting obstacles in the course of therapy, the therapist is less apt to be thrown by these obstacles to treatment, less likely to engage in power struggles with the family, less likely to collude with the

299

system's dysfunction, and more likely to have realistic expectations of the family.

The ways in which members of the therapy process sabotage treatment are infinite and can show great creativity. Each participant contributes to getting stuck in the therapy process. A therapist may lose a systemic understanding of the family and interpret anger, lack of trust, and skepticism as "resistance" or a refusal to change. The fact that someone is seeking help conveys that, at some level, a part of that system is open to change — if it does not cost too much. If the therapist can join with the proactive part of the system, it will be easier to maneuver around those impediments to growth.

Obstacles to treatment are perceptions, not necessarily realities. Often a therapist can remove obstacles by perceiving that the family members have some good reasons to be acting the way they are. This will allow the therapist to join, rather than battle, the family. It is important to assess the reality base for families' anger and "resistance." Many families have encountered several mental health and health professionals who have not offered useful advice, have blamed them for their daughter's or son's eating disorder, or have taken advantage of their desperateness. Given the type of treatment some individuals and families have received, it is remarkable that they are open to pursuing help.

## OBSTACLES POSED BY THE THERAPIST

*Therapy Not on the Therapist's Terms*

One of the most important rules to remember in working with bulimic families is to set up therapy on your terms. This cannot be overemphasized. We have learned that when this does not happen, the therapist becomes subsumed into dysfunctional family pattern, the therapy feels out of control, and you are forced to ask, "Why isn't this working?" The chapter on treatment of the overprotective family (Chapter 19) illustrates the advantages of establishing therapy on the therapist's terms.

Very clear terms regarding all aspects of treatment must be established. Terms may include policies about cancellations, individual consultation outside of the session, who needs to attend, fee payment, and who needs to call for the appointment. These conditions are established before starting the family therapy and changed or reiterated when a new phase of treatment begins. For example, therapy enters a new phase when we shift from seeing the whole family to seeing the bulimic in individual therapy. When done correctly, this shift can support second-order changes in the family system.

It also provides flexibility for the individual to emotionally and psychologically separate from her parents. At this point, we renegotiate how often therapy will take place and what the focus of therapy will be.

## Lack of Experience Working With Bulimic Families

These families are difficult even when the therapist is experienced. The difficulties rest in the rigidity of patterns, avoidance or lack of resolution regarding conflict, pseudo-cooperation, intense anger, multiple problems, high expectations, and dysfunctional protection of family members. An inexperienced therapist will frequently lose a systemic perspective and too frequently succumb to pressure by families to buy their world view and see only the individual.

We recommend that anyone doing family therapy with an eating-disordered family have experience working with other types of families, particularly other psychosomatic families. Here one gains experience creating intensity and keeping a systemic focus even when the family seems so "perfect" or "nurturing" or "cooperative." The therapist learns to recognize how these family systems are different from many other dysfunctional families.

## Therapist's Family-of-Origin Issues

We come to each family carrying with us our own family. A therapist's family-of-origin issues should be appreciated for both their helpful and hindering functions. Thus, we get worried when we hear such therapist statements such as, "I am aware of all my issues," or "I've spent years in therapy myself to work through my personal issues; they don't come into therapy with me." These are obvious signals of impending sabotage. Therapists are most vulnerable to becoming part of the family's dysfunctional system when they do not consider this a possibility.

Engaging in family therapy assumes that the therapist joins with the family. The therapist inevitably becomes part of, hopefully, a new system. The therapist's awareness and control of her/his role in this new system are crucial to therapeutic leverage. Merely becoming part of the system without an awareness of its purpose is likely to incapacitate the therapist.

Therapists should be aware of the following about their own families of origin: the role they played and continue to play, how conflict was avoided or resolved, how boundaries were respected, if the children were triangulated into parental issues, who had the power in the family, how independence was fostered, how anger was expressed, whether communication was direct or indirect, how limits were set, and how individuals "left home."

These are the issues that bulimic families test therapists with daily. Many of these families rapidly engulf the therapist who remains comfortable with triangulation and avoids conflict. Reflecting on closed cases also helps to provide some hindsight into how family-of-origin issues may have surfaced in the therapy.

Before accepting a family into treatment, we suggest that the therapist ask her/himself the following questions to determine how family-of-origin issues may surface with the family:

1) What are the issues that are still operative from my family of origin?
2) How is this bulimic family similar to my family of origin?
3) How does this family offer something that was missing in my own family?
4) Whom do I sympathize with most? Why?
5) Why do I like this family? (We assume that you will not work with families that you do not like.)
6) Which member do I like the most? The least?
7) Am I impressed by any one particular family member?
8) Who in the family intimidates me?
9) If this family decides not to seek therapy from me, what do I think will be the basis for its decision?
10) Which of my own issues may be aroused by this family and how?

The therapist is most likely to become part of the family's dysfunctional system when the system is similar to the therapist's own family of origin (or provides something her/his own family of origin did not). The therapist may then lose a systemic perspective and do any of the following: protect certain family members, speak for family members, feel powerless or helpless, be triangulated in conflicted interactions, feel extremely angry at one parent, avoid talking about important issues (e.g., alcoholism or a parent's depression), actively side with factions within a family, or become engaged in a power struggle in the family.

To interrupt this process, the therapist can often benefit from close supervision, obtain live consultation, take a break from the therapy, or videotape sessions. Each of these interventions carries with it certain risks. Some therapists feel threatened bringing in another therapist to see the family. Yet consultation provides a second opinion that is based on actual case material and can help the therapist remove blinders. Supervision may be an alternative, especially when conducted by someone who knows the background of the therapist and is aware of how family-of-origin issues could be triggered in the treatment process. We have found that videotaping sessions creates some objectivity, almost as if a second person were present. It also helps the therapist and supervisor/consultant evaluate the process of therapy. Lastly, we suggest that the therapist allow her/himself to take a break from therapy with that family. While a break can be threatening in several ways, it can allow the therapist to regain objectivity, remotivate the family, and activate the system.

Related to family-of-origin issues are issues that emerge due to the sex of the therapist. The literature differs as to the preferred sex of the therapist for eating-disordered clients (Boskind-Lodahl, 1976; Rampling, 1978; Selvini Palazzoli, 1978; Szyrynski, 1973). Rather than making a generalization, we would like to point out the different issues that pertain to either a female or male therapist. The female therapist can provide a valuable role model to the family if she is able to model a powerful and empathic response to each family member. She can also identify with the client, although it is important not to overidentify. A female therapist may be particularly effective in soliciting information about and facilitating working-through of victimization experiences. Yet a woman, because of the socialization process, may have difficulty with increasing conflict in the family and dealing with anger and rage, unless she has effectively worked this through in her own life.

A male therapist can also provide a valuable role model, both for the appropriate expression and resolution of conflict in the family and for the expression of nurturing. However, the male therapist must be sensitive to the powerful position he may hold with the family and the client. As both male and therapist, he occupies a double one-up position. He may also be more likely, due to his socialization process, to ignore issues of caretaking and nurturing.

One final comment pertains to persons with a history of eating disorders who now do therapy with individuals with eating disorders. Having had an eating disorder does not qualify a person to work with persons with eating disorders any more than being a recovered alcoholic automatically makes one a good alcoholism counselor. While someone who has recovered from bulimia has much to offer the bulimic family or person in terms of the experience of having an eating disorder and some of the process of recovery, the recovering bulimic does not have the emotional distance and objectivity necessary to facilitate family therapy. We believe that the ex-bulimic or ex-anorectic can be most effective as a therapist when she no longer needs to identify herself as "a recovered bulimic" or "a recovered anorexic." Developing this identity takes time — often years. It is also important to obtain breadth in professional training by working with persons and families who do not have eating disorders.

## OBSTACLES AND SABOTAGE POSED BY THE FAMILY

Although we use the terms "obstacles" and "sabotage," we want to reiterate that this does not mean the family is "bad." Rather, as we have mentioned earlier, these are indications of the family's creativity and manifest different ways each family chooses to cooperate with treatment.

Sabotage seems to be a signal that structural changes are imminent, that uncomfortable issues have been broached, and that family rules have been challenged. It can be very threatening for family members to consider that they are part of what seems to be the individual's problem. Despite our statement to them that "it is no one's fault," it may feel as though their whole world is caving in. It is important when reading this section to recognize that the obstacles posed by bulimic families are not unique to them, but are predictable and common across dysfunctional families and lend themselves to management. From the initial contact, the therapist can assess how difficult therapy with the family might be and assess whether family members have the requisite skills or energy for therapy.

### Partner or Parent Calling to Make Appointment for Partner or Adult Child

When someone else calls for the symptomatic person, it suggests a dysfunctional aspect of one or more of the significant relationships that cannot be ignored. A mother, for instance, calls desperately seeking help for her daughter. Often, she has made several phone calls to reach you, read literature, and talked with friends and other family members. There is every indication that she is determined to get help for her daughter. But where is the daughter? Especially in overprotective families, this help-seeking behavior further perpetuates dysfunctional roles. Warning bells should go off when you hear explanations of the call, such as, "My daughter was too afraid to call," "I was so relieved that she was open to help that I didn't want to push my luck by asking her to call," "She said she would go only if I made the call," or, "It's just so embarrassing for her to talk about her problem."

Setting up an appointment for a daughter if the parent calls can be a way to support the belief that she is not competent to make the call herself. This is not therapy on the therapist's terms for several reasons:

1) The symptomatic person may see you as colluding with other family members to control her.
2) The bulimic may feel forced or coerced to come in for the appointment and thus determined not to get anything out of it.
3) The bulimic is being treated as a child when in fact she is an adult.

4) The bulimic is able to maintain control in a way over the family members.

In this situation, joining with the bulimic individual will be extremely difficult.

Valuable information is obtained by determining why a particular person is making the call instead of the symptomatic person. The first intervention involves telling the caller that the bulimic person also needs to call for the appointment. It may be appropriate to offer the parent or spouse a consultation without the symptomatic member, but not vice versa.

### Client Not Wanting Family Involved

There are variations on this theme: "I don't want my family (or partner) to know," or, "My family does not want to be involved in the therapy." The therapist can end up colluding with the individual to keep this secret and inadvertently make it difficult to conduct therapy. Following the individual's wish that family not be involved sets up many obstacles, including:

1) Therapy is not on the therapist's terms.
2) The individual may be closed to seeing the importance of family patterns in the development and maintenance of bulimia.
3) The bulimic is protecting family members in a way that may make it impossible for her to recover.
4) The therapist is supporting a dysfunctional pattern of family secrets, overprotection, or a lack of support (particularly in chaotic families).

The therapist must be firm, letting the individual know that recovery will involve looking at family patterns. This does not mean that the therapist must insist upon complete family involvement from the initial contact or consultation. The therapist can go slowly, while repeatedly interpreting interactions in terms of family patterns and functions. In this way the individual can start to understand how her family is important to recovery. We support a request for an individual appointment if we suspect any physical or sexual abuse. However, if abuse remains a secret in the family, therapy will be stuck.

If the family is reluctant to be involved in the therapy, it is important for the therapist to separate causality from treatment. Determining that mom and dad need to be involved in treatment does not mean they caused the eating disorder. In fact, determining a single cause is usually impossible because bulimia is complex. Let the family members talk about their guilt and fear about seeing a therapist.

It is important to spread the symptoms around. A routine question we ask here is, "Whom in the extended family does she remind you of?" This usually generates at least one other symptomatic person in the family. More often than not, bulimic families have had symptomatic members throughout their life-cycle. The symptoms in chaotic families are more obvious — for example, alcohol abuse, suicide attempts, hospitalizations, and nervous breakdowns. Asking previously symptomatic persons about their symptoms can take the focus off the bulimic person, while enabling the therapist to join with other family members. These strategies will be helpful in enabling the family to observe that it has had a need for symptoms in one or more members at times throughout its life-cycle.

Do not get involved in trying to convince family members that they need family therapy. Simply offer your observations as to why family therapy is indicated; for example, you might point out how certain cycles and problems seem to repeat through generations. The therapist may slightly reinterpret objections in a way that is both supportive and paradoxical, e.g., "I realize the family's objections are a way of insisting that I provide Chris with some privacy." Remember that it is the family members' choice to be in therapy and your choice to work with them.

## Client Insisting That She Does Not Have a Problem

There are many reasons why a person may insist that she does not have a problem even though she is bingeing and purging. It is possible that the symptomatic individual may be experimenting with bulimic behaviors and does not have bulimia. Other explanations are:

1) She feels that she cannot have a problem in her family.
2) She feels that her privacy is being invaded.
3) She is angry or rebellious at attempts directed towards fixing her.
4) She is fearful of what looking at the problem may expose in the family.

This last reason is often seen in overprotective families or in families where there has been abuse. If the bulimic insists that she does not have a problem, do not try to convince her otherwise. Most likely, her partner or parents have already tried to do this. The therapist can suggest that she try some personal experiments to determine if a problem exists, e.g., go one month without bingeing or purging, or see if she can allow herself to gain two pounds without panicking.

The therapist may have the most difficult time joining with the bulimic individual "who doesn't have a problem." Acknowledge the sacrifice she has made to be at the appointment, particularly when she does not feel she has a problem. The client is usually relieved to have someone be aware of her internal conflict and feelings about being at the appointment. Determine what, if anything, she would like from the consultation even if it does not seem related to the family's goals.

You may predict what can happen with the bulimia if it really is a problem. This does not force the symptomatic person to admit to having a problem, but provides her with information that may allow her to seek help in the future.

### Not All Designated Members Show for First Appointment

This is an obvious signal of coming difficulties. The absent person is often a peripheral or estranged member, but nevertheless an important person to include in the family assessment. This exclusion may be self-selected, as in the case of someone worried that she/he will be assigned a parental role, as has happened in the family for years, or of a person who fears his alcohol problem will be exposed.

You may want to spend some time with the family to find out why various members who did attend think others did not. Ask them how they can get absent members to come in. Offer to reschedule the appointment and be flexible in offering appointment times. Be firm about needing the designated members to be present. Do not talk about the symptomatic person if she is not there; instead, talk with the other members about their difficulty in communicating with the bulimic individual or their helplessness and powerlessness and begin their process of realizing their own roles in the system.

### Erratic Family's Attendance

Cancellations, missed sessions, and missing family members can all be signs of sabotage. As sabotage, these behaviors most commonly occur because:

1) The most likely explanation is that the absence of a certain family member maintains homeostasis in the family.
2) There has been an intense family session which has brought out family secrets or conflict.
3) The family is no longer in a crisis state and is disengaging from the symptomatic member.
4) Family members may be discouraged from attending by others because they may bring up conflict or disclose secrets.

Cancellations are unlikely to occur while the family is still desperate and panicked. Anticipate them after about the third or fourth session, as relationships are calmer and the family settles into its usual patterns. To avoid cancellations, it is a good idea to predict from the beginning of therapy that the family members will probably wonder if they really need therapy after they get through the crisis. They can use this as a signal that they are probably getting close to some of the issues that will have to be considered for the symptomatic member to recover. After an intense session, predict that the family may want to cancel or come in late for the next session. Ask them what it would mean if they did cancel after the session they just completed. Be clear about your terms and limits for therapy. If the family has a pattern of cancellations, even with these types of interventions, the therapist may need to consider how he or she may be contributing to the problem.

It is important to explore the reasons for the erratic attendance. Direct the family members to talk about ways in which they could discourage different family members from attending. Ask someone in the family to be responsible for helping the absent member get to the session, e.g., by picking him or her up or running errands.

### Family Extremely Cooperative in Session, But Expected Changes Not Occurring

Usually this form of sabotage occurs in the perfect family. Signals are family members' saying, "Everything is going great except for her bulimia; she'd be riding on top of the world except for that." Besides telling you that the family members still see the bulimia as an individual problem, this statement shows a lack of motivation to change. The family does not see the connection between the symptoms and family patterns. This statement also reflects the lack of insight common in these families. It is important to remember that insight makes it uncomfortable to repeat old patterns — but change is also risky and uncomfortable. We also suggest that the therapist explore ways in which she or he may be contributing to the lack of change in family patterns or in the bulimic behavior — this may not be a signal of sabotage on the part of the family.

### Family Attempting to Recover Perfectly

Initially, you may feel fortunate to have a family that is so cooperative, hardworking, and "perfect." Beware — the perfect family is likely to be repeating patterns of behavior which contributed to the eating disorder developing in the first place. Each session you may hear, "The last session was so helpful. Since then we have just turned things around and are doing things totally different," or, "We've made some more progress this week." A family attempting a perfect recovery puts covert pressure on the symptomatic person to get over her symptoms quickly and without any relapse.

In order to differentiate a dysfunctional "perfect" recovery (first-order change) from recovery (second-order change), the therapist can intensify sessions or prescribe relapses. How the family responds to these interventions enables the therapist to assess if necessary second-order change has occurred.

The creative therapist can anticipate predictable "obstacles to treatment" so that therapist and family can work collaboratively without constantly struggling over the meaning of someone's coming late to a session, or falling back into old patterns. Throughout treatment, we use repetitious observations and questioning to help family members understand the connections between their interactions and the symptoms of bulimia. Listen to the family members — to what they say and to what they do. Try different interpretations of their behavior; do not immediately assume that the family is setting up obstacles to treatment. They may instead be offering valuable feedback that the therapist can benefit from hearing.

In dealing with sabotage during treatment, our first intervention is to tell our clients that we expect them to sabotage treatment several times. Confront family members about their sabotage both in the session and outside of it. Have them talk about *how* they are doing it rather than *whether* they are doing it.

Our second intervention is to have the family members talk about the possible ways they may sabotage treatment. For example, we ask, "Knowing what you do about yourself, your role in the family, and the family, how do you think the family will get stuck?" or "Under what conditions do you think the family will drop out of treatment?" Make sure everyone gets a chance to offer some ideas.

Asking family members to anticipate how they can and will create obstacles to treatment begins their education to the process of change. It also normalize sabotages rather than pathologizing it as resistance. This intervention helps the family members link their reactions to each other and their feelings to their behaviors. When sabotage does occur, the family and the therapist can feel less out of control, less likely to engage in a power struggle, and more likely to recognize the obstacle to treatment. We find it helpful to reflect with the family on sabotage during the course of therapy as well. Having talked about sabotage at the beginning of treatment makes this possible.

For everyone's well-being, therapists must set up therapy on their terms. Being able to assertively set out the terms for therapy is a statement of experience, knowledge of personal limits, and understanding of bulimic family systems. Secure therapists are also willling to examine their own family-of-origin issues. This work will facilitate family therapy as well as therapists' own personal growth. Whatever the therapist's level of experience, consultation and supervision can be valuable aids in avoiding and recognizing sabotage.

# References

Abraham, S. F., & Beumont, P. J. V. (1982). How patients describe bulimia or binge-eating. *Psychological Medicine, 12,* 625–635.

Abraham, S. F., Mira, M., & Llewellyn-Jones, D. (1983). Bulimia: A study of outcome. *International Journal of Eating Disorders, 2*(4), 175–180.

Ackerman, N. W. (1980). *Treating the troubled family.* New York: Basic Books Inc.

Altshuler, K. Z., & Weiner, M. F. (1985). Anorexia nervosa and depression: A dissenting view. *American Journal of Psychiatry, 142*(3), 328–332.

American Psychiatric Association. (1980). *Diagnostic and Statistical Manual of Mental Disorders* (3rd ed.) Washington, DC: Author.

Anderson, A. E., & Mickalide, A. D. (1983). Anorexia nervosa in the male: An underdiagnosed disorder. *Psychosomatics, 24*(12), 1066–1075.

Andolfi, M., Angelo, C., Menghi, P., & Nicolò-Corigliano, A. M. (1983). *Behind the family mask.* New York: Brunner/Mazel.

Aono, T., & Kumashiro, H. (1983). Psychophysiological studies of eating disorders by means of visual evoked responses. *Psychotherapy and Psychosomatics, 39* 36–46.

Bateson, G. (1972). *Steps to an ecology of mind.* New York: Ballantine.

Beck, A. T. (1976). *Cognitive therapy and the emotional disorders.* New York: New American Library.

Benjamin, M. (1983). General systems theory, family systems theories, and family therapy: Towards an integrative model of family process. In A. Bross (Ed.), *Family therapy.* (pp. 34–88). New York: Guilford.

Beumont, P. J. V., Abraham, S. F., & Simson, K. (1981). The psychosexual histories of adolescent girls and young women with anorexia nervosa. *Psychological Medicine, 11,* 131–140.

Beumont, P. J. V., George, G. C. W., & Smart, D. E. (1976). "Dieters" and "vomiters" and "purgers" in anorexia nervosa. *Psychological Medicine, 6,* 617–622.

Black, C. (1981). *It will never happen to me!* Denver: M.A.C. Printing and Publications Division.

Boskind-Lodahl, M. (1976). Cinderella's stepsisters: A feminist perspective on anorexia nervosa and bulimia. *Signs: Journal of Women in Culture and Society, 2,* 342–356.

311

Boskind-Lodahl, M., & Sirlin, J. (1977, March). The gorging purging syndrome. *Psychology Today*, pp. 49.

Boskind-Lodahl, M., & White, W. C. (1978). The definition and treatment of bulimarexia in college women-a pilot study. *Journal of American College Health Association*, 27, 84–86.

Boskind-White, M., & White, W. C. (1983). *Bulimarexia: The binge/purge cycle*. New York: W. W. Norton.

Bowen, M. (1960). A family concept of schizophrenia. In D. D. Jackson (Ed.), *The etiology of schizophrenia* (pp. 346–370). New York: Basic Books.

Bowen, M. (1978). *Family therapy in clinical practice*. New York: Aronson.

Bowlby, J. (1979). *The making and breaking of affectional bonds*. London: Tavistock.

Brady, W. F. (1980). The anorexia nervosa syndrome. *Oral Surgery*, 50(6), 509–516.

Briere, J. (1984, April). *The effects of childhood sexual abuse on later psychological functioning: defining a post-sexual-abuse syndrome*. Paper presented at the Third National Conference on Sexual Victimization of Children, Washington, DC.

Brodsky, A. M., & Hare-Mustin, R. T. (Eds.) (1980). *Women and psychotherapy: An assessment of research and practice*. New York: Guilford.

Brotman, A. W., Herzog, D. B., & Woods, S. W. (1984). Antidepressant treatment of bulimia: The relationship between bingeing and depression symptomatology. *Journal of Clinical Psychiatry*, 45(1), 7–9.

Broverman, I. K., Broverman, D. M., Clarkson, R. E., Rosenkrantz, P. & Vogel, S. R. (1970). Sex-role stereotypes and clinical judgments of mental health. *Journal of Consulting Psychology*, 34, 1–7.

Brownmiller, S. (1975). *Against our will: Men, women, and rape*. New York: Simon and Schuster.

Bruch, H. (1973). *Eating disorders: Obesity, anorexia nervosa, and the person within*. New York: Basic Books.

Bruch, H. (1978). *The golden cage: The enigma of anorexia nervosa*. Cambridge: Harvard University Press.

Burgess, A., & Holmstrom, L. (1974). Rape trauma syndrome. *American Journal of Psychiatry*, 131, 980–986.

Carter, E., & McGoldrick, M. (Eds.) (1980). *The family life cycle*. New York: Gardner.

Casper, R. C., Eckert, E. D., Halmi, K. A., Goldberg, S. C., & Davis, J. J. (1980). Bulimia: Its incidence and clinical importance in patients with anorexia nervosa. *Archives of General Psychiatry*, 37, 1030–1035.

Chesler, P. (1972). *Women and madness*. New York: Avon Books.

Crisp, A. H. (1981). Therapeutic outcome in anorexia nervosa. *Canadian Journal of Psychiatry*, 26(6), 232–235.

Crisp, A. H. (1981-2). Anorexia nervosa at a normal weight! The abnormal normal weight control syndrome. *International Journal of Psychiatry in Medicine*, 11, 203–234.

Crisp, A. H., Harding, B., & McGuiness, B. (1974). Anorexia Nervosa. Psychoneurotic characteristics of parents: Relationship to prognosis. A quantitative study. *Journal of Psychosomatic Research*, 18, 167–173.

Crisp, A. H., Hsu, L. K. G., & Harding, B. (1980). The starving hoarder and voracious spender: Stealing in anorexia nervosa. *Journal of Psychosomatic Research*, 24, 225–231.

Crisp, A. H., Kalucey, R. S., Lacey, J. H., & Harding B. (1977). Long-term prognosis in anorexia nervosa: Some factors predictive of outcome. In R. A. Vigersky (Ed.), *Anorexia Nervosa*, (pp. 55–65). New York: Raven Press.

Dally, P. (1969). *Anorexia vervosa*. New York: Grune & Stratton.

Dell, P. F. (1982). Beyond homeostasis: Toward a concept of coherence. *Family Process, 21*. 21–41.

Doyle, J. A. (1983). *The male experience*. Dubuque, Iowa: Wm. C. Brown Co.

Dwyer, J. T., Feldman, J. J., Seltzer, C. C., & Mayer, J. (1969). Body image in adolescents: Attitudes toward weight and perception of appearance. *American Journal of Clinical Nutrition, 20*, 1045–1056.

Edelman, B. (1981). Binge eating in normal weight and overweight individuals. *Psychological Reports. 49*, 739–746.

Elkin, M. (1984). *Families under the influence*. New York: Norton.

Ellis, A., & Harper, R. A. (1974). *A new guide to rational living*. Hollywood: Wilshire Book Company.

Fairburn, C. (1982). Binge eating and its management. *British Journal of Psychiatry, 141*, 631–633.

Fairburn, C. G., & Cooper, P. (1982). Self-induced vomiting and bulimia nervosa; an undetected problem. *British Medical Journal, 284*(4), 1153–1155.

Fairburn, C. G., & Cooper, P. J. (1983). The epidemiology of bulimia nervosa: Two community studies. *International Journal of Eating Disorders, 2*(4), 61–67.

Fallon, A. E., & Rozin, P. (1985). Sex differences in perceptions of desirable body shape. *Journal of Abnormal Psychology, 94*(1), 102–105.

Fallon, P. & Root, M. P. P. (1983). *Relapse, prolapse, and collapse*. (Unpublished manuscript.)

Fallon, P. & Root, M. P. P. (1985). *A family typology guide to the treatment of bulimia*. (Manuscript submitted for publication.)

Ferreira, A. (1963). Family myths and homeostasis. *Archives of General Psychiatry, 9*, 457–463.

Framo, J. (1981). *Explorations in marital and family therapy: Selected papers of James L. Framo*. New York: Springer.

Friedrich, W. N., & Pollock, S. (1982). Extreme interpersonal sensitivity in family members. *American Journal of Family Therapy, 10*(4), 27–34.

Garfinkel, P. E. (1981). Some recent observations on the pathogenesis of anorexia nervosa. *Canadian Journal of Psychiatry, 26*, 218–223.

Garfinkel, P. E., & Garner, D. M. (1982). *Anorexia nervosa: A multidimensional perspective*. New York: Brunner/Mazel.

Garfinkel, P. E., Moldofsky, H., & Garner, D. M. (1980). The heterogeneity of anorexia nervosa: bulimia as a distinct subgroup. *Archives of General Psychiatry, 37*, 1036–1040.

Garner, D. M., & Bemis, K. M. (1982). A cognitive-behavioral approach to anorexia nervosa. *Cognitive Therapy and Research, 6*(2), 123–150.

Garner, D. M., & Garfinkel P. E. (1981). Body image in anorexia nervosa: Measurement, theory and clinical implications. *International Journal of Psychiatry in Medicine, 11*(3), 263–284.

Garner, D. M., Garfinkel, P. E., & Bemis, K. M. (1982). A multidimensional psychotherapy for anorexia nervosa. *International Journal of Eating Disorders, 1*, 3–46.

Garner, D. M., Garfinkel, P. E., Schwartz, D., & Thompson, M. (1980). Cultural expectation of thinness in women. *Psychological Reports, 47*, 483–491.

Gerner, R. H., & Gwirtsman, H. E. (1981). Abnormalities of dexamethasone suppression test and urinary MHPG in anorexia nervosa. *American Journal of Psychiatry, 138*, 650–653.

Gillies, J. (1984, February). Feeling fat in a thin society. *Glamour Magazine*, pp. 198–201, 251–252.

Gilligan, C. (1978). In a different voice: Women's conception of the self and of morality. *Harvard Educational Review, 47*, 481–517.

Glassman, A. H., & Walsh, B. T. (1983). Link between bulimia and depression unclear (letters to the editor). *Journal of Clinical Psychopharmacology, 3*(3), 203.

Goldner, V. (1985). Feminism and family therapy. *Family Process, 24*(1), 31–48.

Graham, J. R. (1977). *The MMPI: A practical guide.* New York: Oxford University Press.

Gray, S. H. (1977). Social aspects of body image: Perception of normalcy of weight and affect of college undergraduates. *Perceptual and Motor Skills, 45*, 1035–1040.

Gull, W. W. (1874). Apepsia hysterica: Anorexia nervosa. *Transcripts of the Clinical Society of London, 7*, 22–28.

Gwirtsman, H. E., Roy-Byrne, P., Yager, J., & Gerner, R. (1983). Neuroendocrine tests in bulimia. *American Journal of Psychiatry, 140*, 559–563.

Haley, J. (1973). *Uncommon therapy.* New York: Norton.

Haley, J. & Hoffman, L. (1967). *Techniques of family therapy.* New York: Basic Books, Inc.

Halmi, K. A., Falk, J. R., & Schwartz, E. (1981). Binge eating and vomiting: A survey of a college population. *Psychological Medicine, 11*, 697–706.

Halmi, K. A., Goldberg, S. C., Casper, R., Eckert, E. L., & Davis, J. M. (1979). Pretreatment predictors of outcome in anorexia nervosa. *Journal of Psychiatry, 134*, 71–78.

Hathaway, S. R., & McKinley, J. C. (1967). *The Minnesota Multiphasic Personality Inventory manual.* New York: Psychological Corporation.

Hatsukami, D. K., Mitchell, J. E., & Eckert, E. D. (1984). Eating disorders: A variant of mood disorders? *Psychiatric Clinics of North America, 7*(2), 349–363.

Hatsukami, D., Owen, P., Pyle, R., & Mitchell, J. (1982). Similarities and differences on the MMPI between women with bulimia and women with alcohol or drug abuse problems. *Addictive Behaviors, 7*, 435–439.

Hawkins, R., & Clement, P. (1980). Development and construct validation of a self-report measure of binge eating tendencies. *Addictive Behaviors, 5*, 219–226.

Headley, L. (1977). *Adults and their parents in family therapy.* New York: Plenum.

Herman, J. L. (1981). *Father-daughter incest.* Cambridge: Harvard University Press.

Herzog, D. B. (1982). Bulimia: The secretive syndrome. *Psychosomatics, 23*, 481–483; 487.

Herzog, D. B., Norman, D. K., Gordon, C., & Pepose, M. (1984). Sexual conflict and eating disorders in 27 males. *American Journal of Psychiatry, 141*(8), 989–990.

Hoffman, L. (1981). *Foundations of family therapy.* New York: Basic Books.

House, R., Crisius, R., Bliziotes, M., & Licht, H. (1981). Perimolysis: Unveiling the surreptitious vomiter. *Oral Surgery, 51*(2). 152–155.

Hsu, L. K. G. (1984). Treatment of bulimia with lithium. *American Journal of Psychiatry, 141*, 1260–1262.

Hsu, L. K. G., Crisp, A. H., & Harding, B. (1979). Outcome of anorexia nervosa. *Lancet, 1*, 61–65.

Hudson, J. I., Laffer, P. S., & Pope, H. G. (1982). Bulimia related to affective disorder by family history and response to dexamethasone suppression test. *American Journal of Psychiatry, 139*, 685–687.

Hudson, J. I., Pope, H. G. Jr., Jonas, J. M., & Yurgelun-Todd, D. (1983). Family history study of anorexia nervosa and bulimia. *British Journal of Psychiatry, 142*, 133–138.

Huenemann, R. L., Shapiro, L. R., Hampton, M. C., & Mitchell, B. W. (1966). A longitudinal study of gross body composition and body conformation and their association with food and activity in a teenage population. *American Journal of Clinical Nutrition, 18*, 325–338.

Hurst, P. S., Lacey, J. H., & Crisp, A. H. (1977). Teeth, vomiting and diet: a study of the dental characteristics of seventeen anorexia patients. *Postgraduate Medical Journal, 53*, 298–305.

Jakobovits, C., Halstead, Pl, Kelley, L., Roe, D. A., & Young, C. M. (1977). Eating habits and nutrient intakes of college women over a thirty-year period. *Journal of the American Dietetic Association, 71*, 405–411.

Johnson, C., & Berndt, D. j. (1983). Preliminary investigation of bulimia and life adjustment. *American Journal of Psychiatry, 140*, 774–777.

Johnson, C., Connor, M., & Stuckey, M. (1983). Short-term group treatment of bulimia: A preliminary report. *International Journal of Eating Disorders, 2*(4), 199–208.

Johnson, C. L., Stuckey, M. K., Lewis, L. D., & Schwartz, D. M. (1982). Bulimia: A descriptive survey of 316 cases. *International Journal of Eating Disorders, 2*(1), 3–16.

Jones, D. J., Fox, M. M., Babigan, H. M., & Hutton, H. E. (1980). Epidemiology of anorexia nervosa in Monroe County, New York: 1960–1976. *Psychosomatic Medicine, 42*, 551–558.

Kanfer, F. H. (1975). Self-management methods. In F. H. Kanfer & H. P. Goldstein (Eds.), *Helping people change*. New York: Pergamon Press.

Kaplan, A. S., Garfinkel, P. E., Darby, P. L., & Garner, D. M. (1983). Carbamazepine in the treatment of bulimia. *American Journal of Psychiatry, 140*(9), 1225–1226.

Karpel, M. A., & Strauss, E. S. (1982). *Family evaluation*. New York: Gardner Press.

Kegan, R. (1982). *The evolving self*. Cambridge: Harvard University Press.

Keyes, A., Brozek, J., Henschel, A., Michelson, O., & Taylor, H. L. (1950). *The biology of human starvation* (Vol. 1). Minneapolis: University of Minnesota Press.

Kirkley, B. G., Schneider, J. A., Agras, W. S., & Bachman, J. A. (1985). Comparison of two group treatments for bulimia. *Journal of Consulting and Clinical Psychology, 53*(1), 43–48.

Klesges, R. C. (1983). An analysis of body-image distortions in a nonpatient population. *The International Journal of Eating Disorders, 2*(2), 35–42.

Kolbenschlag, M. (1979). *Kiss sleeping beauty good-bye*. New York: Bantam Books.

Kurman, L. (1978). An analysis of messages concerning food, eating behaviors and ideal body image on prime-time American network television. *Dissertation Abstracts International, A*, 1907–1908.

Lacey, H. (1983). Bulimia nervosa, binge eating, and psychogenic vomiting: A controlled treatment study and long term outcome. *British Medical Journal, 286*(21), 1609–1613.

Laing, R. D. (1969). *The self and others*. 2nd edition. New York: Pantheon Books.

Laing, R. D., & Esterson, A. (1964). *Sanity, madness, and the family*. Baltimore: Penguin Books.

Laseque, C. (1964). De l'anorexie hysterique. In R. N. Kaufman and M. Heiman (Eds.), *Evolution of psychosomatic concepts. Anorexia Nervosa: A paradigm* (pp.

141–155). New York: International Universities Press. (Original work published 1873).

Lenihan, G. O., & Sanders, C. D. (1984). Guidelines for group therapy with eating disorder victims. *Journal of Counseling and Development, 63,* 252–263.

Levin, P. A., Falko, J. M., Dixon, K., Gallup, E. M., & Saunders, W. (1980). Benign parotid enlargement in bulimia. *Annals of Internal Medicine, 93,* 827–829.

Levitan, H. L. (1981). Implications of certain dreams reported by patients in a bulimic phase of anorexia nervosa. *Canadian Journal of Psychiatry, 26*(6), 228–231.

Libow, J. A., Raskin, P. A., & Caust, B. L. (1982). Feminist and family therapy systems therapy. *The American Journal of Family Therapy, 10*(3), 3–12.

Lidz, T., Fleck, S., & Cornelison, A. (1965). *Schizophrenia and the family.* New York: International Universities Press.

Madanes, C. (1981). *Strategic family therapy.* San Francisco: Jossey-Bass, Inc.

Mahler, M. S., Pine, E., & Bergman, A. (1975). *The psychological birth of the human infant.* New York: Basic Books.

Mazel, J. (1981). *The Beverly Hills diet.* New York: Macmillan.

McGoldrick, M. (1980). The joining of families through marriage: The new couple. In E. A. Carter & M. McGoldrick (Eds.), *The family life cycle* (pp. 93–120). New York: Gardner.

Minuchin, S. (1974). *Families and family therapy.* Cambridge: Harvard University Press.

Minuchin, S., & Fishman, H. C. (1981). *Family therapy techniques.* Cambridge: Harvard University Press.

Minuchin, S., Rosman, B. L., & Baker, L. (1978). *Psychosomatic families.* Cambridge: Harvard University Press.

Mitchell, J. E., Hosfield, W., & Pyle, R. L. (1983). EEG findings in patients with the bulimia syndrome. *International Journal of Eating Disorders, 2*(3), 17–23.

Moos, R. & Moos, B. (1981). *Manual for the Family Environment Scale.* Palo Alto: Consulting Psychologist Press.

Morgan, H. G., & Russell, G. F. M. (1975). Value of family background and clinical features as predictors of long-term outcome in anorexia nervosa: Four-year follow-up study of 41 patients. *Psychological Medicine, 5,* 355–371.

Nash, M., & Baker. E. (1984, February). Trance encounters: Susceptibility to hypnosis. *Psychology Today,* pp. 72–3.

Neuman, P. A. & Halvorson, P. A. (1983). *Anorexia nervosa and bulimia: A handbook for counselors and therapists.* New York: Van Nostrand Reinhold Company.

NiCarthy, G., Merriam, K., & Coffman, S. (1984). *Talking it out: A guide to groups for abused women.* Seattle: The Seal Press.

Nichols, M. (1984). *Family therapy: Concepts and methods.* New York: Gardner Press.

Norman, D. K. & Herzog, D. B. (1983). Bulimia, anorexia nervosa, and anorexia nervosa with bulimia: A comparative analysis of MMPI profiles. *International Journal of Eating Disorders, 2,* 43–52.

Okun, B. F., & Rappaport, L. J. (1980). *Working with families: An introduction to family therapy.* North Scituate: Duxburry Press.

Orbach, S. (1978). Social dimensions in compulsive eating in women. *Psychotherapy: Theory, Research and Practice, 15*(2), 180–189.

Palmer, R. L. (1979). The dietary chaos syndrome: A useful new term? *British Journal of Medical Psychology, 52,* 187–190.

Papp, P. (1983). *The process of change.* New York: Guilford.

Paykel, E. S., Mueller, P. S., & de la Vergne, P. M. (1973). Amitriptyline, weight gain and carbohydrate craving: A side effect. *British Journal of Psychiatry, 123,* 501–507.

Perron, M. & Endres, J. (1985). Knowledge, attitudes, and dietary practices of female athletes. *Journal of the American Dietetic Association, 85*(5), 573–576.

Polivy, J., & Herman, C. P. (1985). Dieting and binging: A causal analysis. *American Psychology, 40*(27), 193–201.

Pope, H. G. & Hudson, J. I. (1984). *New hope for binge eaters: Advances in the understanding and treatment of bulimia.* New York: Harper & Row.

Pope, H. G., Hudson, J. I., Jonas, J. M., & Yurgelun-Todd, D. (1983). Bulimia treated with imipramine: A placebo-controlled, double-blind study. *American Journal of Psychiatry, 140*(5), 554–558.

Pope, H. C., Hudson, J. I., Yurgelun-Todd, D., & Hudson, M. S. (1984). Prevalence of anorexia nervosa and bulimia in three student populations. *International Journal of Eating Disorders, 3*(3), 45–52.

Pyle, R., Mitchell, J., & Eckert, E. (1981). Bulimia: A report of 34 cases. *Journal of Clinical Psychiatry, 48*(2), 60–64.

Pyle, R. L., Mitchell, J. E., Eckert, E. D., Halvorson, P. A., Neuman, P. A., & Goff, G. M. (1983). The incidence of bulimia in freshman college students. *International Journal of Eating Disorders, 2*(3), 75–85.

Rampling, D. (1978). Anorexia nervosa: Reflections on theory and practice. *Psychiatry, 41,* 296–301.

Radloff, L. (1975). Sex differences in depression: The effects of occupation and marital status. *Sex Roles, 1,* 249–269.

Reto, C., Root, M. P. P., & Fallon, P. (1985). *Incidence of suicide in a bulimic population.* Paper presented at Washington State Psychological Association, Vancouver, B. C., 1985.

Ritterman, M. (1983). *Using hypnosis in family therapy.* San Francisco: Jossey-Bass.

Root, M. P. P. (1983). *Bulimia: A Descriptive and Treatment Outcome Study* (Doctoral Dissertation, University of Washington, Seattle, Washington).

Root, M. P. P. & Fallon, P. (1983a). *Physiological Consequences in Bulimia.* (Unpublished manuscript).

Root, M. P. P. & Fallon, P. (1983b). *Bulimia and Related Eating Disorders Screen.* Seattle, Washington.

Root, M. P. P. & Fallon, P. (1983c). *Personal Monitoring Journal for Bulimia.* Seattle, Washington.

Root, M. P. P. & Fallon, P. (1985). *Victimization Experiences as Contributing Factors in the Development of Bulimia in Women.* (Manuscript submitted for publication).

Root, M. P. P., & Friedrich, W. N. (1985). Heterogeneity in a bulimic sample: Diagnostic and therapeutic implications. (Manuscript submitted for publication).

Rost, W., Neuhaus, M., & Florin, I. (1982). Bulimia nervosa: Sex role attitude, sex role behavior, and sex role related locus of control in bulimarexic women. *Journal of Psychosomatic Research, 26*(4), 403–408.

Russell, G. (1979). Bulimia nervosa: An ominous variant of anorexia nervosa. *Psychological Medicine, 9,* 429–448.

Saba, G., Barrett, M. J., & Schwartz, R. (1983). All or nothing: The bulimia epidemic. *Family Therapy Networker, 7,* 43–44.

Sabine, E. J., Yonace, A., & Farrington, A. J., Barrett, K. H., & Wakeling, A. (1983). Bulimia nervosa: A placebo-controlled, double-blind, therapeutic trial of mianserin. *British Journal of Clinical Pharmacology, 15,* 195–202.

Sargent, J., Liebman, R., & Silver, M. (1984). Family therapy for anorexia nervosa. In D. M. Garner & P. E. Garfinkel (Eds.) *Handbook of psychotherapy for anorexia nervosa and bulimia.* (257–279). New York: Guilford Press.

Sargent, J., & Liebman, R. (1984). Outpatient treatment of anorexia nervosa. *Psychiatric Clinics of North America, 7*(2), 235–245.

Schultz, D. A. (1979). *Human sexuality.* New Jersey: Prentice-Hall, Inc.

Schwartz, B. (1982). *Diets don't work.* Houston, Tx: Breakthru Publishing.

Schwartz, R. (1982). Bulimia and family therapy: A case study. *International Journal of Eating Disorders, 2,* 75–82.

Schwartz, R., Barrett, M. J., & Saba, G. (1984). Family therapy for bulimia. In D. Garner and P. Garfinkel (Eds.), *Handbook of psychotherapy for anorexia and bulimia.* New York: Guilford.

Schwartz, D. M., Thompson, M. G. & Johnson, C. L. (1982). Anorexia nervosa and bulimia: The socio-cultural context. *International Journal of Eating Disorders, 1,* 20–36.

Seligman, M. E. P. (1974). Depression and learned helplessness. In R. J. Friedman & M. M. Katz (Eds.), *The psychology of depression: Contemporary theory and research* (pp. 83–108). Washington, DC: V. H. Winston and Sons.

Selvini Palazzoli, M. (1978). *Self starvation.* New York: Aronson.

Selvini Palazzoli, M., Boscolo, L., Cecchin, G., & Prata, G. (1978) *Paradox and Counterparadox.* New York: Aronson.

Simpson, M. A. (1973). Female genital self-mutilation. *Archives of General Psychiatry, 29,* 808–819.

Society of Actuaries & Association of Life Insurance. (1979). *Build and blood pressure study.* Chicago, IL: Author.

Sontag, S. (1978) *Illness as metaphor.* New York: Farrar, Straus, & Giroux.

Sours, J. A. (1983). Case reports of anorexia nervosa and caffeinism. *American Journal of Psychiatry, 1450*(2), 235–236.

Speck, R. & Attneave, C. (1973). *Family networks.* New York: Pantheon.

Spencer, J. A., & Fremouw, W. J. (1979). Binge eating as a function of restraint and weight classification. *Journal of Abnormal Psychology, 88*(3), 262–267.

Stangler, R. S., & Printz, A. M. (1980). DSM-III: Psychiatric diagnosis in a university population. *American Journal of Psychiatry, 137,* 937–940.

Stanton, D. & Landau-Stanton, J. (1984). Self-destructive families: A systems approach to treating suicide, substance abuse, and bereavement. Workshop presented at AAMFT Annual Conference, San Francisco, CA.

Stanton, M. D., & Todd, T. C. (Eds.) (1982). *The family therapy of drug abuse and addiction.* New York: The Guilford Press.

Steinglass, P. (1978). The conceptualization of marriage from a systems theory perspective. In T. J. Paolino & B. S. McCrady (Eds.), *Marriage and Marital Therapy.* New York: Brunner/Mazel.

Steinglass, P. (1980). A life history model of the alcoholic family. *Family Process, 19,* 211–225.

Stern, S. L., Dixon, R. N., Nemzer, E., Lake, M. D., Sansone, R. A., Smeltzer, D. J., Lant, S., & Schrier, S. S. (1984). Affective disorder in the families of women with normal weight bulimia. *American Journal of Psychiatry, 141*(10), 1224–1227.

Stierlin, H. (1973). A Family perspective on adolescent runaways. *Archives of General Psychiatry, 12,* 56–62.

Strober, M., Salkin, B., Burroughs, J., & Morrell, W. (1982). Validity of the bulimia-restricter distinction in anorexia nervosa. Parental personality characteristics and family psychiatric morbidity. *Journal of Nervous and Mental Disease, 170*(6), 345–351.

Swartz, C. M., & Dunner, F. J. (1982). Dexamethosone suppression testing of alcoholics. *Archives of General Psychiatry, 39,* 1309–1312.

Szyrynski, V. (1973). Anorexia nervosa and psychotherapy. *American Journal of Psychotherapy, 27,* 492–505.

Tavris, C. (1982). *Anger. The misunderstood emotion.* New York: Simon & Schuster, Inc.

Tomm, K. (1984). One perspective of the Milan Systemic Approach: Part II. Description of session format, interviewing style and interventions. *Journal of Marital and Family Therapy, 10,* 253–271.

Walker, L. E. (1979). *The battered woman.* New York: Harper & Row.

Wallach, J. D. & Lowenkopf, E. L. (1984). Five bulimic women. *International Journal of Eating Disorders, 3*(4), 53–66.

Wallechensky, D., Wallace, I., & Wallace, A. (1977). *Book of lists.* New York: Morrow.

Walsh, B. T., Croft, C. B., & Katz, J. L. (1981–82). Anorexia nervosa and salivary gland enlargement. *International Journal of Psychiatry in Medicine, 11*(3), 255–261.

Walsh, B. T., Stewart, J. W., Wright, L., Harrison, W., Roose, S. P., & Glassman, A. H. (1982). Treatment of bulimia with monoamine oxidase inhibitors. *American Journal of Psychiatry, 139*(12), 1629–1630.

Walsh, F. (1978). Concurrent grandparent death and birth of schizophrenic offspring: An intriguing finding. *Family Process, 17,* 457–463.

Wardle, J., & Beinart, H. (1981). Binge eating: A theoretical review. *British Journal of Clinical Psychology, 20,* 97–109.

Watzlawick, P., Beavin, J. H., & Jackson, D. D. (1967). *Pragmatics of human communication.* New York: Norton.

Watzlawick, P., Weakland, J. H., & Fisch, R. (1974). *Change.* New York: Norton.

Weiss, S. R., & Ebert, M. (1983). Psychological and behavioral characteristics of normal-weight bulimics and normal weight controls. *Psychosomatic Medicine, 45*(4).

Weissman, M. M. (1980). Depression. In A. M. Brodsky & R. T. Hare-Mustin, (Eds.), *Women and psychotherapy: An assessment of research and practice* (87–112). New York: Guilford.

Weissman, M. M., & Klerman, G. L. (1977). Sex differences and the epidemiology of depression. *Archives of General Psychiatry, 34,* 98–111.

Wells, T. (1977). Up the management ladder. In E. I. Rawlings & D. K. Carter, *Psychotherapy for women: Treatment toward equality.* Springfield, IL: Charles C. Thomas.

White, W. C., & Boskind-White, M. (1981). An experiential-behavioral approach to the treatment of bulimarexia. *Psychotherapy: Theory, Research and Practice, 18*(4), 501–507.

Williams, G. J. & Money, J. (Eds.) (1980). *Traumatic abuse and neglect of children at home.* Baltimore: Johns Hopkins University Press.

Wooley, O. W., & Wooley, S. (1982). The Beverly Hills eating disorder: The mass marketing of anorexia nervosa. *International Journal of Eating Disorders, 1*(3), 70–75.

Wooley, S., & Kearney-Cooke, A. (In press). Intensive treatment of bulimia and body image disturbance. In K. Brownell, & J. Foreyt (Eds.), *Physiology, psy-*

*chology, and the treatment of eating disorders.* New York: Basic Books.

Wooley, S., Wooley, O., & Dyrenforth, S. (1979). Theoretical, practical, and social issues in behavioral treatments of obesity. *Journal of Applied Behavior Analysis, 2*, 3–25.

Wynne, L. L., & Ryckoff, L., Day, J., & Hirsch, S. I. (1958). Pseudo-mutuality in the family relationships of schizophrenics. *Psychiatry, 21*, 205–220.

Yalom, I. D. (1975). *The theory and practice of group psychotherapy* (2nd ed.). New York: Basic Books.

# Index

abandonment, loyalty and, 23–24
Abraham, S. F., 3, 7, 17
abuse, *see* battering, rape, and sexual abuse
Ackerman, N. W., 183
Agras, W. S., 194, 201
Al-anon, 268, 281
alcoholism, 8, 11, 12, 57, 89, 148
  in chaotic families, 120, 121, 271, 272
  in group therapy, 196
Altshuler, K. Z., 209, 212
American Psychiatric Association, 6, 17, 23
amenorrhea, 15
amitriptyline, 211
Anderson, A. E., 9
Andolfi, M., 40, 42
Angelo, C., 40, 42
anger:
  in chaotic families, 116, 123, 273
  depression linked with, 11
  in individual therapy, 177–78
  in overprotective families, 106
  in perfect families, 92, 244, 246, 247
  women and, 21–22
anorectic families:
  parent-child coalitions in, 80
  triangulation in, 80
anorexia nervosa:
  bulimia vs., 16–19, 79–81
  family interactions related to, 79–80
antidepressant medication, bulimic clients
  and, 208, 209, 211–13
Aono, T., 18
Attneave, C., 39
autonomy:
  as balance in childhood, 68–69, 72

  in chaotic families, 115
  in overprotective families, 100–101, 263

Babigan, H. M., 5
Bachman, J. A., 194, 201
Baker, E., 114
Baker, L., 32, 80, 112, 185
Barrett, K. H., 209
Barrett, M. J., 80, 112, 249
Bateson, Gregory, 48, 49
battering, 9–10, 25, 34
Beavin, J. H., 181, 227
Beck, A. T., 176, 211
Beinart, H., 7
Bemis, K. M., 11, 80, 209
Benjamin, M., 39, 64
Bergman, A., 119
Berndt, D. J., 3, 7
Beumont, P. J. V., 7, 17, 18
*Beverly Hills Diet, The* (Mazel), 27–28
bibliotherapy, bulimic families and, 223, 268
binge-eating, dieting prior to, 29
binge-purge behavior, 3, 7, 88, 92, 106, 123, 172, 174, 192, 199, 201
  antidepressant medication and, 209
  collapse and, 194, 203, 204
  control issue and, 13
  guidelines for, 154
  prolapse and, 203, 204
  relapse and, 194, 203, 204, 242–43, 294
bipolar affective disorder, 211, 212
birth order, 42
  in chaotic families, 114–15, 140
  in overprotective families, 104–5

(*continued*)
  in perfect families, 89
Black, C., 112
Bliziotes, M., 14, 15
body-image, dissatisfaction with, 28–29
Boscolo, L., 137
Boskind-Lodahl, M., 6, 18, 26, 29, 194, 303
boundaries:
  adolescent and parent, 71
  in chaotic families, 114–15, 150
  enmeshed, 33, 256
  in family assessment, 133–35
  impermeable, 34, 133
  in individual assessment, 140
  in individual therapy, 164
  intrusive, 33, 34
  joining and, 220
  in overprotective families, 99, 105
  in perfect families, 84
  permeable, 33–34, 59, 133
Bowen, M., 41, 46, 53–55
Bowlby, J., 121
Brady, W. F., 14
Briere, J., 34, 212
Brodsky, A. M., 25
Brotman, A. W., 11, 209
Broverman, D. M., 25–26, 30
Broverman, I. K., 25–26, 30
Brownmiller, S., 25
Brozek, J., 9, 209
Bruch, H., 16, 26, 29, 80, 112
bulimia:
  as alternative form of affective disorder,
    11, 208–10
  anorexia vs., 16–19, 79–81
  assessment of, 131–49
  behavioral symptoms of, 7–9
  chronicity of, 12, 13, 15
  definitions of, 5–6
  development of, 3–15
  individual symptoms of, 7–15, 35
  obstacles to treatment of, 299–310
  onset of, 3, 65
  physiological symptoms of, 14–15
  psychological symptoms of, 9–13
  psychopharmacological issues in, 208–15
  recognition of problem, 3
  set of beliefs in, 173, 176, 177, 201
  stereotypes associated with, 4–5
  treatment of, 131–215
  *see also* couples therapy; group therapy;
    individual therapy
Bulimia and Related Eating Disorders
    Screen, 131
  group therapy and, 199
  individual assessment and, 141–49

  sections of, 141–49
  as treatment for bulimia, 149
bulimic families:
  adolescence and, 70–72
  adolescence vs. mid-life crisis in, 70–71,
    72
  bibliotherapy and, 223, 268
  boundary problems in, 33–34, 81
  circular conceptualization in, 40
  clinical conceptualization in, 40
  consultation with, 150–60
  contradictory communications in, 226–
    27, 234, 235
  designing interventions for, 222–25
  divorce and, 40, 71–72
  emotional distance regulators in, 183, 248
  expression of feeling and, 35–36
  family systems concepts applied to, 39–51
  genograms of, 60, 93, 109, 125, 250
  guidelines of recovery for, 156–58, 223
  impact of secrets on, 59–60
  individuation in, 32–33
  inexperienced therapists and, 301
  joining with, 220–22
  launching in, 72–75, 222
  life-cycle transitions in, 65–75
  loyalty in, 35, 84
  members of, 39–40
  multigenerational patterns in, 56–58
  obstacles posed by, 304–9
  organization in, 34–35
  personal space in, 105
  recycling of symptoms in, 225
  relationships in, 12–13
  remarriage in, 75
  resistance and, 300
  resolution of issues in, 36
  sabotage and, 304–9
  separation in, 32–33
  single parents and, 75
  stuckness and, 64, 74, 81, 82, 132, 300
  systemic issues in, 32–36
  treatment approach for, 219–25
  types of, 79, 81–82
  *see also* chaotic families; overprotective
    families; perfect families
bulimic marriages:
  enmeshment in, 183, 184
  intimacy in, 182–84
  power imbalances in, 181–82
Burgess, A., 212
Burroughs, J., 6

carbamazepine, 11
Carpenter, Karen, 83, 158
Carter, E., 57, 64, 66

Casper, R. C., 6, 17, 18
Cecchin, G., 137
chaotic families, 4, 112–28
    affection and nurturance in, 116, 123
    age of onset of bulimia in, 120
    alcoholism in, 120, 121, 271, 272
    anger in, 116, 123, 273
    autonomy in, 115
    birth order in, 119–20
    boundaries in, 114–15, 140
    case histories of, 124–28, 267–95
    conflict resolution in, 118
    creation of emotional distance in, 123
    dissociation from reality in, 123
    drug abuse in, 120, 121, 272, 273
    expression of conflict in, 137
    expression of feelings in, 116–17
    family-of-origin issues in, 120–21
    first-order changes in, 139
    functions of bulimic behavior in, 122–24
    grief in, 117
    identity in, 115
    launching in, 74, 122
    life-cycles in, 121–22
    loss in, 117
    messages in, 117–18
    multigenerational patterns in, 57
    perspective on, 118–20
    powerlessness in, 116
    predictability in, 124
    relinquishing responsibility in, 123
    second-order changes in, 139
    self-abuse in, 123
    sexual abuse in, 120
    substance abuse in, 112
    therapy in, 112–14
    third chair exercises in, 278–81, 282, 294
    triangulation in, 44–45
Chesler, P., 22, 23, 24, 25
childhood:
    autonomy as balance in, 68–69, 72
    in conflict-detouring, 43
    onset of bulimia in, 67–70
Clarkson, R. E., 25–26, 30
Clement, P., 6
coercion, 304
    and individual therapy, 165
Coffman, S., 25, 212
cognitive restructuring:
    in group therapy, 201
    in individual therapy, 175
cohesion-enhancing, 121
collapse, binge-purge behavior and, 194, 203, 204
communication, 49–51
    axioms of, 49–50

symmetrical vs. complementary relation-
    ships in, 50, 51
conflict-detouring:
    children's role in, 43
    in overprotective families, 249, 257
conflict resolution, 68, 169
    in chaotic families, 118
    family assessment and, 135–37
consultation:
    assessment in, 153, 168
    case history using, 154–60
    education and, 154
    as family-initiated, 150–51
    goals of, 152–54
    individual focus shifted to family focus
        in, 153
    joining in, 153
    as professional-initiated, 152
    as therapist-initiated, 151–52
control, self-image and, 13
Cooper, P. J., 6, 15
couples therapy, 180–93
    boundary delineation in, 187–88
    decision making in, 189
    delayed intervention in, 192–93
    immediate intervention in, 189–92
    as primary therapeutic modality, 180
    rebalancing in, 185–87
    techniques of, 184–93
Crisius, R., 14, 15
Crisp, A. H., 5, 6, 8, 14, 15, 18, 80
Croft, C. B., 15

Dally, P., 26
Darby, P. L., 11, 209
David, J. J., 6, 17, 18
Davis, J. M., 17
Day, J., 183
dehydration, 15
de la Vergne, P. M., 211
Dell, P. F., 64
dental symptoms, 14
depression, 8, 10–11, 173
    anger linked with, 11
    bulimia-related, 208–9
    women and, 22–23, 212
dexamethasone suppression test (DST), 11,
    208, 209
*Diagnostic and Statistical Manual of Men-
    tal Disorders* (DSM-III), 6, 17, 147
dieting, 27–30, 56, 172
    statistics on, 28–29
Differentiation of Self Scale, 54
diuretic abuse, 7, 15
Dixon, K., 15
Dixon, R. N., 11, 209

double-binds, 25–26, 41
Doyle, J. A., 30
drug abuse, 8
    in chaotic families, 120, 121, 272, 273
    in group therapy, 196
Dunner, F. J., 11, 209
Dwyer, J. T., 28, 29
Dyrenforth, S., 26

Ebert, M., 8, 10, 12, 15
Eckert, E. D., 3, 5, 6, 7, 8, 15, 17, 18, 23,
    26, 29, 209
Edelman, B., 6
electrolyte imbalance, 15
Elkin, M., 118, 120
Ellis, A., 176
Endres, J., 29
enmeshment, 33, 46–47
    boundary violations and, 46, 47
    in bulimic marriages, 183, 184
    in chaotic families, 285
    in perfect families, 247
    emotional resonance in, 47
    in overprotective families, 249, 256,
        257, 266
entropy, 41
Esterson, A., 53
expression of feelings, 10–11, 184
    in chaotic families, 116–17
    incongruent smiling and, 36, 227
    in overprotective families, 101
    in perfect families, 85

Fairburn, C. G., 6, 15
Falk, J. R., 6, 17, 29
Falko, J. M., 15
Fallon, A. E., 28
Fallon, Patricia, 7, 8, 9, 14, 34, 141, 163,
    172, 182, 199, 201, 209
families:
    bulimia supported by, 3
    bulimic's symptoms mirrored by, 4
    gender inequity mirrored in, 23
    grief in, 10, 36
    as homeostatic systems, 48
    types of, summarized, 4
    *see also* bulimic families; chaotic fami-
        lies; overprotective families; perfect
        families
family assessment, 131–39
    boundaries in, 133–35
    conflict resolution and, 135–37
    family protection in, 138
    likelihood of change in, 138–39
    therapists and, 131–33

Family Environment Scale, 133
family-of-origin issues, therapists and,
    301–3
family-of-origin therapy, 53, 186, 187
family projection process, 54–55
family systems concepts, as applied to
    bulimic families, 39–51
family therapy, 40
    spreading the symptom around in, 40,
        306
Farrington, A. J., 209
feedback, 41, 48, 85
Feldman, J. J., 28, 29
Ferreira, A., 58
first-order changes:
    in chaotic families, 139
    in perfect families, 235, 309
Fisch, R., 132, 138, 192, 235, 299
Florin, I., 3
Fonda, Jane, 83
Fox, M. M., 5
Framo, J., 53
free fatty acids (FFA), 43
Fremouw, W. J., 29
Friedrich, William N., 8, 10, 12, 13, 23, 26

Gallup, E. M., 15
Garfinkel, P. E., 3, 5, 6, 11, 12, 17, 18,
    26, 27, 80, 81, 209
Garner, D. M., 3, 5, 6, 11, 12, 17, 18, 26,
    27, 80, 81, 209
George, G. C. W., 18
Gerner, R. H., 11, 17, 209
Gillies, J., 29
Gilligan, C., 183
Glassman, A. H., 11, 209, 210
Goff, G. M., 6
Goldberg, S. C., 6, 17, 18
Goldner, V., 23, 24
Gordon, C., 26
Gray, S. H., 29, 30
grief:
    in chaotic families, 117
    in overprotective families, 101
    in perfect families, 86
group therapy, 194–205
    absence of family and, 196
    alcohol abuse in, 196
    Bulimia and Related Eating Disorders
        Screen and, 199
    client readiness in, 197–98
    cognitive restructuring in, 201
    contraindications for, 196–98
    as cost-effective, 195
    dissimilar clients in, 197

dropouts in, 198
drug abuse in, 196
family drawings and, 202
family therapy vs., 197
goals in, 199, 200
increased readiness for, 195
indications for, 195–96
sabotage by client in, 199–201
structure of group in, 198–202
termination of, 202–5
therapeutic aspects of, 194–95
victimization and, 195–96
Gull, W. W., 79
Gwirtsman, H. E., 11, 17, 209

Haley, J., 41, 49, 224
Halmi, K. A., 6, 17, 18, 29
Halstead, P., 29
Halvorson, P. A., 6
Hampton, M. C., 28
Harding, B., 5, 6, 8, 18, 80
Hare-Mustin, R. T., 25
Harper, R. A., 176
Harrison, W., 11
Hathaway, S. R., 26
Hatsukami, D. K., 8, 209
Hawkins, R., 6
Headley, L., 60
Henschel, A., 9, 209
Herman, C. P., 29–30
Herman, J. L., 25, 34, 212
Herzog, D. B., 11, 18, 23, 26, 209
Hirsch, S. I., 183
Hoffman, L., 39, 40, 41, 43, 45, 46, 48,
  52, 54
Holmstrom, L., 212
homeostasis, 47–49
  imbalance and, 48, 49
  mechanisms of, 49
homosexuals, bulimia stereotypes and, 5, 31
Hopkins Symptom Checklist, 18
Hosfield, W., 17
House, R., 14, 15
Hsu, L. K. G., 6, 8
Hudson, J. I., 8, 11, 17, 208, 209
Huenemann, R. L., 28
Hurst, P. S., 14
Hutton, H. E., 5

identity:
  in chaotic families, 115
  in overprotective families, 100
  in perfect families, 84–85
imipramine, 209, 211
individual assessment, 140–49

boundaries in, 164
Bulimia and Related Eating Disorders
  Screen and, 141–49
joining in, 140–41
victimization and, 141
individual therapy, 161–79
  absence of family members and, 164
  anger in, 177–78
  boundaries in, 164
  coercion and, 165
  cognitive restructuring in, 175
  cognitive set of family in, 175–76
  contraindications for, 165–67
  dysfunctional protection of family and,
    165–66
  facilitating ownership in, 175
  family patterns in, 176–78
  indications for, 162–64
  launching and, 164
  nutritional consultants and, 174
  premature termination of, 168–69
  as preparation for family therapy, 164
  significant others and, 166
  symptom control as goal in, 171–74
  teaching symptom control in, 162
  termination of, 178–79
  victimization and, 163–64
  writing as intervention in, 170–71
I-position, 46, 54

Jackson, D. D., 181, 227
Jakobvits, C., 29
Johnson, C. L., 3, 7, 8, 15, 17, 18, 26
joining:
  acceptance of family views and, 221
  acknowledgement of family effort in,
    221–22
  boundaries and, 220
  with bulimic families, 220–22
  in consultation, 153
  family rules and, 220
  in individual assessment, 140–41
  positive relabeling and, 221
Jonas, J. M., 8, 11, 17, 209
Jones, D. J., 5

Kalucey, R. S., 5, 18
Kanfer, F. H., 199
Kaplan, A. S., 11, 209
Karpel, M. A., 66, 68, 70
Katz, J. L., 15
Kearney-Cooke, A., 81, 82
Kegan, R., 64, 68, 70, 73, 115, 182–183
Kelley, L., 29
Keyes, A., 9, 209

Kirkley, B. G., 194, 201
Klerman, G. L., 22
Klesges, R. C., 28, 29
Kolbenschlag, M., 21
Kumashiro, H., 18
Kurman, L., 26, 27

Lacey, J. H., 5, 14, 15, 18
Laffer, P. S., 11, 209
Laing, R. D., 53, 58
Lake, M. D., 11, 209
Landau-Stanton, J., 65, 138
Lant, S., 11, 209
Laseque, C., 79
launching:
    in bulimic families, 72–75, 222
    in chaotic families, 74, 122
    individual therapy and, 164
    in perfect families, 246, 247
laxative abuse, 7, 15
Lenihan, G. O., 194
Levin, P. A., 15
Levitan, H. L., 17
Lewis, L. D., 3, 7, 8, 15, 17, 18
Licht, H., 14, 15
Liebman, R., 80
life-cycle transitions, 57
    in bulimic families, 65–75
    types of, 71–72, 73–74
Lithium, 209, 211–12
Llewellyn-Jones, D., 3, 17
loss:
    in chaotic families, 117
    in overprotective families, 101
    in perfect families, 86
loyalty, abandonment and, 23–24

McGoldrick, M., 57, 64, 66, 67
McGuiness, B., 80
McKinley, J. C., 26
Madame Tussaud's Wax Museum, 27
Madanes, C., 80
Mahler, M. S., 119
marriage:
    differentiation in, 64–65, 66
    integration in, 66–67
Mayer, J., 28, 29
Mazel, J., 27–28
men, socialization of, 30–31
Menghi, P., 40, 42
menstruation, 15
Merriam, K., 25, 212
metacommunications, 50, 51
    punctuation in, 50–51
mianserine, 209
Michelson, O., 9, 209

Mickalide, A. D., 9
Minnesota Multiphasic Personality Inventory (MMPI), 8, 10, 26, 199
Minuchin, S., 32, 33, 41, 80, 98, 112, 181, 185, 249
Mira, M., 3, 17
Mitchell, B. W., 28
Mitchell, J. E., 3, 5, 6, 7, 8, 15, 17, 18, 23, 26, 29, 209
Moldofsky, H., 3, 6, 18
Money, J., 212
monoamine oxidase inhibitor (MAOI), 209, 211
mood swings, 8–9, 209
Moos, B., 133
Moos, R., 133
Morgan, H. G., 5, 18
Morrell, W., 6
mother-daughter relationships, 23–24, 75, 134
    in overprotective families, 249, 256
    repetition compulsion in, 58
Mueller, P. S., 211
multigenerational issues, 40, 52–63
    in overprotective families, 102–3, 250
    schizophrenia in, 53, 58
multigenerational transmission process, 53–55

Nash, M., 114
Nemzer, E., 11, 209
Neuhaus, M., 3
Neuman, P. A., 6
NiCarthy, G., 25, 212
Nichols, M., 131, 132
Nicolò-Corigliano, A. M., 40, 42
Norman, D. K., 23, 26

Okun, B. F., 48
O'Neil, Cherry Boone, 83
Orbach, S., 20, 23, 27
overprotective families, 4, 98–111
    age of onset of bulimia in, 105
    anger in, 106
    autonomy in, 100–101, 263
    birth order in, 104–5
    boundaries in, 99, 105
    case histories of, 107–11, 249–66
    conflict-detouring in, 249, 257, 266
    expression of feelings in, 101
    family-of-origin issues in, 102–3, 260–62
    identity in, 100
    grief in, 101
    homeostatic functions in, 106
    launching in, 73–74, 263–65
    life-cycles in, 103–5

loss in, 101
messages in, 101–2
mother-daughter relationships in, 249, 256
multigenerational issues in, 102–3, 250
parents in, 106
perspectives on, 105–6
therapy for, 98–99
triangulation in, 42, 43
Owen, P., 8

Palmer, R. L., 17
parent-child coalitions:
  in anorectic families, 80
  triangulation as, 41–42, 44, 45
Paykel, E. S., 211
Pepose, M., 26
perfect families, 83–97
  age of onset of bulimia in, 89–90
  anger in, 92, 244, 246, 247
  birth order in, 89
  boundaries in, 84
  bulimia functions in, 91–93, 96–97
  case histories of, 93–96, 226–48
  client as prior anorectic in, 89
  distance regulation in, 248
  expression of feelings in, 85
  family-of-origin issues and, 56, 90, 241
  first-order changes in, 235, 309
  grief and loss in, 86
  identity and self-image in, 84–85
  launching in, 246, 247
  life-cycles in, 90–91
  messages in, 86–87
  multigenerational patterns in, 56
  perspectives on, 87–89
  powerlessness in, 85–86
  rules in, 88
  second-order changes in, 242, 246, 309
  therapy in, 83–84, 169
  treatment of, 226–48
  triangulation in, 45–46
Perron, M., 29
perverse triangle, 41–42
*Peter Pan* (Barrie), 54
Pine, E., 119
*Playboy*, 21
Polivy, J., 29–30
Pollock, S., 12
Pope, H. G., 8, 11, 17, 208, 209
powerlessness, 9–10
  in chaotic families, 116
  in perfect families, 85–86
Prata, G., 137
premature termination, 168–69
Printz, A. M., 6

prolapse, binge-purge behavior and, 203, 204
psychopharmacological issues:
  medical consultation and, 208
  psychiatric consultation and, 208, 210–11
*Psychosomatic Families* (Minuchin, Rosman and Baker), 43, 185
purging, 7, 88, 92, 106, 123, 201
Pyle, R. L., 3, 5, 6, 7, 8, 15, 17, 18, 23, 26, 29

Radloff, L., 23
Rampling, D., 303
rape, 9–10, 25, 34
Rappaport, L. J., 48
relapse, binge-purge behavior and, 194, 203, 204, 242–43, 294
Reto, C., 8
rigid triads, 41
Ritterman, M., 57
Roe, D. A., 29
Roose, S. P., 11
Root, Maria P. P., 3, 7, 8, 9, 10, 13, 14, 15, 17, 18, 23, 26, 34, 141, 163, 168, 172, 182, 194, 199, 203, 209
Rosenkrantz, P., 25–26, 30
Rosman, B. L., 32, 80, 112, 185
Rost, W., 3
Roy-Byrne, P., 17
Rozin, P., 28
Russell, G., 3, 5, 6, 7, 8, 15, 17, 18
Ryckoff, L., 183

Saba, G., 80, 112, 249
Sabine, E. J., 209
sabotage:
  appointment-making and, 304–5
  bulimic families and, 304–9
  denial of bulimia as, 306–7
  erratic attendance as, 307–8
  family exclusion as, 305–6
  in group therapy, 199–201
  perfect recovery as, 308–9
  unchanged family patterns and, 308
Salkin, B., 6
Sanders, C. D., 194
Sansone, R. A., 11, 209
Sargent, J., 80
Saunders, W., 15
Schneider, J. A., 194, 201
Schrier, S. S., 11, 209
Schultz, D. A., 26
Schwartz, B., 172
Schwartz, D. M., 3, 7, 8, 15, 17, 18, 26, 27
Schwartz, E., 6, 17, 29

Schwartz, R., 80, 112, 249
second-order changes:
  in chaotic families, 139
  in perfect families, 242, 246, 309
self-abuse, in chaotic families, 123
self-esteem, 12
self-image, 12, 13, 27
  in perfect families, 84–85
Seligman, M. E. P., 22
Seltzer, C. C., 28, 29
Selvini Palazzoli, M., 9, 26, 80, 99, 137,
    165, 209, 221, 303
sexual abuse, 9–10, 12, 34, 58–59, 163
  in chaotic families, 120
sex-role behavior, feminine, 10
Shapiro, L. R., 28
shoplifting, 8
significant others:
  before and after bulimia is revealed, 4
  individual therapy and, 166
Silver, M., 80
Simpson, M. A., 18
Simson, K., 17
Sirlin, J., 26, 29
Smart, D. E., 18
Smeltzer, D. J., 11, 209
smiling, incongruent, 36, 227
"smiling depression," 10, 50, 84
social classes, bulimia stereotypes and, 5
Society of Actuaries and Association of Life
    Insurance, 27
Sontag, Susan, 21
Sours, J. A., 8
Speck, R., 39
Spencer, J. A., 29
Stangler, R. S., 6
Stanton, D., 65, 138
Stanton, M. D., 112, 118, 121
Steinglass, P., 39
Stern, S. L., 11, 209
Stewart, J. W., 11
Stierlin, H., 44, 118
Strauss, E. S., 66, 68, 70
Strober, M., 6
structural family therapy, 41, 43
Stuckey, M. K., 3, 7, 8, 15, 17, 18
stuckness, bulimic families and, 64, 74, 81,
    82, 132, 300
substance abuse, 8, 35, 148
  in chaotic families, 112
suicide, 8–9
superwoman syndrome, 25–26
Swartz, C. M., 11, 209
symptom control:
  education in, 172
  as goal in individual therapy, 171–74

teaching in individual therapy, 162
systemic conceptualization, advantages of,
    40
systemic symptoms, 32
Szyrynski, V., 303

Tavris, C., 22
Taylor, Elizabeth, 27
Taylor, H. L., 9, 209
teenagers, bulimia stereotypes and, 5
therapist-client relationship, 167–68
  chaotic, 168, 295
  overprotective, 167, 265
  perfect, 167
therapists:
  and family assessment, 131–33
  family-of-origin issues and, 301–3
  inexperienced, and bulimic families, 301
  male vs. female, 303
  as obstacles, 300–303
  recovered anorectics as, 303
  recovered bulimics as, 303
"therapist shopping," 168
therapy modalities, *see* couples therapy;
    group therapy; individual therapy
thinness, cultural preference for, 26–27
Thompson, M. G., 26, 27
"three-way matrimony," 80, 99
Todd, T. C., 112, 118, 121
Tomm, K., 137
triangulation, 41–46, 135–36, 223
  in anorectic families, 80
  detouring-attacking triad in, 42, 273
  detouring-supportive triad in, 42, 273
  dyads vs. triads in, 41
  as parent-child coalition, 41–42, 44, 45
  as system stabilization, 41
tricyclic medications, 11, 209, 211, 212
Twiggy, 27

undifferentiated family ego mass, 54

victimization:
  and group therapy, 195–96
  and individual therapy, 163–64
  of women, 25
Vogel, S. R., 25–26, 30
vomiting, 7, 15

Wakeling, A., 209
Walker, L. E., 25, 34, 212
Wallace, A., 27
Wallace, I., 27
Wallechensky, D., 27
Walsh, B. T., 11, 15, 209, 210
Walsh, F., 58

Wardle, J., 7
Watzlawick, Paul, 49, 132, 138, 181, 192,
  224, 227, 235, 299
Weakland, J. H., 132, 138, 192, 224, 235,
  299
Weiner, M. F., 209, 212
Weiss, S. R., 8, 10, 12, 15
Weissman, M. M., 22
Wells, T., 26
White, W. C., 6, 18, 26, 194
whites, bulimia stereotypes and, 5
Williams, G. J., 212
women:
  anger and, 21–22
  average vs. idealized, 27
  bulimia stereotypes and, 5
  depression and, 22–23, 212

learned-helplessness hypothesis and, 22
power and, 24
socialization process and, 20–29, 303
social-status hypothesis and, 22
superwoman syndrome and, 25–26
victimization of, 25
Woods, S. W., 11, 209
Wooley, O. W., 26, 27, 29
Wooley, S., 26, 27, 29, 81, 82
Wright, L., 11
Wynne, L. L., 183

Yager, J., 17
Yalom, I. D., 194, 195
Yonace, A., 209
Yurgelun-Todd, D., 8, 11, 17, 209

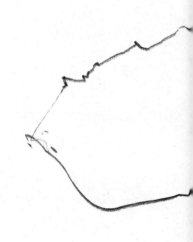